Narratives of the Mind

A New Perspective on Mental Disorders

Dr. Rakesh Khanna MBBS, MD, FRANZP

THIS BOOK IS DEDICATED TO MY PARENTS

MY EXISTENCE WAS CONTINGENT UPON THE EXISTENCE OF MY PARENTS AND MY CHILDREN BEAR TESTIMONY TO MINE.

WE ARE ALL JUST ONE LINK IN A LONG CHAIN OF HUMANITY

CONTENTS

INTRODUCTION

This book comes from the desk and keyboard of a psychiatrist with four decades of experience in the speciality. Psychiatry is one of the newest specialities of medicine. Every clinical consultation in medicine commences with 'history taking.' After introductory information, a typical medical consultation starts with the enquiry: 'What is your story?' Story in the clinical setting can be defined as "an account of past events in someone's life or in the development of something." It is also seen as 'a particular person's representation of the facts of a matter.'

Psychiatrists have a keen interest in all aspects of the person including the history of their present illness, their life history, their socio-cultural history, and their sense of the totality of their situation that brings them for consultation. The more detailed the history, the better the understanding of what makes this person a unique individual who is seeking help at a given time.

Here is a story of stories; the story of we humans, as we came to exist and how we lived and evolved through the passage of time. The authenticity of many of these 'facts' may still be subject to our beliefs rather than being scientifically and unequivocally proven. They may at best be seen as "good enough hypotheses."

We are better adapted at seeing life and its vicissitudes in the form of stories. Concepts as stories, rather than strings of facts, make it easier to understand and retain. Religious texts (initially in oral form and later in writing) are splendid examples. They have been around for thousands of years, all telling stories with an implied meaning and message. They have had a powerful influence on human lives for a long time and will remain relevant for all times to come. There are themes and variations in our stories, but across time and space they always remain relevant to each of us.

For thousands of years, people have been telling stories to each other. They told stories around the campfire, caves or whenever and wherever they could sit together and had time to spare after meeting the needs of life. They travelled from town to town, state to state and across nations, and continents telling stories from where they came from, and what life there was all about. Storytelling seems to have played a significant role in all human interaction. Their role may be far more significant in human memory than simply being just one of the several kinds of human interaction.

The reason that we constantly relate stories to each other is that all memory is essentially memory of stories. We remember them by having heard them or by composing them. Once these stories are there, they are relied upon for all that we can say and understand. The more stories we share, the closer our sense of kinship. We tell and read stories to kids. Initially storytelling was possible only in the oral form. Then we invented symbols to express language and means of writing. Still later we invented paper and printing. We write fiction and non-fiction. We hold libraries at homes, in educational centres, and in the community. Storytelling and transmission became even easier with the advent of offset printing, radio, transistor, internet, and smart phones.

Estimates of how long our species has existed remain contentious. Numbers vary from about 75,000 to 200,000 years. Unfortunately, such discrepancies may never be resolved since a large part of human history is irreparably lost to us. At least some of these variations are the result of uncertainty in separating modern humans (Homo Sapiens) from some of our immediate ancestors (Neanderthal man and Homo Erectus). They were roaming the earth together for some time. We can, at best, hope to create an account of how humans developed over the last 25 to 30 thousand years. It is much easier to have a broad consensus on how human societies grew since the advent of farming about 13 to 15 thousand years ago.

One example illustrates our limitation well. Even the term 'prehistory' only came into common use after the discoveries at the Devon in 1858, when stone axes, which could only have been fashioned by humans, were found alongside remains of a cave bear, woolly rhinoceros, and other extinct species, all together under a sealed casing of rock. This, and subsequent archaeological findings, sparked a complete rethinking of existing evidence. 'Suddenly, the bottom dropped out of human history' (Graeber and Wengrow 2021).

We further our understanding by forming hypotheses and then try to find evidence confirming and refuting the hypotheses. One view largely accepted is the evolution of species. Simpler forms of organisms have evolved into more complex forms. The evolutionary process is slow. Nature is still evolving and so are we. Natural selection consists of competition among genes to be represented in the next generation.

As children, we first acquire words by associating them to objects. Then we learn about increasingly complex objects and their uses. With evolving vocabulary and experiences, we come to gradually understand emotions and interpersonal relationships. We develop connections with parents, siblings, larger family members and people who make our interpersonal world. As complexities of our lived-experience expands, we can grasp more facts which are woven into our life-stories. They include stories about self, family, community, food, religious beliefs, and concepts constituting our community, nation, the world we live in and beyond.

The view prevailing for thousands of years revolved around what has been termed as **"Essentialism."** It postulated that there is 'an essence of life': a set of core properties created even prior to human existence. That meant a purpose in life was granted to an individual even before he or she was born. It was an immensely popular view given weight by religious thinking which emphasised the presence of an omnipresent God who created everyone with a particular plan in mind.

These views were challenged by: (1) **Enlightenmen**t: "human-kind's emergence from its self-incurred immaturity", its "lazy and cowardly" submission to the "dogmas and formulas" of religion and political authority (Kant 1784/1991). (2) The theory of evolution as propounded by Charles Darwin. He pointed out the uniqueness of every individual, not only in the human species, but for every sexually reproducing species of animal. Darwin is credited with killing essentialism not only in biology and religion but also in philosophy. (3) **"Existentialism"** which refers to the way in which people relate to and make sense of themselves and their situation. "Existence precedes essence."

An extension of this stream of thought receiving increasing recognition is **"Enactivism":** a form of embodied cognition. Enactivists argue that the organism and the world are dynamically coupled (Varela, Thompson and Rosch 1991). Living beings are self-organising units actively maintaining their own boundaries by interacting with their environment. They rely on making sense of their environment for survival. This implies that sensemaking in its basic form is about distinguishing (perceiving) what is supportive of one's existence and what entails threat. It is inherent to all living beings. It is in this sense that our body, cognition, and emotion are part of a continuum.

Karl Jaspers (1913/1997) believed that the study of psychiatry required an understanding of philosophy. Without a basic understanding of philosophy, we can only create psychopharmacologists and not proper psychiatrists.

Philosophy without a grounding in physiology is good for curious minds but of limited benefit to humanity at large. Incorporating philosophy in medicine and psychiatry enriches both.

Philosophy is not merely a doctrine or a system of thought. It is also a way of life. Philosophers advocated attitudes and practices thought to foster health and happiness. Existentialism as a tradition of philosophical enquiry explores 'the nature of human existence.' It draws from the diversity of interests: the metaphysical, the moral and political. "Existentialism emphasises the whole gamut of human experience – in his feeling, thinking, and behaving. The existential position emphasises a kind of basic conflict that flows from the individual's confrontation with 'the givens of existence.' These 'givens' signify the intrinsic properties that are an inescapable part of the human being's existence in the world" (Yalom, 1980).

The word "exist" implies differentiation ("ex-ist" = "to stand out"). Existence is not used here just as a metaphysical concept. It is firstly based in our body (anatomy and physiology). Existence is always particular and individual. It involves my existence, your existence and their existence. As humans we share some aspects with all other humans, some qualities with a more limited group of people, but we are all unique individuals. We are born under a certain unique set of circumstances and grow up in varying circumstances confronted with diverse possibilities or alternatives. The choices we make, to a substantial extent, determine the trajectory of our lives, though many of these choices themselves are partly determined by the circumstances in which we live in and by our life experiences.

Freedom is of supreme value in existentialism and its primary virtue is authenticity. The existentialist project is about becoming an individual. Authenticity is a feature of the existentialist individual. To be truly authentic is to have realized one's individuality and vice versa. The person avoiding choice becomes a mere face in the crowd and fails to become authentic. This book is not an in-depth analysis of existentialism, though some aspects relevant to the theme developed herein are discussed specifically in a later section and referred to throughout different sections.

Our biological building block consist of the double helix of our DNA, but the real-life building blocks of life, as we live it, is the triple helix: the physiological, the experiential, and the social-cultural. The various systems of the body including our brain and mind are in constant flux and go on a merry go-round with our social and cultural milieu which is influenced by our historical past. Every person is a unique individual born in a unique set of circumstances and goes through a kaleidoscope of familial, social, and cultural milieu determining the trajectory of their life. Echoes of these factors can be discerned both in health and sickness. During our attempts at 'making sense' of our existence, we are prone to revise our social, cultural, and even historical stance depending on our prevailing mental set.

The stories we relate to and believe in also shape our life and its successes and failures. Over time, humans developed storytelling into an art form.

In the life of the nomads and even in the early part of living in small communities, there was not much to do once darkness fell. Life was precarious most of the time. Talking about where they found sources essential to sustain life (food, water etc) must have been one important theme. The other most frequently occurring theme may have been the dangers faced through the day. The nomadic gathering and hunting humans would have been quite frequently confronted with death. Besides their own sense of insecurity, they must have struggled with the death of others from their tribe. Think of a person who was just like you and sharing life with you who is now lying dead. He or she neither sees nor hears nor participates in anything like they did before that minute. How would the survivors have coped with that? Looking at the sky and saying the person must have gone to one of the myriads of stars in the sky could be the first story ever invented, told, and retold.

Life and death are inextricably linked. Death anxiety is often considered as the basic source of all anxiety. It is one of the major driving forces for all human achievement but may also be a major source of all forms of psychopathology. All primates were primarily concerned with their immediate safety and finding sources of sustenance and means of survival. This basic need for safety we share with them. But humans were able to think beyond their immediate needs. They developed the cognitive ability to look beyond the here and now. They were able to plan for their future. They could grow, prepare, and store food. They were able to master fire, clean forests, and communicate with increasingly large numbers of people.

Life can be likened to a long movie occupying several decades, and our lifespan has kept getting longer with the passage of time. It unfolds slowly. "A life is not an unrelated series of actions or projects or states of being. Every life has, we might say a trajectory. It is lived in a temporal thickness. Even if my life's trajectory seems disjointed at times or lacks continuity, it is *my life* that is disconnected in its unfolding, not elements of several other lives" (May 2011). May further adds: "If life has a trajectory, then, it can be conceived narratively. A human life can be seen as a story or a series of stories that are related." This does not mean that the person, whose life it is, must, conceive of it or live it narratively. Reflecting on life, one can see it in terms of various story lines, whether parallel, intersecting, or distinct.

Humans show an intense interest in other people, from the first days of life as infants learn scents and sounds of the adults around them. We review past experiences and often gain useful insight. We make social connections with people who are on the same wavelength. We prefer to be with others who look like us, speak the same way, and hold similar interests and beliefs.

Evolution provided us with the cognitive and emotional faculties helping us to develop over hundreds of thousands of years. Changes in the way we lived life were slow and therefore easier to adapt. The pace of change started to accelerate since industrialisation and has reached an avalanche over the last fifty years or so. What worked in more traditional societies may not be as effective at a time of increasing demands of the fast-changing contemporary life. We are bombarded with information and overloaded with emotional material that we can witness anywhere in the world, almost live, and round the clock. This rapid pace has potentially overwhelmed the adaptive capacity of many people. This may account for the marked increase in the incidence and prevalence of mental disorders.

The first half of my life in psychiatry was as a trainee and then as a teacher and researcher with some administrative responsibilities. I saw myself as an average teacher, a replicative and head-counting kind of researcher (none of the research or publication would be of much value outside my curriculum vitae), and I did not particularly like the role as an administrator. I finally chose to get into an office based private practice, at first part-time and from 2002 onwards into full time practice. The success of private practice depended on every session being of sufficient value for the patient/client for them to want to return for next visit.

I felt the need to further my understanding about what it means to be a human and their sufferings. I realised some of the limitations of my understanding of psychiatry. I knew my diagnostic manuals, psychopharmacology, and standard therapies, yet they seem inadequate in providing a true understanding of the situations with which I was dealing. I was now able to see the same patients one on one, over extended periods even beyond the abatement of their acute symptoms. Resolution of symptoms was different from full remission and beyond. Something more was required to achieve a degree of integration of the patient to achieve a more fulfilling life.

I started reading more widely to increase my understanding of the patient as a person who may have presented at one point in time with a certain set of symptoms warranting a particular diagnosis. In the process I came to know about Irvin Yalom and his writing which I found interesting. I read *When Nietzsche Wept*, then *The Spinoza Problem*, and *The Schopenhauer Cure*, followed by *Staring at the Sun*, *Existential Psychotherapy*, and every book he wrote. These readings furthered my interest in philosophy. Over the last several years I have read more extensively than ever before. Finally, I decided to draft this book based on my readings, experience as a psychiatrist and my understanding of what human existence is all about and how distinct aspects of our existence influence our mental condition.

I love reading and the process of drafting this book continued to get staggered. Finally, Einstein's quote grabbed my attention: "There comes a point in your life when you need to stop reading other people's books and write your own."

To understand ourselves it is important to visit our history. We are the product of the stories we are born into, stories we created over time and stories we live in the here and now. It is useful to understand our very distinct ancestors, as far back and in as fine a detail as possible. Besides history we also need the help of archaeology, as well as palaeontology. "For the real human story, history makes no sense without prehistory, and prehistory makes no sense without biology." (Wilson 2012). One of the fascinations of ancient and mediaeval history is that it gives us an illusion of having all the facts at our disposal within the manageable compass.

Human beings are an exceptional story of survival and we have flourished so well that we seem to have increasing sway over every other species that ever lived. As soon as we are born, the world gets to work on us and transforms us from merely biological into social units. Every human being at every stage of history or pre-history is born into a society and from his earliest years is moulded by that society (E. H. Carr 1961).

In this book I wish to explore the biological, developmental, socio-cultural, and existential context in which we live our lives and then look at the ways these impact on the development of various mental disorders. A wider understanding of these aspects of life will lead to better treatment strategies.

If there is an 'essence that precedes existence,' that essence is more likely to be biological, ontological, historical, experiential, and socio-cultural. In order to understand life in contemporary times, a passing look at our evolutionary biology and historical and cultural anthropology is of significance on several counts. Humans did not emerge suddenly. "The concrete world of the individual always develops *historically*. It stands within a tradition and always exists in society and community" (Jaspers 1959). It is generally accepted that our body, as it exists in modern times, evolved over 50,000 years ago. A historical and developmental perspective reminds us that the present emerged out of the past. The way we live life also evolved over time. Every change has its pros and cons. There are important lessons to be learnt from a close examination of these changes.

Invention of electricity had a profound influence on our circadian rhythms. The circadian system is adapted to ensure daily synchronization with seasonally-varying daylength vis light information and other Zeitgebers. The circadian system is phylogenetically older and more pervasive than sleep and thus provides an oscillatory function upon which the sleep system functions. Electricity extended our hours of activity and the reduction of sleep hours, irrespective of seasons. Further advances in technology (with radio, TV, internet, and the likes) made exposure of the eyes to bright light even more likely, and thereby reducing the secretion of melatonin, the sleep hormone.

We were always curious to know about people, things, and events beyond the sphere of our senses. Widespread availability of news went through a protracted process and was a major advancement. News is now readily available almost real time and in a life-like format. They may have far reaching consequences to the emotional overload that we carry. News has now also been viewed as toxic. The book further explores these issues in the form of stories and looks at their implications with regard to causation, treatment, and prevention of mental disorders.

We have put lots of effort into automations of distinct kinds. We live life in ways vastly different from how our physiology developed a long time ago. We live in oversized houses, consume more than we need and, in the process, cause harm to our body and environment. We have stretched our days out by use of electricity, we use fossil fuel to warm our houses and wear shorts and tee shirts even in winter while we cool them in summer to a level so low we need blankets. We are now alarmed by the potentially dire consequences of climate change due to our huge carbon footprint.

We eat more than we require, use all kinds of remotes to save energy, and then go to gym to burn calories. Jobs, as we know them today, have only existed since the industrial revolution, and yet so much of our self-esteem and self-worth is tied to this. We have developed amazing modes of communication and yet loneliness is a major problem in contemporary society. We live in many ways richer and more comfortably than ever but appear to have an epidemic of anxiety and depression. Suicide rates remain stubbornly high despite greater availability of care for mental disorders.

Part one of the book, 'Narratives of the Mind," takes a brief look at the origins of the human species and how we have evolved to become story tellers. Included here are some of the basic changes making humans unique creatures. The development of our communication skills and the ability to create stories and disseminate widely is of particular interest in this narrative. It helped us to become social animals like none other. An outline of the development of emotions and cognitions, followed by an exploration of human adaptation provides a better understanding of our historical roots and its impact. These include the adaptation to an agrarian life, a shift towards science and technology, the rise of industries, and our ever-expanding adaptive needs. I end part one with the story surrounding 'the birth of the individual.' We must first come to 'existence' before we can start the process of separation and individuation and go on to create our own stories.

Part two of the book is about stories humans have created over time. It helps to keep into consideration the concrete world from which the patients come from, and how they have continued to change over time. I describe the various instruments of communication we have developed to be able to tell and disseminate our stories more effectively. The importance of cultural, social, and political realities on the development of individual personalities is highlighted. I provide a review of existing literature on the psychological basis of life including making sense of death, making affective bonds, existential isolation, and seeking meaning in life. This section ends with an overview of major religious scriptures and some of the significant philosophical issues relevant to defining existence and the impact of these on contemporary life.

Part three begins with an analysis of our physiology and the importance of our physical environment. Understanding emotions is a vital part of understanding what it means to be human. I consider 'the happiness deficit' in our contemporary society and factors related to it. I then proceed to the story of mental illness which includes the evolution of the two major international classification systems, the limitations of current diagnostic concepts and categories, and the rise and fall of different diagnostic models. Finally, I summarise the invention of medications used to treat mental disorders and the limitations of biological studies.

Part four, 'When stories go haywire,' covers some necessary insight into a few common mental disorders such as affective disorders (depression and anxiety), post-traumatic stress disorder and attention deficit disorder. I focus on the limitations of the way we currently tend to view these disorders. For example, the artificial distinction between anxiety and depression, and the use of trauma and attention deficit as a 'catch-all' explanation for many disorders, which actually lie on a complex continuum.

Part four also centres on the ideas surrounding what it means to be a person and the impact of personality on mental disorders, followed by an analysis of the continuum of psychopathology across mental disorders. No account of mental disorders can be complete without an awareness of the personality attributes of those who develop particular illnesses. Much of the ground that is explored here is to increase our understanding of humans as they exist at this time and in these surroundings.

The last section of part four deals with treatment considerations from an existential and enactive perspective. An Existential-based formulation of mental disorders is suggested which involves a four-dimensional model of existence: 1) a physiological self, 2) an experiential self, 3) a socio-cultural self, and 4) an existential self. The existential dimension is in effect the art of sensemaking and stance taking.

Treatment measures such as psychotropic medications, cognitive behaviour therapy and mindfulness-based therapies used for mental disorders often cut across diagnostic labels and are successfully applied to a range of disorders. While a treatment relying too heavily on psychopharmacology may lead to remission of symptoms, it may not lead to full recovery nor effectively prevent relapse. The therapeutic model I propose combines existing forms of therapy with a deeper understanding of existential issues, which I believe can lead to better outcomes for those suffering from mental disorders.

Part five provides some concluding remarks. The crux of the problems in current day psychiatry is a constant attempt to find simple solutions to complex problems. Rather, a true understanding of the interwoven dimensions of the patient must take centre stage in the clinical practice of psychiatry.

Narrative approaches have played a prominent part in the evolution of psychiatry over the years. Freud, Freudians and Neo Freudians made spectacular contributions in bringing 'mind' to the centre of our understanding of mental disorders. Psychoanalytic thinking has even changed our understanding and description of everyday life. Psychanalysis held sway for decades and was later overtaken by psychodynamic psychotherapy. Gradually, more structured, and briefer forms of therapy gained currency. Managed care and its various incarnations have no doubt played a role in bringing about these changes. Every form of therapy has its place in the practice of psychiatry. Each have their proponents and, no doubt, have helped many.

In Narrative Based Medicine doctor and patient together are 'co-constructors' of a shared reality in which the history and expectations of each play a significant role in determining the outcome (Holmes 2000). "It is the nature of science that all knowledge is partial: no scientific theory can have validity outside of their chosen scope" (Karl Jaspers). The approach herein is more in Jaspers' methodological mode rather than Freudian or Kraepelinian. As Nietzsche rightly said: "You have your way. I have my way. As for the right way, the correct way, and the only way, it does not exist."

In contrast to Freud, Karl Jaspers likened direct, accessible psychic experiences to the foam on the sea's surface. He disputed whether unconscious psychic events exist. It may be that psychic events though they may have been actually experienced were unnoticed or not reviewed by the individual. These unnoticed psychic events can be discussed clinically by producing favourable circumstances in which the reality of that story or stories can be established. Existence-based therapy outlined here is yet another way to structure therapy. It attempts to bridge the gap between a "mindless" or "brainless" psychiatry. I have found this approach useful in clinical practice and it has provided me with greater work satisfaction. It is the narrative of the person that makes each of us a unique individual. Devoid of that personal story, a diagnosis conceals much more than it reveals. It is the goodness of the fit between the one seeking help and the one providing it which is of crucial importance.

Authoring this book has helped me to organise and synthesise my own thoughts. *Narratives of the Mind* is an attempt to provide a bird's eye view of the various aspects of life forming the basis of what it means to be a human living in contemporary times, how we interact with the world around us, and how they affect the mental disorders we come to suffer from. It does not claim to cover any of these areas exclusively or exhaustively.

The book is primarily addressed to the general interested reader touched by mental disorders in some way. Given their prevalence, it is likely that everyone in contemporary society has come across it in one way or the other. Hopefully, it may help the reader broaden their understanding of humans as individuals by discussing common mental disorders and their treatment. They may be able to play with the idea of an Existential formulation before engaging with their preferred specialist to work on making greater sense of their condition. It may also be of interest to people working with those with mental disorder if they are in initial stages of their career or have felt the need to see it in a broader context.

The discussion of those matters is prefaced by an account of how we humans got here to even contemplate having minds let alone problems with them. Something goes awry with each of us at some time and I think there's considerable value in running through the history of how we came about. Describing the progress of humankind from amoeba-like fragments to hosting complex neuroses informed often by the very sophisticated ways we communicate with each other seems a worthwhile introduction to an analysis of the ways psychiatrists try to relieve the often-burdensome mental consequences of existence.

PART I

STORIES WE ARE BORN WITH

Our earth is estimated to be about 4.5 billion years old. Bacteria were the first life form to evolve and are believed to have existed for about 3.5 billion years. Hundreds of millions of years lapsed with no sign of change until cyanobacteria used the energy of visible incoming solar radiation to convert carbon dioxide and water into new organic compounds which released oxygen (Herrero and Flores 2008). This created a radical shift leading to the creation of earth's oxygenated atmosphere.

The atmosphere of our world now is vastly different to the atmosphere of the earth in which life first developed. It has been almost fully reconstituted by the bacteria, vegetation and other life forms that have acted upon it over this vast span of time. Bacteria are still the most numerous and varied life form to exist on earth. Strangely, our body has more bacteria than there are human cells of our body. In the human gut alone, there are usually around one hundred trillion bacteria, compared to about ten trillion of their own cells. Mostly, bacteria and human cells live in harmonious symbiosis.

Bacteria are thought to be quite intelligent creatures despite being cells without nuclei and in the absence of a nervous system. They display varieties of perception, memory and a limited ability to communicate. They sense conditions in their environment and react in ways that are essential to their survival if not ours. They communicate among themselves using chemical and electrical networks. Bacterial cells can also cooperate with other cells to create the organelle of more complex cells. The mitochondria of our cells are examples of such organelles.

They were followed, about two billion years later, by nucleated cells and about 700 to 600 million years ago multicellular organisms evolved. Some of our own cells began by incorporating bacteria in their structure. The process of cooperation was necessitated by the need to maintain homeostasis (a relatively stable equilibrium between interdependent elements, especially as maintained by physiological processes).

The nervous system evolved around 540 to 600 million years ago. Its emergence was a significant enabler of life for elaborate multicellular organisms. Nervous systems interact closely with the body in an entirely different way from those it holds with the environment surrounding the organism. The emergence of the nervous system opened the way for homeostasis to be neuronally mediated. On the way to accomplishing the complex task of making life possible in a complex body, the nervous system developed strategies, mechanisms, and abilities that not only took care of vital homeostatic needs but also influenced the environment.

Once nervous systems emerged, brains and then minds became possible and, within them, feelings along with all the images representing the exterior world and its relation to the organism. Mind encompasses feelings, subjectivity, memory and reasoning all intricately linked to the development of verbal language and creative intelligence. After the development of conscious minds capable of feeling and creative intelligence, the way was open for the creation, in the social and cultural space, of complex responses transcending homeostatic needs to gain considerable autonomy; therein is the beginning of our cultural lives (Damasio 2017).

Mind depends on the presence of nervous system charged with running life efficiently in its respective bodies while hosting and guiding complex interactions of the nervous system and the body.

Just over four million years ago many four-legged animals emerged and awkwardly walked on two legs. Gradually, this form of locomotion because the norm for these ape-like beings who began spending more time on land than on trees. The detailed evolution from unicellular organisms to human beings has been a long and convoluted process and outside the purview of this book.

HOW DID WE EVOLVE TO BE STORY TELLERS?

Humans are members of a large family of animals called the great apes. From the humble beginnings of the naked ape, we transformed into clothed and bejewelled creatures who now live a life increasingly technologically driven. The pace of change was initially slow but over the last two hundred years it picked up pace. The last fifty years has been a time of such rapid change that can truly be called exponential. We have reached a stage of technical knowhow, wherein every invention has the capability of changing life radically.

Despite all the obvious differences between humans and other apes, the underlying differences are tiny. Molecular biologists Sibley and Ahlquist (1984) published the results of their long-term DNA studies of humans and apes. The genetic makeup of orangutans and humans were found to differ by about 3.6%, gorilla and humans by about 2.3%, and chimpanzees and humans (and baboons and humans) by about 1.6%. The likely genetic difference between Homo sapiens and Pan troglodytes is astonishingly small. Thus 98.4% of the human DNA is chimpanzee DNA. How such a small difference could afford such a massive advantage over other apes is quite intriguing. Every advantage sets a cascade of multiplying degrees of further advantage.

Mammals give affection, they want affection, and they respond to our emotions the way we do to theirs. Female chimpanzees have been seen to drag reluctant males toward each other to make up after a fight while removing weapons from their hands. High ranking male chimpanzees often act as impartial arbiters to settle community disputes in the light of community concerns they value. We can see in these behaviours evidence about creating affective bonds among primates.

In the 1920s, Emile Devau (a Frenchman) and Louis Bolk, (a Dutch) independently found the possible mechanism accounting for the human brain's remarkable development. Both pointed out that man, in contrast to other primates is not fully developed at birth and remains in the foetal stage far longer than other mammals. They are thus highly receptive to learning. While the brains of all other mammals grow more slowly than their body after birth, in man it continues to develop at almost the same pace as in the womb. The cerebellum and the cerebral cortex, in particular, profit from this continued growth. And within the cerebral cortex, are the regions important for orientation in space, musicality, and powers of concentration which continue to develop (Precht 2011).

Early birth solved one problem, but it caused others. The human brain is only 25% of adult size, as opposed to 40-50% for an infant chimp (Wong 2012). Humans emerge from the womb like molten glass from a furnace and remain reliant on the parents and other care providers for many years. The duration of the human child's dependence has continued to grow due to a multitude of social and cultural factors. No other animal sleeps on beds, eats cooked food, learns to use complex tools, or goes to school for education.

When standing, the human centre of gravity lies approximately anterior to the second sacral vertebra. However, human beings are not locked in this anatomical position so the centre of gravity changes constantly with every new arrangement of the body and limbs. To achieve just the basic locomotive skills as compared to any other animal requires much more time.

The brain accounts for about 2 to 3 percent of the body weight of humans, averaging 1.200 to 1,400 cubic centimetres. It consumes about 25 per cent of the body's energy when the body is at rest. It also receives 25 percent of the blood supply. The singular evolution of this bigger brain allowed humans to collect more information about the world so to reason about it in a more sophisticated manner while deploying a greater variety of actions to achieve its goals.

Some researchers suggest that the great apes, including humans, use most of their intelligence for complex social interaction. Dealing with members of our own species is often our main preoccupation. We may ordinarily use only a fraction of our brain capacity because intelligence comes into play only when we reach an impasse. The human brain is impressive, but mostly runs at a low level (a common throwaway line is that we use only 10% of our brains capacity). As human life became increasingly organised, our society took greater care of individual needs. Human consciousness was shaped largely by the attempt to survive and move ahead, creatively and profitably, through the sophisticated foresight and consequent avoidance of error our large brains provided.

Despite biological similarities, people in various parts of the world grew differently. Jarred Diamond (1997) pointed out, "In the 13000 years since the last Ice Age, some parts of the world developed literate industrial societies with metal tools, other parts developed only nonlinear farming societies, and still others retained societies of hunter gatherer with some tools". He added, "History followed different courses for different peoples because of differences among peoples' environments, not because of biological differences among people themselves."

The appearance of novel ways of thinking is thought to have started between 70,000 to 30,000 years ago and was associated with new ways of communicating. Accidental genetic mutation may have changed the inner wirings of the brains of humans enabling us to communicate using increasingly sophisticated language. Evolution is conservative, only building on what nature has already produced. New features may be added, and the old may undergo some alteration, but most things remain the same. Evolution laid down the cornerstone of basic physiology long ago (Peterson 2018). The wide variation in time estimates (70,000 to 30,000 years) exemplifies uncertainties about our knowledge. We must opt for best plausible 'stories' rather than pretend these propositions are factual statements.

One of the keys to the mystery of biology is what force was it that lifted prehuman social behaviour to human level. The central tenet of one explanation, the 'Kin selection theory' (also called 'inclusive fitness theory'), is that interacting organisms may have evolutionary advantage by helping each other (or at least not hurting each other) if they share the genes. The degree of incentive is heightened by the degree of relatedness between them.

Alternatively, the 'multilevel (or group) selection theory' supposes selection not only acts on individuals but (simultaneously) on multiple levels of biological organization, including cells and/or groups. This view suggests that even if behaviours benefiting other individuals are selectively disadvantageous at the individual level, they might still evolve, if they are advantageous at – and hence selected, for a higher level of the biological hierarchy (e.g., the group or colony level). It has most likely played a powerful role of group-to-group competition and forged advanced social behaviour – including that of humans.

These two theories aim at explaining the evolution of social behaviours. Kramer and Meunier (2016) believe the two theories can offer complementary approaches to the study of social evolution. Their different perspectives might be fruitfully combined to promote understanding of our evolution in group structured populations. These evolutionary processes required other significant changes greatly enhancing the opportunities for humans compared to all other animals.

THE BASICS OF WHAT MADE HUMANS SO UNIQUE:

There were three seemingly small but incredibly significant evolutionary changes providing humans with a distinct advantage over other animals:

A. A BIPEDAL STANCE AND A MORE DISTAL THUMB:

The mating systems of great apes are characterised by intense male-male competition in which conflict is resolved through force or the threat of force. Great apes mostly fight from bipedal posture, striking with both the fore- and hindlimbs. Sexual selection contributed to the evolution of habitual bipedalism in hominins.

The bipedal human can strike with 40–50% higher force and energy compared to the quadrupedal posture and imparts more than 200% greater energy when striking downward than upward. The increase in work done in downward and upward strikes when subjects switched from quadrupedal to bipedal posture likely reflects the difference in the range of motion of the arm in these two postures (Carrier 2011).

Humans adopting an upright position accorded them other significant advantages. As a result of the upright stance, their hands were not constantly rubbing against the earth. This made it possible for hands to be deployed more freely and effectively. Evolutionary process helped develop an increased concentration of neurons and finely tuned small muscles of the palm and fingers. These changes in turn allowed them to produce and use increasingly sophisticated tools.

The thumb took a more distal position that enabled even greater dexterity to our hands. The oppositional movement accorded by the uniquely placed thumb allowed us a greater ability to use different tools. This provided a crucial advantage in making us so successful as a species.

The bipedal stance also made us more effective in covering spaces otherwise difficult such as climbing hills and steps. It afforded us a dexterity in moving at different speeds while still being able to use our hands to do other exploratory activities. The head which contains four of the five special senses (vision, hearing, smell, and taste) being at a higher level is able to provide better sensory input, thereby providing increased anticipation of danger.

The cascade of advantage that these changes brought about were of great significance indeed.

B. OUR UNIQUE EAR APPARATUS

The human ear contains an elastic drumhead vibrating in response to the variations in air it encounters, a bony lever that multiplies the vibration's force, a piston that impress the vibration into the fluid in a long tunnel (conveniently coiled to fit inside the wall of the skull), a tapering membrane that round down the length of the tunnel that physically separates the waveform into harmonics and an array of cells with tiny hairs that are flexed back and forth by the vibrating membrane which in turn sends a train of electrical impulses to the brain.

Such an extraordinary arrangement of delicately balanced bones in unison with membranes, and fluid which allows the brain to register patterned sound is truly remarkable. Even the fleshy outer ear – asymmetrical top to bottom and front to back and crinkled with ridges and valleys – is shaped in a way that sculpts the incoming sound to inform the brain whether the sound maker is above or below, in front or behind (Pinker 2018).

This unique human ear apparatus brilliantly enhances our communication compared to any other species. Ears afford the ability to perceive objects and events outside our visual fields, even when dark thus providing warnings about approaching risks. and multiplying our ability to communicate with others, The ear was an essential cornerstone to effective collaboration using vocal symbols.

EVOLUTION OF VOCAL SKILLS

Sound is one of the fundamental properties of nature. Natural forces and most animals emit sounds. Every sound originates as a vibration propagated as a wave of pressure passing through mediums such as a gas, liquid or solid. It is produced by the movement of physical objects and events such as the falling trees and branches, the rustling leaves, the falling rain, and the blowing wind. We can appreciate sound through the reception of such waves by the ear apparatus and interpretation by the brain. Humans can only hear sound waves as distinct pitches when the frequency lies between about 20 Hz and 20 kHz. Other animals have different range of hearing abilities.

Every animal has different linguistic abilities. Many animals including all apes have vocal languages. Whales and elephants have impressive vocal abilities too. Parrots can copy a large variety of sounds, words, and phrases. All individuals are born producing species-specific vocalization and they also react to them in a way that is typical to the species. One explanation is that animals may have started vocalizing as an attempt to imitate the physical world around them. Later they may have started to use it for communicative purposes. Humans started using more sophisticated ways of creating music as they evolved and could use tools generating notes and sounds at will.

Upon hearing someone vocalize, primates try to locate the vocaliser. They also try to identify their emotional state and to understand the circumstances leading to that emotional state. Humans, like all other primates, are social by nature. Among the more than two hundred species of apes, not even one lives in complete isolation. Like humans, apes also use a complex system of sounds to communicate. They too have Wernicke's area in the temporal lobe (for the comprehension of speech), and Broca's area in the prefrontal cortex (to produce speech).

Reptiles, amphibians, and mammals all have a larynx and a voice box at the top of the throat. It serves to protect the lower airways, facilitates respiration, and plays a key role in phonation. Folds of tissue there—the vocal cords—vibrate to enable humans to talk, pigs to grunt, and lions to roar. From a structural point of view, protective function of the adult human larynx is precarious by virtue of its low position in the neck.

The compromise in the protective function of the lower position of the larynx affords an advantage for the richness of human vocal abilities because the lower situated larynx may provide a larger column of air to produce larger number of vocalizations. With this ability to produce many more distinct sounds than any other animal, humans could develop language. As with humans, primate intelligence arose from the necessities of social behaviour. We can connect a limited number of sounds and signs to produce an infinite number of sentences, each with a distinct meaning. We can imbibe, store, and communicate vast amounts of information using these vocal and linguistic skills.

It is quite likely that a more advanced neurological system combined with greater communicative needs helped develop greater dexterity of the muscles involved in creating sounds. Regular exercise of this function gradually improves muscle growth and development. Singers spend ages developing their vocal skills. Human beings did, at some point, gain control over their vocalization. What comes naturally to humans is to direct others' attention visually in space through some form of action such as looking or pointing, based on the tendency of all primates to follow the direction of the gaze of others.

DEVELOPMENT OF COMMUNICATION SKILLS

Communication is the physical and behavioural characteristic influencing the behaviour of others. The communication signals chosen by individual organisms are used flexibly and strategically to achieve a particular goal. They can be adjusted in many ways depending on circumstances.

The different sense organs of our bodies are unique to each species and provide data for the mind. Our conscious experience is to a considerable extent determined by the linguistic concepts we use to understand the world around us. These concepts help us categorize our experiences which, in turn, allows us to relay it coherently and effectively to others. Ability to communicate effectively with each other is a central part of living involving both verbal and nonverbal modes of communication.

A. PRIMATE COMMUNICATION:

Primates communicate through vocal and non-vocal (gestural) means.

a. **VOCALIZATION:** Within any species of ape all individuals have the same basic vocal repertoire with essentially no individual differences. Among nonhuman primates, vocalizations are mostly very tightly tied to emotions and are often associated with especially urgent functions. They do not give alarm calls so long as they themselves are not at risk (Cheney and Seyfarth 1990b).

b. **GESTURES:** Two basic types of great ape gestures have been suggested: (1) ***Inattention movements***: these occur when an individual performs only the first step of a normal behavioural sequence, often in abbreviated form. This is enough to elicit a response from the recipient. (2) ***Attention getting gestures*** are such things as ground-slap, poke-at, throw-stuff, which serve to attract attention of the recipient to the communicator. These are unique to primates or even great apes. Once learned, an attention getting gesture is used quite widely for many social goals such as play, grooming, nursing etc.

Gestural communication mostly takes place in the visual channel and is directed towards a single individual. It is effective only if the recipient is visually attending.

B. HUMAN COOPERATIVE COMMUNICATION:

Michael Tomasello (2008) believes that it would have been evolutionarily impossible to jump from ape gestures and vocalizations to arbitrary linguistic conventions directly. It must have passed through intermediate stages of nonconventional, action based, naturally meaningful, cooperative gestures that could act as a kind of natural grounding.

a. POINTING

Our most fundamental type of communication gesture is pointing. Infants begin using pointing and iconic gestures in complex ways before acquiring language. Deaf children, very early on and without any vocal or signed language invent iconic gestures to communicate in extremely rich and complex ways. According to Grice (1956, 1975) our communication is fundamentally a cooperative enterprise, operating most naturally and smoothly within the context of a mutually assumed common conceptual ground and mutually assumed cooperative communication protocols.

When infants need food or comfort, their cry typically results in a helpful adult response. The infant learns to associate his or her crying to the adult's response thus improving their behavioural repertoire. Within the first few months of life, infants also engage and share emotions. Most infants acquire language in the months around their first birthday. During the second year of life, they start using conventional gestures learnt by imitating adults. These iconic gestures are later replaced by novel gestures and linguistic acquisition.

OUR LANGUAGE:

Sharing of memories is made possible by language developed in accordance with our needs as we explore new dimensions of life. As Quine (1960) put it: "Language is a social art. In acquiring it, we depend entirely on intersubjectively available cues as to what to say and when." The first native language is learned unconsciously and then 'aped' in social situations through collaborative and communicative activities which became possible by the increasing tolerance and generosity in sharing the spoils of group activities (e.g., meat of the prey of group hunting). This allowed people to participate in joint goals. Mass communication takes place with and between unrelated and unknown people. Social norms in the context of symbols and formal institutions provide the template for these interactions. We invented cultural practices and institutions whose existence depends on the collective agreement of all group members.

One way of expressing solidarity with others is to behave like them through similarities in dressing, talking, and holding the same attitudes. We discriminate against people or groups who are dissimilar and go to great lengths to find ways to make it obvious who belongs and who does not. We also want to be liked by others so sharing emotions and attitudes about the world within the group forms the basis for group identity.

Most of what makes our communication so powerful is the psychological infrastructure already present through forms of gesturing, such as pointing. Language builds upon this infrastructure. We focus to a much greater extent than apes on the actual actions performed. This is a result of our unique vocal modality which enables communication at a longer distance and in darkness so enhancing our effective reach? We have ways of referring to absent or unknown objects and events and marking such things as who did what to whom (including third parties) expressed in a manner understandable to the listener. Objects of reference must be in space, and events located in time, including in imagined time.

The same applies in modern sign languages where gesture structures communication to make clear who did what to whom. Each different language has its own syntactical and grammatical conventions for structuring utterances to solve various problems raised by the need for communication. Becoming a skilful narrator requires mastery of a set of devices to provide coherence and cohesion across events. The ability to tell a relevant story is highly variable and much valued. The ubiquitous smile on seeing someone is thought to have originated millions of years ago. The 'Fear-Grin' used by monkeys and apes showing the unclenched teeth signifies they mean no harm - clenched teeth was their best offensive threat display weapon.

There are many variations in the ways humans greet each other when meeting. A handshake, a hug with kisses a particular number of times or sequence are the most frequent greeting gestures. In India people fold their hands close to their chest to greet each other (Namaste), but younger people touch the feet of elders as a mark of respect. Japanese use the deep bow and Chinese a bow followed by a handshake. A bow is used in other cultures in front of Royalty or the Court.

THE EVOLUTION OF LANGUAGE

Recent genetic research indicates that one of the genes responsible for articulate human speech (The FOXP2 gene) emerged in the human population no more than 150,000 years ago. (Enard et al 2002) about the same time as we began colonising the globe. This gene allows incredibly fine-grained motor control for speech giving us a massive competitive advantage over other species. We have about six thousand different human languages, each with unique communication conventions.

Mind depends on the presence of a nervous system charged with running life efficiently in respective bodies while hosting and guiding complex interactions. For millions of years, we could store all relevant information just in our brains, but their capacity was limited, and information stored in peoples' brains also died with them. Our brain had adapted to store and process only particular kinds and quantity of information. The Hebrew Bible, the Greek Iliad, the Hindu Mahabharata, and the Buddhist Tipitaka all began as oral works and were transmitted orally and would have survived even if writing never evolved. An extension of Price's law: 90% of communication occurs using just five hundred words. (Peterson 2018)

Agrarian development led to increasingly complex societies. New types of information were generated and in larger amounts meaning that the silo of the human brain was now neither big enough nor sufficiently dependable. Between the years 3500 to 3000 B.C. ancient Sumerians invented a system to store information outside the brain. The data-processing system invented by the Sumerians was called "writing." They did so by combining two types of signs pressed into clay tablets. One type represented numbers and the other catalogued people, animals, merchandise, territories, dates and so forth. Such writing was limited to data and used only for record keeping. Between 3000 BC and 2500 BC increased signs were added to the Sumerian system.

Gradually, writing evolved into a full script that we now call cuneiform. About the same time, Egyptians developed hieroglyphics. Other full scripts were invented in China around 1200 BC and Central America around 1000 and 500 BC. From these initial centres, full scripts spread everywhere, taking on various new forms and novel tasks. What is crucial to learning language is that toddlers imitate what they hear. Like chimpanzees in the wild, people use only about three dozen different sounds to construct complex sentences.

For chimpanzees, each sound has a specific meaning but not for us. Sounds like 'ba' or 'do' gradually lose their meaning and became mere syllables. We combine meaningless sounds to form meaningful words and then connect a limited number of sounds and signs to produce an infinite number of sentences, each with a distinct meaning.

Communicative needs determine language. In cross-cultural psychology, the most popular and widely analysed dimension of cultural values is between individualism and collectivism. Individualistic cultures in which individuals view themselves as independent tend to show greater detachment from relationships and community. In contrast, collectivist cultures stress the primacy of relationships, roles and status within the social system. In the more individualistic societies, the word 'uncle' is used for people related to the person on either side of their parents. In more collectivist societies, for example, India, the father's brothers (Chacha), father's sisters' husband (Fufa), mother's brother (Mama) are separately designated. There are often different words used for father's elder and younger brother. Similar differentiation occurs for aunts (Chachi, Fufi or Bua, and Masi respectively).

THEORIES OF LANGUAGE DEVELOPMENT

Like all primates, we are social animals. Informing fellow beings about sources of food and water and alerting them to lurking danger is hard wired. Other primates are limited by the complexity of their life experiences, inner thought process and language. Most information shared by our early ancestors would have been mostly about other members of the social group, nearby threats and provisions. Linguistic skills enabled gossip over extended periods often focusing on the wrongdoing of others. Gossip helped *homo sapiens* form larger and more stable communities up to a practical maximum of about 150 individuals. Most people can neither intimately know, nor gossip effectively about more than that number.

After discovering cowpox vaccine in 1796 it took 175 years to reach smallpox zero in 1975 while only a fraction of that time elapsed from the discovery of radio technology to it becoming the ideal vehicle for spreading stories and, hence, gossip throughout the world using increasingly portable means to make it possible. That speed may indicate gossip to be a core human activity possibly even more important to us than our health.

The 'gossip theory' of language development does not eliminate the equally plausible proposition that language evolved mainly to allow communication about the basic need for survival. Humans are uniquely dependent on socially transmitted information to cope with their physical and social needs. An important class of emotions are those mediating the acquisition, use and dissemination of cultural information.

On a larger scale, conformity to cultural values and beliefs makes behaviour more predictable thereby allowing complex coordination and collaboration. Our vocabulary has found or invented words for radical innovations, discoveries, social processes, ways of living and the harnessing of resources. The need to communicate with people living further and further apart gave rise to common languages for international communication such as the overwhelming use of short form English for air traffic control.

"There is no greater agony than bearing an untold story inside you." (Maya Angelo 1970). Loneliness by depriving us of our ability to tell our stories, and the stories of others to people close to us is a demonstrably significant contributing factor to depression.

STORY TELLING BEYOND THE PERSONAL

Everyday survival preoccupied all primates. After the nomadic period, our concerns about the future became an even greater part of life. We eventually created fiction describing imaginary events and people, a unique feature of our language enabling us not only to imagine things but to do so collectively. We weave mutually accepted terms of engagement or rules, providing us with the ability to cooperate with more people. We create stories, believe in them and try to make others believe them too. The irony is that we may be trapped by our own stories. Disputes and wars are often caused by stories created by one group being in conflict to those created by another group.

Mutually accepted stories, commonly labelled as myths, are usually a symbolic narrative of unknown origin and, at least partly, traditional. They often relate to actual events and are especially associated with religious or cultural beliefs. They are shared stories, to an extent, imaginative or fictitious but devised for a particular purpose and governed by certain well understood rules of engagement. Substantial numbers of strangers may cooperate successfully by believing in shared stories.

Societies are rooted in collective stories of their uniqueness and superiority. Churches/Temples/Masjids/Synagogues follow from the common religious beliefs of that religion. The common national identity of States enables people to join armies and lay down their lives for the nation, quite strategically dubbed as 'the ultimate sacrifice.' Judicial systems share belief in what is seen as right and wrong by a society at a particular time but always subject to change. Beliefs and cultures are dynamic in nature and continually evolving. Sport fans are rooted in common beliefs in the ability of their preferred sports and teams. None of the above binding forces exist outside the stories that people invent and propagate among themselves (Harari 2014).

The long tradition of storytelling passed from generation to generation over many thousands of years across all cultural groups. The earliest written records of them were not found till extremely late in the history of humankind. Story telling is an art, and by no means an easy one. There are at least two selves within us: an 'experiencing self' and a 'remembering or narrating self.' The experiencing self - immersed in events or situations, tells no stories. Memories are obtained from our experiencing self which does not aggregate experiences, it averages them. Most critical choices (such as partners, careers, holidays) are taken by the narrative self with whom most of us identify. Walter Fisher (1987) sees us as being innate storytellers.

When given a message, we do not appreciate it in a straightforward rational or emotional way but slot the message into a story of some kind and consider how convincing it is overall. Stories are our way of making sense of things. The "narrative paradigm" we create is to structure our thoughts around these narratives rather than in logical folders.

All our memory, knowledge and social communication are based on three important propositions as articulated by Schank and Abelson (1995): (1) Virtually all our knowledge is based on stories constructed around past experiences; (2) New experiences are interpreted in terms of old stories; (3) The content of the memories depends on whether and how they are told to others and these reconstituted memories form the basis of the individual's "remembered self".

Human memory is a collection of thousands of stories remembered through experience. Such stories are obtained by hearing them, experiencing them or composing them (Schank and Abelson 1995). Once there, they are relied upon for all we can say or understand. For a listener, understanding means trying to find out how the speaker's stories compare to his or her own stories. Different people understand the same story differently precisely because the stories they already know are different. What someone is doing when he understands is to figure out what story to tell. People constantly question themselves and each other to discover why someone has done what he has done and what the consequences are likely to be. 'Understanding' means retrieving stories and applying them to new experiences.

INCREASING DEMANDS / EVOLVING VOCABULARY

There has been a gradual increase in our need to find novel words and expressions to describe things that did not exist before. A whole new vocabulary exists that our ancestors would find hard to understand. Every new generation uses words and terms alien to the previous generation.

For most of history, humans knew nothing about 99.99% of the organisms on this planet, namely microorganisms. In 1674, with the advent of the microscope, for the first time a human saw a microorganism, and that soon became common knowledge.

A crucial link in the spreading timetable system was public transportation. In 1784 a carriage service with a published schedule began operating in Britain. Initially the timetable specified only the hour of departure of the train but not arrival since each British City and town had its own local time differing from London by up to half an hour. The first commercial train service operated between Liverpool and Manchester from 1830. Ten years later, the first train timetable was issued. In 1847 all train timetables were calibrated to Greenwich observatory times.

More institutions followed the lead. Finally, in 1880, the British government legislated that all timetables in Britain must follow the Greenwich time. When the broadcast media (Radio and Television) and later increasing international travel ensued, humans entered a world of universal timetables.

On the 16th of July 1945 for the first time a human detonated an atomic bomb. With the blink of an eyelid a whole new world was generated for us requiring a new set of words and language had to expand to effectively communicate about it.

Desktop computers became increasingly available to people from the early 1990s with a gradual shift towards more affordable and transportable laptops. Increasingly efficient computers and faster internet changed the lives of most of our population. Mobile phone technology took off with a bang and the advent of smart phones around 2004 made information readily available and easily accessible to the vast majority. The rise of social media created its own benefits, but a unique set of challenges as well. Increasing length and breadth of knowledge in different disciplines makes it increasingly hard to follow the rapid changes.

NEED FOR INCREASING COOPERATION AND COLLABORATION

Through sharing of stories, we can cooperate in extremely flexible ways with countless number of strangers. Many pursuits in life we undertake are the result of our ability to invent rules and convey it effectively to others who may wish to participate in similar collaborative ventures. We developed the right kind of language to convey such ideas/rules. Many of these ideas were entirely imaginary but had to be shared and agreed upon. Thus, we found ways to play diverse kinds of games. 'Olympic games' and 'world cups' of various kinds of sports are massive international ventures.

No animal other than humans engages in trade, and all trade networks are based on fiction. Trade cannot exist without trust, and it is exceedingly difficult to trust strangers. The global trade network is based on trust in such fictional entities as the dollar, Federal Reserve Bank, and the totemic trademarks of cooperation (Harari 2014). Humans are constantly reinventing their languages. Human communication is open and dynamic, and those involved in communication are constantly adjusting to one another to communicate as effectively as possible to accomplish their goals.

Communication is a two-way street. A small number of languages have now been adopted to serve the purpose of international communication. The general principle is that the more the common ground between those engaged in communication the less the number of utterances required and more effective it is. Thanks to the large numbers of efficient and effective means of communication, we are now truly living in a global village.

THE EVOLUTIONARY TRAJECTORY

There are proponents of both an evolutionary and a revolutionary theory of the development of human behaviour. Those who believe in the 'revolutionary theories' claim that modern human behaviours arose suddenly and simultaneously throughout the world around 40 to 50 thousand years ago. This was possibly due to the reorganisation of the brain and the origin of language. African archaeological records, however, suggest a gradual assembling package of modern behaviours in Africa and its later export to other regions of the old world (McBrearty and Brooks 2000).

Kim Sterelny (2011) proposed the 'theory of niche construction' which postulates that agents individually and collectively shape their environment. Selection results in the adaptation of agents to their environments, but agents also adapt their environments to their own prototype. In modifying their own environment, many organisms also engineer the developmental environment of their offspring. It is believed that cumulative evolution depends on the high fidelity of inheritance which in turn depends on sending developmental signals across the generation with high fidelity.

The theory of niche construction proposes that humans became 'behaviourally modern' when they could reliably transmit accumulated informational capital to the next generation and transmit it with sufficient precision for innovation to be preserved and accumulated. In turn, the reliable accumulation of culture depends on the construction of learning environments. This offers a possible explanation for the major time-lag (at least 100,000 years) between the origin of anatomically modern humans and the appearance of typically human cultural behaviour.

On the balance of probabilities evolutionary rather than revolutionary perspective is more plausible.

THE EVOLUTION OF EMOTION

The term 'emotion' grew out of the work of Thomas Willis, a 17th century London doctor who identified and named many brain structures. Emotion was derived from the Latin word *movere* or to move. The modern use of the term first appeared in a set of lectures published in 1820 by an Edinburgh professor, Thomas Brown.

Charles Darwin applied his observational studies on evolution and natural selection to study human communication in his 1872 work, *The Emotions in Man and Animals.* He proposed that, as with animals, emotions also evolved and were adopted over time with some degree of similarity as shown by the facial expressions of certain animals when stressed.

A common view is that facial expressions initially served a noncommunicative adaptive function. The widespread wrinkled eyes associated with fear increased the visual field and the speed of moving the eyes which helped find and follow threats. The wrinkled nose and mouth with disgust limit the intake of foul-smelling dangerous particles in the air. Later, such reactions became increasingly more distinctive and exaggerated to fulfill a primarily social communicative function of influencing the behaviour of other members of the group.

Cross-cultural studies and studies of the congenitally blind have found they display the same expression of shame and pride related to social status. These expressions have clear similarities to displays of submission and dominance by other primates. Emotions so displayed evolved as an aid to tuning mental operations to the specific circumstance nature delivered. It is a system evolved over many millions of years, works well most of the time but is not foolproof. According to Carroll Izard (2009) discrete emotional experiences emerged in ontogeny before language or conceptual structures framing the qualia. Thus, discrete emotion feelings are acquired. Becoming capable of expressing ourselves with language contributed to our emotional evolution. Not only could we then articulate and share emotions but were able to use our experiences to foresee and act on future experiences.

THE EVOLUTION OF COGNITION

Cognitive evolution enabled humans to revise their behaviour in accordance with changing needs. They were also able to transmit the new behaviour to future generations without the necessity of genetic or environmental changes. This helped *homo sapiens* outstrip all other human and animal species. Humans acted on their material environment as well as their informational environment. This informational engineering had important consequences for cognition and culture and, of course, psychiatry. In acting on our informational environment, we sometimes enhance individual cognitive capacity. The invention of numerals and their notation enabled us to think about quantity in ways previously impossible. Material symbols enhanced memory.

Behavioural modernity emerged when a stabilised system of interaction made the accumulation of cognitive capital shareable with larger groups thus highlighting the differences between us and our more primitive ancestors. Having spread to every corner of the world acquiring the technologies, the organisational skills and the vision to explore further avenues and places, even other galaxies which the Webb telescope allows us to see from millions of light years away we seem to be a colossus striding over the world. How apt now seems Hamlet when Shakespeare had him say: "What a piece of work is man, how noble in reason, how infinite in faculty."

Survival of the fittest and elimination of the weak plays a key role in understanding both the growth and decay of many aspects of our life. Evolution left us no small burden since our cognitive, emotional, and moral faculties were adapted to individual survival in an archaic environment, not in our universally thriving modern, competitive world. To prosper and even just survive, we must deal with our evolved cognitive faculties and emotional capacity. These worked well enough in traditional societies but are now infested with bugs for whose elimination, or muting, medicine and particularly psychiatry searches for a fix (Pinker 2018).

Our neurological apparatus determines that each person plays a substantial role in the creation of his or her own reality. We have several inbuilt mental categories (for example quantity, quality, cause, and effect) which come into automatic play when confronting sensory data thereby enabling us to personally constitute the world unconsciously.

None of us are immune to "cognitive dissonance." When reality clashes with our deepest convictions, we recalibrate reality rather than amend our world view. Rigidity of beliefs is greater than before (Bregman 2017). Smart people do not use their intellect to draw the correct answer, they use it to obtain what they want to be the answer (Ezra Klien 2014).

Kahneman (2011) sees humans as a product of our evolutionary environment and in many ways ill-equipped to deal with a rational, science-based, logical world. Worse, we are at constant risk of repeating the same cognitive errors and biases, easily manipulated, and riven by irrational beliefs and fears. In reality that is dominated by science and statistics most humankind lacks the basic knowledge and experience to thrive. In fact, a tiny minority with those capabilities manipulate the others and command great wealth.

No one person invented these technologies, yet they are the most significant and far-reaching developments ever. Our computing ability continues to multiply exponentially as does internet speed and reach thanks to the cooperation of multitudes around the world. This is a revolution built on previous evolutions and has once again changed the fundamentals of how we live and survive through the rapidly changing course of life. What Artificial Intelligence may be able to achieve is overwhelming indeed.

THE VARIOUS FORMS OF ADAPTATION

Humans have not only evolved physically but also over time. by adapting to new ways of living. These adaptations were partly made by choice to improve our prospects of survival and comfort and partly dictated by the force of nature and circumstances.

ADAPTATION TO AN AGRARIAN LIFE

For most of history our ancestors lived by foraging and hunting. The end of the last Ice Age led to an increase in temperature, so people began carrying seeds to their abodes for processing and eating. Some fell on the way. Over time, more grains were spilled in transportation, and grew along the human trail.

Different people acquired food production skills at different points in time. By selecting and growing these few plants, humans learned to satisfy their nutritional requirements and grow in numbers.

Clearing the forests not only helped through increased availability of farming land, but enhanced safety for themselves and their cattle which provided a useful source of meat (protein) besides helping with agriculture. Wheat, rice and potatoes were easy to grow and store and all this culminated in the so called "Agriculture revolution,' a transition begun in the hill country of southeastern Turkey, western Iran and the Levant. Wheat and goat were domesticated approximately 9000 BC; peas and lentils around 8000 BC; horses by 4000 BC, and grapevines in 3500 BC. By the first century AD we humans across the world were mostly living on agriculture.

With the certainty of a food supply through agriculture, we gradually abandoned our nomadic way of life and settled near fields. The rise of farming gradually spread over millennia with changes occurring in stages, each involving just a small alteration in daily life.

When forests burned through natural events and/or human effort thus allowing more space for wheat and other grains, we attended to the surface and began ploughing, weeding, watering and fertilising the fields. The foragers became farmers.

Cultivation provided much more food than required. We started saving for the future, had more time at our disposal which was spent on pleasure activities including sex which caused populations to rise rapidly. The advent of village life secured us against wild animals while shared power cleared more forests. The complexities of living collectively needed greater collaboration so to provide larger houses for food storage and animal welfare. We raised more animals and increased our ability to survive the vagaries of weather while learning methods of long-term storage enabling food and prosperity over our lifetime and even for future generations.

Before adopting an agrarian lifestyle, most peoples were hunter/gatherers looking for food. They were isolated within their own band of about one hundred people who encountered in their whole life not more than a few hundred other people. When food sources were particularly rich, groups settled down in seasonal and even permanent camps.

Agriculture made the future far more important than ever. Their concern about the future was rooted not only in seasonal cycles of production, but also in the fundamental uncertainty of an agriculture at the mercy of fire, droughts, floods and pests. To build reserves, they produced more than they could immediately consume thus intensifying worries about the future. Fear, therefore, soon became a major player in the theatre of the human mind. Peasants worried about the future not only because they had more cause for worry, but also because they were able to plan for their future by clearing more land, digging another irrigation canal and sowing more crops.

Food surplus enabled a large supporting team of full-time workers such as artisans, bureaucrats, officialdom and professional soldiers. They allowed populations to acquire other comforts of life such as pursuing ways to keep warm (by making wearable materials) and living more comfortably in better and larger houses. These gains made life increasingly complex.

Population increase required more food and increased crop yields of agriculture followed. Better irrigation, better fertilizers, larger tracts of lands, automation in farming techniques all contributed to the ongoing agriculture revolution. Genetic alterations to wheat and rice in recent times have been a boon to a vastly increased population.

Since our species came into existence, there have been only two sustained periods of warm climate sufficiently supportive of an agriculture economy to leave traces in the archaeological record (Richardson, Boyd, and Bettinger 2001). The first was the Eemian interglacial around 130,000 years ago and the second, beginning around 12,000 years ago. By then, people were already present on all continents and in many kinds of environment. Geologists call this period the Holocene (Greek *holos* meaning entire and *Kainos* meaning new).

Ecological factors played a significant factor in the formation of cities. At the beginning of the Holocene, the world's great rivers were mostly wild and unpredictable. Then around seven thousand years ago, flood regimes changed, giving way to more settled flows creating the wide and highly fertile floodplains associated with the first urban civilizations.

Parallel to this, the melting of polar glaciers slowed down during the Middle Holocene thus allowing sea levels the world over to stabilize to a greater degree than ever before. Thus, those great fan-like deltas having well-watered soils, annually sifted by river action, and rich wetland and waterside habitats favoured by migratory game and waterfowl. These deltaic environments were major attractions for neolithic farmers who gravitated to them, along with their crops and livestock.

A SHIFT TOWRDS SCIENCE & TECHNOLOGY

Harari (2014) claimed that 'the great discovery that launched the 'scientific revolution' was the realization that humans do not know the answer to their most important questions'. Curiosity was the precursor of invention. In his later work, *Homo Deus* (Harari 2015) he took a more moderate position by quoting physicist Max Planck who famously said that "science advances one funeral at a time – only when one generation passes away do new theories have a chance to root out the old ones". A more likely middle ground suggests: 'Knowledge that does not change behaviour is useless. Equally knowledge that changes behaviour loses its relevance' (Harari 2015).

Magellan's 1522 expedition from Spain took three years to circumnavigate the world: a feat achievable today in just 48 hours. Francis Bacon (1620) published *The New Instrument* in which he argued that "knowledge is power." The real test of knowledge is whether it empowers us. A theory enabling us to do new things constitutes knowledge.

Technology developed gradually one step at a time, with frequent pauses. The first step was the development of stone tools about two and a half million years ago. The evolution of our body permitting an erect posture, the oppositional movement made possible by the configuration of the thumb relative to other fingers, and the brain structures provided a major impetus for rapid growth. A more sedentary life following the agriculture revolution contributed towards this growth.

Jared Diamond (1997) challenged the cliché: 'Necessity is the mother of invention'. "In fact, many or most inventions were developed by people driven by curiosity or by a love of tinkering, in the absence of any initial demand for the product they had in mind. Once a device was invented, the inventor then had to find an application for it. Only after being used for a considerable time did consumers feel, they needed it. Still other devices, invented to serve one purpose, eventually found most of their use for other, unanticipated purposes." Hence invention is the mother of necessity rather than the other way around.

Thomas Edison built his first phonograph in 1877 to be used, he thought, for preserving the last words of dying people, recording books for the blind, announcing clock time etc. He thought his invention of little commercial value but later marketed it for office dictating machines. Twenty years later the phonograph was first used to record and play music, its main and much wider utility.

Nikolaus built his first gas engine in 1766 but its capacity was weak while also being unwieldy at seven feet tall. In 1885 the design improved sufficiently to allow installation on Gottfried Daimler's motorcycle. Finally installed in the first truck in 1896, it took until World War I for people to be convinced they should replace their horse drawn carts. Inventors tinkered for a long time because early models performed poorly. Cameras, typewriters, and televisions were also of inferior quality till further inventions made them less cumbersome and more portable.

Diamond (1977) further pointed out that the "heroic theory of invention" was encouraged by 'patent law', because patent applications had to prove novelty of inventions submitted. Technology develops cumulatively, rather than through isolated heroic acts and finds most of its uses after invention, rather than meeting a foreseen need.

THE RISE OF INDUSTRIES

The rise of industries marked the change from an agrarian and handicraft economy to one dominated by machine manufacturing. These technological changes introduced novel ways of working and living and fundamentally transformed society. It was associated with the French revolution of the 18th century, strangely spearheaded by affluent lawyers, not famished peasants.

The term *Industrial Revolution* was first popularized by the English economic historian, Arnold Toynbee to describe Britain's economic development from 1760 to 1840. Subsequently, the term has been more broadly applied to a process of economic transformation rather than as a period in a particular setting.

From the beginning of civilisation until the advent of industries a man could, as a rule, live adequately by working at tasks paying little more than required for the subsistence of himself and his family. The wife worked too, and children added their labour as soon as they were old enough to do so. The small surplus above bare necessities were not left to those who produced it but often misappropriated by warriors and priests.

Harnessing the power of steam was the first step towards the industrial revolution. The industrial use of steam power started with Thomas Savery in 1698. He constructed and patented in London the first engine, which he called the "Miner's Friend" since he intended it to pump water from mines. The first practical mechanical steam engine was introduced by Thomas Newcomen in 1712. Their common principle was burning coal to use the resulting heat to produce steam which expands and pushes a piston moving anything connected to it. The efficiency of steam engines gradually improved.

The use of tools, machinery and automation has vastly changed our lives. Many of the benefits emanating from the industrial revolution remained unfulfilled (Bregman 2017). Keynes (1930) predicted that by 2030 humankind would be confronted by the greatest challenge it had ever faced: what to do with an ocean of spare time. Benjamin Franklin (1868) predicted that four hours of work a day would eventually suffice. Karl Marx (1844) had similarly looked forward to the day when everyone would have the time "to hunt in the morning, fish in the afternoon, raise cards in the evening, criticize after dinner…without ever becoming hunter, fisherman, herdsman or critic." From about 1850 some prosperity created by the industrial revolution began trickling down to the lower classes. And money is time. In 1855, the stonemasons of Melbourne secured an eight-hour workday. In 1926, Henry Ford implemented a five-day workweek at the Ford Motor Company. Famed science fiction writer Isaac Asimov (1964) was worried about 'the spread of boredom" in fifty years (about 2014).

Bernard Shaw (1927) predicted workers in the year 2000 would be clocking just two hours a day. In 1956 Richard Nixon promised Americans they would only have to work four days a week "in the not-too-far-distant future." Those predictions did not exactly come true. We are not bored to death; we are instead 'working ourselves to death', because of the long work hours being commonplace. The army of psychologists and psychiatrists are fighting not the advance of ennui but an epidemic of stress.

TIMES ARE A CHANGING FASTER.

The past two centuries have seen explosive growth in both population and prosperity worldwide. The global economy is now 250 times bigger than before the industrial revolution – when nearly everyone, everywhere was still poor, hungry, dirty, afraid, stupid, sick, and ugly (Bregman 2017).

The very concept of the passage of time has changed. We traverse distances that many of our ancestors did not travel over weeks, months, years or even a lifetime. Rapid modes of transportation enabled us to move further, more frequently and over shorter periods of time. Modern communication allows interaction with more people over a wider space and longer time, and technology provides vivid images and sounds emanating from all parts of our world. No other generation of humanity has had such tremendous capabilities. That has also made us even more time-poor. The emotional cost of these advances may be enormous.

THE BIRTH OF AN INDIVIDUAL

Our children are the product of a biological process. But each child is born into a social matrix existing prior to its conception and birth. They must navigate this complex matrix throughout life by forming various psychological connections evolving across a life span.

No child can choose their parents yet so much of the future is determined at the very point of conception. The place where one is born (for example Western Europe as opposed to Africa) is also a major determinant of future possibilities as is the physical, emotional and financial state of the parents. This plays a significant role in the attachment made with the child and will influence its sense of security or the lack of it. The family of birth also supplies the first language learned, food preference, kind of neighbourhood and a host of other influences in life which together establishes a complex interaction between personal abilities, circumstances, aspirations, social expectations and cultural perspective.

The newborn baby is totally dependent on others. The baby feels hungry and the mother (and significant others) rush to feed him/her. The crying stops, the anxiety dissipates and there are smiles all around. The baby falls sick thereby causing distress to significant others who seek relief for the baby and that is followed by comfort and joy in the parents and other carers. The close bond between the parents and the child continues even after they part. The next generation bears the imprint of those parents.

Every human is also the product of the times they are born and live in. When a child is born, the primary need is for nutrition, physical and emotional comfort, and all the other ways related to maintaining homeostasis and survival. The baby's needs grow from just nutrition and comfort to developmental needs including multimodal stimulation and emotional needs. How the mother/father/and significant others respond to signals of distress determines the need and intensity of making these signals. The less sensitive the environment to the baby's requirements the greater the need to increase the pitch and intensity of the distress signals and the more distressful it may be for those receiving these signals. Thus, a pattern of interaction can be established determining the 'goodness of the fit' between the child and the significant others in their life.

Does every significant other respond in same way or in diverse ways? What is the goodness of the fit between different adults involved in the care of the child?

We are born at a unique set of time and space to parents who are themselves individuals at a certain stage of their own development. They create distinctive ways of relating to themselves and to the child. Their physical and emotional states and their intellectual abilities play a significant role. Their aspirations and orientation towards their sense of themselves and the world are central to how they deal with the birth of the child and its rearing.

Were we born intact or with the burden of anatomical or physiological problems making us an easy or difficult child? How did the parents cope with issues affecting their sleep and aspects of general functioning? Did the mother or father or both go through biological or psychological role transition issues leading to adjustment problems or post-natal depression? Were they able to seek and access adequate help?

There are myriad questions but what really matters is the presence of a sufficiently safe environment in which the child feels loved and cared for. Absence of stressors overwhelming this safe environment enhances coping skills, self-esteem, and self-confidence. The three Ls of parenting (Love, Limitations, and Let them Grow) is a particularly good guide for parenting. It is often said that 'LOVE for a child is spelt as TIME' or, more appropriately, 'quality time.' Setting adjustable limits repeatedly based on the developmental stages of the child is crucial. 'Letting them Grow' is more about providing appropriate autonomy to explore and become an individual in one's own right. It implies age-appropriate nurturing.

Daniel Winnicott (1953) introduced the idea of the "good enough" mother. Parents often bend over backwards to achieve perfection in meeting every need of their child. He stressed that 'good enough' could in fact be better than perfection by fostering children's healthy adaptation to the realities of human interaction. Some stress is essential to healthy development in a manner analogous to that of immunization providing protection from viruses.

Daniel Kahneman (2011) observed: "The idea that large historical events are determined by luck is profoundly shocking, although it is demonstrably true. It is hard to think of the history of the twentieth century, including its large social movements, without bringing in the role of Hitler, Stalin, and Mao

Zedong. But there was a moment in time, just before an egg was fertilised when there was a fifty-fifty chance that the embryo that became Hitler could have been a female. It is impossible to argue that the history would have been the same in their absence. The fertilisation of these three eggs had momentous consequences, and it makes a joke of the idea that long-term developments are predictable".

PART II

STORIES CREATED OVER TIME

Over tens of thousands of years, we have continued to change ourselves and our environment while creating many 'stories.' Children inherit these stories which constitutes their social and cultural milieu and, to a considerable extent, are shaped by them. Learning these is important since they will significantly affect the way the child thinks, feels and behaves.

INSTRUMENTAL COMMUNICATION

The oral form of communication had significant limitations of time and space. Spoken words could be heard only by the few who were in the speaker's earshot. The listener had also to be receptive enough to retain the information. They required sufficient interest and aptitude to understand and then transmit the message to others. Communication was agonisingly slow until new technology enabled rapid transmission of information and knowledge across the globe.

THE INVENTION OF WRITING

Writing enabled transmission of information, knowledge and wisdom more accurately, with greater precision and over longer distances without the vagaries of word-of-mouth transmission and other human errors. Merchants and rulers could convey more accurate and persuasive commands to outposts. Soon, people viewed being able to write as a matter of pride and a mark of being 'civilised.'

The origin of writing is traced to the Sumerians of Mesopotamia before 3000 BC, Egyptian writing around 3000 BC, Chinese writing by 1300 BC, and Mexican writing is traced to before 600 BC. Thousands of clay tablets were excavated from the ruins of the city of Uruk (an ancient city of Sumer, later known as Babylonia about two hundred miles from modern Baghdad.) They depict the development of the Sumerian language showing the agreed-on visible marks representing actual spoken words. It is probable that other cultures who later developed writing borrowed, adapted, or at least been inspired by the existing Sumerian system (Diamond 1997).

Over hundreds or thousands of years societies took on the established principles, devised other rules and formulated their specific forms of letters to suit the local modes of verbal communication. Early scripts were incomplete, ambiguous and/or complex. Most early writing recorded buying and paying for goods and services. Kings and merchants wanting business transactions recorded used professional writers. Scribes also wrote primitive religious tracts, an aid to indoctrination which further enhanced the rulers' power. Few people learnt to write but the skill became ubiquitous after the written language was eventually simplified and became more expressive and accessible.

PRINTING

Before the advent of printing, we lived in a world where the most common means of communication was face to face talk. Handwritten manuscripts or copies were available to very few people of privilege. Even the most educated would read only a handful of books over a lifetime.

Book printing began earnestly in the 16th century. Print changed the social nature of reading. In mere decades, the production of books rose from hundreds to millions per year allowing ideas to travel further and faster. A library at home was a mark of privilege and aristocracy.

NEWSPAPERS, SHORT STORIES & NOVELS

Newspapers were invented to transmit information to a larger section of the population. Initially they were brief, black-and-white and contained only words. Printing was slow and labour intensive as was distribution though much better than by word of mouth. Eventually came colour and many photos adding life to the news.

Advances in printing technology allowed publication of short stories, novels (fiction), non-fiction, biographies and other forms of thoughts and ideas.

At least in participatory democracies this allowed the population to be more informed and knowledgeable. However, increasing competition and mass advertising, though bringing greater readership, increased the desire of the venal proprietors to influence public opinion for their own commercial or political ends. 'Newsworthy' is no statement about the truth of the reporting. People seek and consume news to enhance their fan experience, not to make their opinions more accurate (Pinker 2018).

RADIO

Radio gave birth to the entire field of electronics. No invention of modern times has delivered so much while initially promising so little. However, Italian inventor Guglielmo Marconi accidentally discovered that grounded antennas could send signals more than a mile instead of a few hundred yards.

But his vision proved limited until 'he took it to the marketplace, successfully utilising it ship to ship, famously with the *Titanic* . . .but he never had the idea of broadcasting' (Susan Douglas 1989). Although its commercial potential today seems obvious, broadcasting was kick-started by amateurs: "By the 19 teens, ham radio operators were everywhere." The first commercial radio station in the United States, went to air in Pittsburgh. July 1, 1941.

FROM IMAGES TO DRAMA

We are endowed with the ability to imagine and from that came images.

Images were carved and painted on rocks thousands and thousands of years ago. Much later we invented canvases allowing a more sophisticated art form but always telling a story. Dramas were performed in all societies for thousands of years by people gathered in one shared space to enact and experience culturally accepted stories.

PHOTOGRAPHY, AND MOVIES

The invention of photography provided a wonderful method of harvesting the past by preserving events and memories. It took several decades to move from still photography to moving images and this took the art of storytelling to another level requiring collaboration of many people with a variety of skills. These ranged from the author to script writer, director, actor, photographer, and many others making it possible to record and project the film. The initial films were black and white silent movies but soon progressed to colour and sound, thus, creating a whole new way of experiencing movies as an art form. There have been spectacular advances in technology since making movies an even more sophisticated way of watching stories unfold.

TELEVISION

Television is one of the greatest inventions of all times bringing the experiential viewing of news and the magic of the movies to everyone's home. It greatly enhanced the quality of everyday life by delivering in colour the dramatized gamut of human experience. It also unveils nature even allowing, via the Webb telescope, the sight of stars colliding and galaxies dying thirteen million light years away.

No medium has ever dominated people's lives as much as television. Nicholas Johnson (2003) observed: "Television is one of the most powerful forces men has ever unleashed upon himself". We cannot underestimate the dramatic changes it has brought to our modern society. Apart from distant space, modern TV cameras can also take breath-taking detailed pictures of the deep sea. The medium makes such abundant use of close-up shots it is often referred to as 'the medium of close-ups.'

Television now introduces children to songs, stories, culture, and traditions affecting how they think of others. From six months, infants notice skin differences, and, by their second year, they begin questioning and knowing about peoples' similarities and differences.

THE ADVENT OF COMPUTER, DESK-TOP PRINTING, AND THE INTERNET

With increasing availability of the internet, and billions of smart phones available around the world, the entire world turned into reporters and correspondents. With widespread availability of morphing and other advanced technology, reporting can be manipulated into a widespread instrument for pushing agendas. Every bit of added information challenges a previous conception, forcing it to diffuse into chaos before becoming something better (Petersen 2018) We have in many ways become victims of the stories created for ourselves. We very passionately believe in them and will defend them with all our might even if war ensues. And very soon artificial intelligence (AI) may bruit its power across all media and all manner of cultural and educational interchange. I doubt, though, that psychiatrists will be supplanted by a machine.

CULTURE AND CIVILIZATION

All cultures have narratives helping define their group as a coherent entity through time. They include creation myths, folk tales, metaphors, parables and the like passed on from generation to generation. Sharing stories expands our common ground with others thus enhancing mutual social acceptance which plays a critical role in the process of cultural selection.

E.H. Carr (1961) wrote: "History has been called an enormous jigsaw with a lot of missing parts in history. Our picture of Greece in the fifth century B.C. is defective not primarily because so many of the bits have been accidentally lost, but because it is the picture formed by a tiny group of people in the city of Athens. We know a lot about how the fifth century Greece looked like to an Athenian citizen, but hardly anything about what it looked like to a Spartan, a Corinthian, or a Theban – not to mention a Persian, or a slave or other noncitizen resident in Athens."

Cultures borrow from each other, but they also define themselves by the ways in which they can define themselves as distinct from them. The way one culture defines itself against another is always, at root, political, since it involves self-conscious arguments about the proper way to live (Graeber and Wengrow 2021).

Changes in culture lead us to accept behaviour that only fifty years ago was unthinkable like "live-in relationships" or "children out of wedlock."

CULTURE AS AN IMMORTALITY PROJECT

Humans are a self-conscious animal. Death and becoming food for worms causes immense anxiety. Culture changes all this and makes man seem important, vital to the universe, immortal in some ways. The entirety of human civilization may be one elaborate defence against death (Ernest Becker 1971)."

Freud speculated that the basic human group was formed out of fear of death. The first humans huddled together from a fear of separateness and what lurked in the dark. We perpetuated the group to perpetuate ourselves and the history taking of the group is a symbolic quest for mediated immortality. United as a group, we could better survive the ever-lurking dangers to life.

Humans are skilled at ascribing meaning to ordinary things. Menzies and Menzies (2021) have elaborated on the idea that culture may also be another clever defence against death. Our own lives become part of a symbolism likely to outlive us. Culture provides meaning in a meaningless world. When buying into a culture, we become part of something greater than ourselves. Martyrs have slavishly followed the demands of a particular culture when pursuing symbolic immortality.

'Love and marriage go together like a horse and carriage' goes the song. And it was no less true of early communes and present-day societies. Marriage relieves sexual tension in an orderly way and provides an optimistic base and method for preserving the group into the future. Many social norms were devised and refined to cement the basis of this primary social unit which requires between the partners sexual attraction, common commercial interests, shared understanding about children, disciplining, social norms and acceptance by the two families of some broader community issues which come into play. The more we share, the better the marital unit.

THE POLITICAL STORY

Politics (from the Greek word *politiká* meaning 'affairs of the cities') means making decisions in groups about power relations among individuals including managing the relative distribution of resources or status. Politics' very chequered history, ranges from control by chieftains, kings, Emperors or oligarchs to moving through various shades of democracy around the world. Nobody is unaffected by the political reality of where they live, work or travel even if oblivious to their impact on everyday life.

The food surplus and new transportation technology enabled increasing number of people to live in ever-expanding groups. Various parts of the world evolved not due to any basic differences in their biology, but because of their geography. Before democracy, power was amassed by the biggest members who sometimes gained favour by invoking some kind of divine backing.

Most countries in the world now tend to consider themselves as democracies. Although the word Democracy suggests it is the people who govern (Greek, *demos* mean people and *kratos* means power), it really works though, as Rousseau said, more as an 'elective aristocracy' because, we are allowed to decide who holds power over us. Any citizen can run for public office, but winning without access to an aristocratic network of donors and lobbyists is very difficult (Bregman 2019). Churchill (1940) quipped: "Democracy is the worst form of government, except for all the others."

Marx believed we make our own history, but not under conditions of our own choosing. The guiding principle of communism was "From each according to his ability, to each according to his needs." Communism is considered unworkable because it depends on a flawed, if romantic, understanding of human nature.

The term fascism denotes a form of ultranationalism (ethnic, religious or cultural) with the nation headed by an authoritarian leader. The most important driving force is a division between 'us' and 'them.' Every mechanism of fascist politics works to create and solidify this distinction while practising the unconstrained targeting of ideological enemies by often violent means. According to fascist ideology, nature imposes hierarchies of power and dominance inconsistent with the equality of respect espoused in liberal democratic theory.

The recent resurgence of fascism, the rise of religious fundamentalism and the thoughts/demands of living according to religious rules of one kind or another is lamentable. The intensely held views and endless media debates are so easily amplified to everyone's smartphone via social media and do often cause significant distress.

THE PSYCHOLOGICAL BASICS OF LIFE

Death is our constant companion and one of the original sources of anxiety since children become aware of death quite early. It persists throughout our lifetime, sometimes consciously but mostly resident in our subconscious.

It is difficult to discover what the very young child knows about death (Klein 1948)) since they lack language and possess only a slight capacity for abstract thinking.

Marie Nagy (1948/1959) asked children from ages 2 to 10 to express their thoughts about death in words and pictures and found the under-fives were curious about what becomes of the body, why the person is buried etc. And then from 5-9 years the child realises death is final and tends to think of death as a person, like a frightening clown or a mysterious figure in the night. From ages 9 and 10 onwards death is not only seen as final, but inevitable and universal. According to Piaget (1954/1972) the children's conceptualisation of death falls into four categories. At first inanimate objects are considered to have life. Around the seventh year the child attributes life only to things that move. From eight to twelve year the child attributes life to self-motivated things and by twelve, the child's view increasingly becomes like that of an adult.

Early life is a time of intense egocentricity whereby the child cannot perceive any boundaries between oneself and other objects and beings. Every demand is satisfied without personal effort, thus providing a sense of specialness which works as a shield against death anxiety. Throughout life at some level, we continue to be convinced of our personal invulnerability and, through that, deny death (Yalom 1980).

Parents constantly rescue their children whenever they are in trouble and so the child develops a sense of being special and sees parents as the ultimate rescuer. This forms the foundation of the defence structure the individual erects against the fear of death.

Every child is exposed to death by encounters with insects, flowers, pets etc. The child's reaction may be overly complex with several issues involved, such as guilt arising from sibling rivalry, loss and fear of one's personal death.

Separation from the mother is catastrophic for the infant. Furman (1974) worked with many bereft children and concluded that during the second year of their life children achieved a basic understanding of death. "Concrete information" about death was occasionally helpful, but the child's task was complicated when the adults wittingly or unwittingly misrepresented or obscured the objective facts. The death of a parent is a similarly catastrophic event for a child as is another child's death by undermining the consoling belief that only old people die. Seven-year-olds are far more inclined than are children of 11 and 12-year-olds to accept death's finality and irreversibility.

During the latency period the child learns (or is taught) to negate reality. Gradually the child develops efficient and sophisticated forms of denial as awareness of death glides into the unconscious, and they stop showing an overt fear of death. Young children are shielded from death. Denial is implanted early in life with tales of heaven, or of return of the dead, or with the assurance that children do not die.

Later, when the child is thought to be ready to cope, adults expose them to reality. Euphemisms such as 'gone to sleep', 'went to heaven', 'is with the angels' continue to be used and the mechanism of denial is incorporated into one's own lifestyle and character structure. Similar euphemisms exist in every language and culture as part of our everyday discourse, not only with children but also between adults.

Otto Rank (1936/1978) believed in a primal fear faced by individuals which is manifested sometimes as a fear of life, sometimes as a fear of death.

By "fear of life" Rank meant anxiety about losing connection with a greater whole. The fear of becoming an isolated being. The prototypical fear was "birth" the original trauma, and the original separation. By "fear of death" Rank referred to the fear of extinction, of loss of individuality, of being dissolved again into the whole. Between these two fear possibilities, these poles of fear, the individual is thrown back and forth all his life. Life anxiety emanating from the defences of specialness is the price we pay for standing out, unshielded from nature.

We each have an intuitive knowledge of death leavened by the individual's tendency to deny death, particularly its finality. When reality intrudes forcibly, the death-denial defences may be inadequate and then allow anxiety to surface. Commonly, adults recall death-laden scenes when asked to produce an 'earliest memory' or go back to their childhood when asked to produce a death memory (Feifel 1977).

"Tragic" and "untimely" usually describes the death of a young person thus making a significant link between age and mortality. Birth, growth, senescence, and then death is our firmly enshrined conception. Any departure from this sequence causes distress. Kastenbaum (1981) dubbed it the "pecking order of death." Epicurus (341 to 270 BC) emphasized that death anxieties are not conscious to most individuals but can be inferred from disguised manifestations: for example, excessive religiosity; an all-consuming accumulation of wealth; a blind grasping for power and honours. All these offer a counterfeit version of immortality.

Charles Wahl (1959) commented on the lack of description of death anxiety in psychiatric literature as perhaps a sign that psychiatrists also have a reluctance to study a problem so closely and personally indicative of the contingency of the human state. This may confirm de La Rochefoucauld's (1945) observation that "One cannot look directly at either the sun or death."

Humans fear their own mortality and every action taken on an individual and societal level is directed by the necessary denial of imminent death (Becker in *The Denial of Death* 1973). Humans use denial to erase the palpability of death so that we do not realize we are reacting to this existential fear.

DEATH AND EXISTENTIAL ISOLATION

The human child goes through a long process of separation and individuation marked by uncertainties. Kaiser termed the tension inherent in this dilemma as a "universal conflict." "Becoming an individual entails, a complete and fundamental, an eternal and insurmountable isolation." Heidegger said: ".. though one can go to his death for another, such 'dying for' can never signify that the other has had his death taken away in even the slightest degree. No one can take the other's death away from him. At the most fundamental level, dying is the loneliest human experience."

Not only do we constitute ourselves, but we perceive a world fashioned so to conceal what we have constituted. Eric Fromm believed isolation to be the primary source of anxiety. Existential isolation is always there but so hidden by layer upon layer of worldly artefacts each imbued with personal and collective meaning, that we experience it only as a world of everydayness and routine activities. We are surrounded in a stable world by familiar objects and institutions, a world in which all objects and beings are connected and interconnected many times over. Having been lulled into a sense of cosy, familiar belongingness (Yalom 1980) the vast existential emptiness and isolation is buried and silenced by the ordinariness of our possessions and routine activities.

The fear of existential isolation is the driving force behind many interpersonal relationships. No relationship can completely eliminate a sense of isolation. We are each the centre of 'our universe with concentric circles of different radii around this centre. Immediately outside 'me' are those closest (usually our birth family we and/or the family we created). Larger family and close friends occupy the next circle. If we keep moving outwards we are part of the society, nation, world and the whole universe. Our personal universe interacts with those of others though we are each alone in existence though love may compensate for the pain of isolation.

Our "universal conflict" is that of striving to be an individual despite this requiring one to endure frightening isolation. Commonly we deal with this through various forms of denial: "I am not alone; I am part of others." Individuals whose major orientation is toward fusion are labelled as "dependent" and escape the terror of death through belief and immersion of oneself in an ultimate rescuer.

A mode of escaping anxiety of existential isolation is by escaping individuation altogether. Identification with the group offers relief from the fear of existential isolation. Similarly, individual members of social, religious, and even more modern cultural and ethical, volunteer groups may also be participating to avoid their fear of existential isolation.

Many rituals of life (religious as well as other routines) may, at least in part, be an attempt to deal with existential isolation. For many, this denial works so effectively we are never even aware of it. The stark reality is that we were born to mortals; we are mortal, and we give birth to mortals.

MAKING AFFECTIVE BONDS:

The type of attachment children develop with key people in their surrounding is of critical importance throughout their life. For Bowlby (1969), the content of the internal working model of self relates to how acceptable, or lovable one is to primary attachment figures. The goal of attachment is the creation of an amenable external environment for children to develop a safe and secure internal model of their self. Secure attachment to the caregiver allows children to explore their world confident that the caregiver is available when needed. It allows development of a positive, coherent, and consistent self-image along with a sense of being worthy of love. The child will then have a positive expectation that significant others will be accepting and responsive. Absence of such secure attachment could lead to psychopathology.

Although Bowlby was primarily interested in young children, he believed in the core functions of the attachment system continuing through one's life. The mental representation of attachment becomes the "internal working model of expectations" about the maternal-child relationship and later self-other relationships. Love is an incredibly special form of affective bond. Plato observed that love is in the one who loves, not in the one who is loved (Alain de Button 2016). To fall in love with someone feels like such a personal and spontaneous process, it can sound strange - and even insulting - to suggest that something else (such as society or culture) plays a covert and critical role in governing our most intimate relationships.

Our love unfolds against a cultural backdrop creating a powerful sense of what is "normal" in love subtly guiding us as to where we should place our emotional emphases. Love has a history, and we ride - sometimes helplessly - on its currents.

Eric Fromm (1963 in *The Art of Loving*) believed the human being's most fundamental concern was existential isolation and to ward it off a quest for interpersonal union with another person in love. He differentiated "symbiotic union" - a form of fallen love - from "mature love." Symbiotic love, consisting of an active (sadism) and a passive (masochism) form, is a state of fusion where neither party is whole or free. Mature love is "union under the condition of preserving one's integrity, one's individuality.

According to Fromm, love is an active, not a passive process. Love is a positive affect; it is giving and not receiving - a "standing in", not a "falling for." For the mature "productive" person, giving is an expression of strength and abundance. In the very act, one expresses and enhances one's aliveness. In addition to giving, mature love implies other basic elements: concern, responsivity, respect and knowledge. To love means to be actively concerned for the life and the growth of another. Too often we make the mistake of considering exclusive attachment to one person as proof of the intensity and purity of the love. Such a love is in Fromm's term, "symbiotic love" or "overinflated egotism."

"You do not love them: what you love is the pleasant sensations love produces in you! You love desire not the desired. We are more in love with desire than with the desired. No one has ever done anything wholly for others. All actions are self-directed, all service is self-serving, all love self-loving. Need-less love is an individual's mode of relating to the world" (Yalom 1980).

Caring for the children is a major factor in prevention of suicide among women. In 2011, the Centre for Disease Control and Prevention (CDC) adopted promoting connectedness as its strategic direction for preventing suicidal behaviour. The CDC defines connectedness as "the degree to which a person or group is socially close, interrelated, or shares resources with other persons or groups."

SEEKING MEANING IN LIFE

Meaning denotes a sense of coherence and searching for it implies a search for coherence. Purpose refers to intention, aim and function. In conventional usage, purpose of life and meaning of life are used interchangeably. A citizen of today's urbanized, industrialized secular world faces life without a religiously based, though often obscure, cosmic meaning-system. There have been alternatives such as being so preoccupied meeting other more basic needs that one eschews the search for 'meaning.' Living close to the earth, feeling a part of nature, ploughing the ground, sowing, reaping, cooking, and naturally and un-self-consciously thrusting themselves into the future by begetting and raising children was sufficient. This was reinforced by a keen sense of belonging to the larger units of family and community thus obviating the need to find a further meaning to life.

Victor Frankl (1946) distinguished two stages of the "meaninglessness syndrome": (1) Existential vacuum or existential frustration, a common phenomenon, characterised by the subjective state of boredom, apathy and emptiness. Free time makes one aware of the fact there is nothing one wants to do. (2) Existential neurosis when, in addition to meaninglessness, the patient develops overt clinical neurotic symptomatology.

Frankl focused exclusively on the role of meaning in psychopathology and therapy. Though stressing that everyone has a meaning no one else can fulfill, these unique meanings fall into three categories: (1) what one accomplishes or gives to the world in term of one's creations, (2) what one takes from the world in terms of encounters and experiences, and (3) one's stand towards suffering, toward a fate one cannot change. (Yalom 1980)

For Wittgenstein there was no answer to the question of the meaning of life and even if life is broken down into components, it is still a perceived reality with which science simply cannot deal. "Whereof one cannot speak, one must be silent" (Wittgenstein 1922).

RELIGIOUS TRADITIONS

Religion seems to have existed forever and signifies a set of beliefs, practices, and language directed towards a search for transcendent meaning in a particular way, generally based upon belief in a perpetual, sometimes originating deity. Religious scriptures are the recorded collective wisdom of generations evolved over hundreds and even a few thousand years encompassing philosophy, ethics, literature and art.

Religion can be seen as an assembly of ignorance and knowledge. The part devoted to God is what is still unknown but what is known no longer needs a supernatural explanation. Believing and praying to a rain God was religious at one time but is now considered ignorant and even foolish. No God is now needed to explain or receive rain.

We feared death which came in many unexpected ways often in abundance through epidemics and the vagaries of nature. Life was more at the mercy of the elements and the concept of a benevolent God helped some through these rigours.

Scholars believe people have always believed in gods and spirits. But, the deities of our nomadic ancestors were not particularly interested in the lives of mere mortals, let alone in punishing their infractions. The emergence of large settlements triggered a significant shift in religious life. Infectious diseases like tuberculosis, cholera and the plague were all unheard of until we traded our nomadic lifestyle for farming. Seeking to explain these catastrophes, we began believing in vengeful, omniscient and omnipresent beings enraged because of something we had done. We developed the notion of sin (Bregman 2019).

Menzies and Menzies (2021) saw all religions as an 'immortality project'. Religious systems promising everlasting life, but also caused more deaths than any other belief systems in our history.

In the Hindu belief system, one's ATMAN is their immortal soul. A Hindu is supposed to follow a life of DHARMA, a moral code of living. KARMA, a cosmic calculation of the moral and immoral deeds committed throughout their life. Their karma determines the kind of afterlife they would be entitled to. The atman never dies, it is just housed in a series of transient and perishable physical bodies. Such a belief system helps with the fear that we are just flesh and bones and are one day destined to turn to dust. Buddhism also emphasises the repetitive nature of Samsara. The symbol most sacred to them is the wheel, which denotes everything being cyclic, including the cycle of birth and death. Buddhists are encouraged to reflect on the perishable and transient qualities of their own bodies.

It is interesting to take note of Charvaka or Lokayat, a philosophical school of materialism developed around 600 BCE in India. It rejected the notion of an after world, karma, liberation (moksha), the authority of the sacred scriptures, the Vedas and the immortality of the self. Being less interesting in terms of a blessed abode after death, Charvaka doctrine had disappeared by the end of the medieval period. However, its importance can be judged by the lengthy attempts made to refute it found in both Hindu and Buddhist philosophical texts.

In the Hebrew Bible, God is seen as the solution to the problem of mortality. Initially, the dominant view was, regardless of how moral or corrupt a life one had led, all souls retired to the same destination. This posed a significant challenge. From the Second Temple period onwards, the Hebrew texts reflected a conceptual shift veering towards resurrection and separation of the righteous and the wicked. Like all religion, it needed to be seen as a moral code of conduct. Otherwise, what would be the point in following a 'good life' rather than enjoying all life's pleasures?

Christianity with over two billion adherents was one of the first religions to promise immortality of both soul and body. The Christian Bible teems with reassuring messages from God about the immortality of the faithful. Death is mentioned 378 times in the New Testament, and heaven 277 times (compared to love 202 and peace 109 times). Jesus was said to resurrect the dead even on this earth.

Islam sees death as a beginning and not the end. 'The faithful do not die. They are moved from here to the hereafter.' 'Death is a blessing to a Muslim' because 'the grave is the first stage of the journey into eternity.' At the heart of both Islam & Christianity is the promise of eternal life. Nearly every page of the Quran refers to the afterlife. Christianity offers an instantaneous one-way trip to heaven whereas followers of Islam must wait until the day of judgement. Muslims who have lived a righteous and devout life are promised to go to Paradise (Jannah) where every wish is fulfilled and youth and beauty are in surplus: splendid gardens, rivers of milk and clean water, beautiful maidens serving unending banquets. And they never age nor suffer.

Being reunited with Allah and deceased loved ones in Jannah is the ultimate goal for every Muslim, the natural endpoint of a lifetime of good deeds and devout worship.

Emile Durkheim placed the roots of religion in collective tribal rituals which unleashed powerful rewarding emotions and feelings. This may have had a stabilizing outcome for the homeostasis of individuals in the group. Karl Marx wrote that religion was" the opium of the people" and combined his rejection of religion with the pragmatic recognition that religion can be a soulful refuge in a dehumanised and soulless world (Damasio 2018).

We are all part believers at best in all our beliefs including religion. There are no hundred percent blacks or whites. We often adjust our thinking to make peace with our doubts and reservations. Hindus kill Muslims; Muslims kill Hindus. Muslims kill Christians and vice versa. The same is true for Jews, Christians, and Muslims. At the same time, high caste Hindus kill lower caste Hindus. Protestants and Catholics kill each other, and Shia and Sunnis kill each other. All that killing occurs in the name of God. Whose God we are talking about? Why is one God better or worse than the other?

Organized religion can be seen as an instrument of manipulation. The king was always the strong warrior who would protect the priest. He used his position as the religious head to help maintain order and discipline in the population by the promise of heaven or condemnation to hell. This spared the king from constantly using force, a cosy and effective arrangement. Of course, the promised afterlife provided compensation for those sacrificing themselves in war for king and country.

This nexus was established and nurtured through the years. Though democracy tried to loosen that grip, politicians have often fostered the codependent relationship between political and religious powers for their own ends.

The great myths and religious stories of the past, particularly those derived from an earlier oral tradition, were moral in their intent rather than descriptive. They were mostly about propriety and an appropriateness of behaviour towards people in the family, neighbourhood, others in the community and the authorities.

Belief in an afterlife provides a degree of solace to the anxious mind and lets believers sleep at night. However, across human history, religious beliefs have created violence on a scale unimaginable. Matthew White has listed thirty religious' conflicts among the worst things that people have ever done to one another, resulting in around fifty-five million deaths (Pinker 2018).

There has been a gradual erosion in Australian religious beliefs. A recent census illustrates how those with no religion increased from about 6% to nearly 40% over the last fifty years even though the census question is so worded as to favour the pro-religious position.

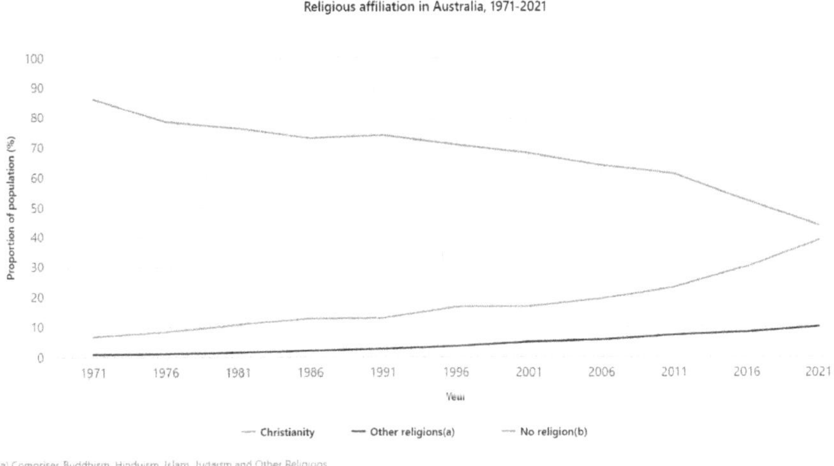

(a) Comprises Buddhism, Hinduism, Islam, Judaism and Other Religions.
(b) Secular Beliefs and Other Spiritual Beliefs and No Religious Affiliation.

Source: Australian Bureau of Statistics, Religious affiliation in Australia 4/07/2022

In Britain a fresh batch of figures from the 2021 census were published by the Office for National Statistics showing that, for the first time, less than half the population of England and Wales consider themselves Christians. Their number fell by 17% in a decade, to 27.5m; the number of people who ticked the "no religion" box rocketed by 57%, to 22.2m.

This erosion in religious affiliation does not translate into humans becoming amoral. The number of people doing yoga and meditation is rising. Interest in mindfulness and stoicism is growing. Many now subscribe to humanism as their new way of thinking. Philosopher A. C. Grayling (2011) wrote *The Good Book: A Secular Bible* as a book of life and practice for a secular age in which many find religion no longer speaks to them.

ENLIGHTENMENT

"Enlightenment consists of humankinds' emergence from its self-incurred immaturity, its lazy and cowardly submission to the dogmas and formulas of religious and political authority" (Immanuel Kant 1784). Enlightenment thinkers were always conscious of our fallibility.

Rousseau was one major figure who is credited with 'ushering in' enlightenment. David Graeber and David Wengrow (2022) provided an elaborate account of how he was heavily influenced by the thought and cultural processes widely practised by Native Americans. This elaborate exploration appears quite plausible and turns a new leaf in our understanding about enlightenment.

The Native Americans saw the French existing in a kind of Hobbesian state of 'war of all against all.' They would have seen the Europeans mainly through missionaries, trappers, merchants and soldiers – that is groups almost entirely male. Having very few women and fewer children around may have made their competitiveness and lack of mutual care even more extreme. Indigenous Americans, on the other hand, lived in generally free societies enjoying the equality of men and women. American women were considered to have full control over their own bodies, and therefore unmarried women had sexual liberty and married women could divorce at will.

Kandiaronk was an Indigenous man from America was engaged in political negotiations with Europeans for years, and regularly ran circles around them by anticipating their logic, interests, blind spots and reactions. Baron De Lahontan (1931) claimed to have based *The Dialogues* on notes jotted down during or after a number of conversations he had had with Kandiaronk. De Lahontan's description of Native Americans was brushed aside as representing the 'noble savages.' Ellingson (2001) concluded there never was a 'noble savage' myth; at least not in the sense of a stereotype of simple societies living in an age of happy primordial innocence. They were most often complicated mix of virtues and vices. It may be called the 'myth of the myth of the noble savage.'

Humans are vulnerable to illusions and fallacies. Our brains, limited in their capacity to process information, evolved in a world without science, scholarship and other forms of fact checking. But reality is a mighty selection pressure, so a species living by ideas must have evolved with an ability to prefer correct ones (Pinker 2018).

HUMANISM

Over the last three hundred years societies have turned increasingly secular in their orientation and the importance of religion, at least in the West, has receded. Humanism promotes a non-supernatural basis for meaning and ethics: Good without God. Spinoza said, "those who are governed by reason desire nothing for themselves which they do not desire for the rest of humankind (Pinker 2018).

According to Socrates, if the Gods have good reason to deem certain acts moral, we can appeal to those reasons directly, skipping the middleman. If they do not, we should not take their dictates seriously. Thoughtful people can give good reason they do not kill, rape or torture other than fear of eternal hell. Spinoza alluded to "the realization that there's nothing magic about the pronouns I and me that could justify privileging my interests over yours or anyone else's."

The moral alternative to theism is humanism in which the central belief is to uphold the preciousness of everyone. The march towards humanism has not been entirely smooth. Inequality has been part of the human race. Most societies and countries had laws discriminating against ethnic or racial minorities and others who differed in the social norms of various kinds. The rights of Gays, Lesbians and transgender people is still a controversial issue in many countries.

The most obvious and sustained discrimination is that based on gender. Sex based discrimination occurs in almost all races at every stratum of society. It has been there probably since humans started having property which, in some societies, included the women. Men, being physically stronger, appointed themselves as heads of the family system.

The Women's Rights movement has been highly effective but needs reinforcement by men teaching their sons to see women as equals while teaching their daughters to fight for their rights.

Humanism does not aim to make everyone equal. A certain level of inequality is part of how nature evolved. Only women can give birth and breast feed. Height is partly genetic and partly nutritional. Many of our physical and physiological attributes are also along a continuum but humanism is devoted to equal opportunities for everyone no matter their genetic constitution.

PHILOSOPHY

Metaphysics was the earlier term used for philosophy and involved an enquiry into the nature of reality and existence. It included all abstract thinking. Later, metaphysics separated into 'moral philosophy' (what is now called philosophy), and 'natural philosophy' (what we now know as 'science'). Philosophy is defined as 'the study of the fundamental nature of knowledge, reality, and existence'. It is also considered as a 'theory or attitude that acts as a guiding principle for behaviour.'

In the words of A. C. Grayling (2019): "We humans occupy a patch of light in a great darkness of ignorance. Each of the special disciplines has its station on the arc of the circumference of that patch of light, straining to see outwards into the shadows to decry shapes, and thereby to push the horizon of light a little further outward. Philosophy patrols the whole circumference, making special efforts on those arcs where there is, as yet, no special discipline, trying to formulate the right questions in order that there might be a chance of formulating answers."

Asking the right question is a crucial task of both philosophy and science. There are philosophical underpinnings for thought and behaviour governing everyone's life. Everyday philosophy may be less eloquent than academic philosophy but remains relevant for the person. If one takes God out of religious texts, they remain as the philosophical traditions of their time.

In a historical context, Jaspers (1913/1997) noted that all the major schools of philosophy we know today emerged – apparently independently – in Greece, India, and China at roughly the same time, between the 8th and 3rd century BC. They emerged in precisely those cities which had recently seen the invention and widespread adoption of coined money. He called it the Axial Age. This age - encompassing the lifetimes of Pythagoras, the Buddha and Confucius – corresponds not only to the invention of metal coinage and new forms of speculative thought, but also the spread of chattel slavery of across Eurasia.

Philosophers have quite differing views about human life. For Socrates in order "to learn to live well, one must first learn to die well". For Seneca "no man enjoys the true taste of life but he who is willing and ready to quit it." For Nietzsche, "a major difference between man and the cow was that the cow knew how to exist, how to live without angst – that is fear – in the blessed now, unburdened by the past and unaware of the terrors of the future. But we unfortunate humans are so haunted by the past and future that we can only saunter briefly in the now."

Philosophy has been the preserve of the privileged and the elite of every society. Sanskrit, the language of commentary on the Vedas and of philosophy in Indian culture, was not spoken by most people but was also positively forbidden to members of the lower castes involved in sustenance activities such as food production. In the Greek context, Aristotle justified the very existence of labourers, including agricultural labourers, by fact that their work enabled a small number of men, like him, to devote their lives to reflection.

Baruch Spinoza, the 17th century Dutch thinker was an eloquent proponent of a secular, democratic society and staunchly supported freedom and tolerance in the early modern period. Spinoza thought the "freedom to philosophise" not only could be granted without detriment to public peace, to piety, and to the rights of the sovereign, but must also be granted if these are to be preserved.

People often wonder why it is that after some three millennium of philosophical activity no dramatic changes seem to have been made to the questions that philosophers ask. The reason is because people keep asking the same questions and are perplexed by the difficulties. Wittgenstein when asked why "Philosophy hasn't made any progress?" His answer was: "If somebody scratches the spot where he has an itch, do we have to see some progress?" Philosophy scratches at the various itches we have, not to find some cure for what ails us, but to search in the right place and begin to understand why we engage in such apparently irritating activity. It testifies that human beings are rightly perplexed by their lives. Wittgenstein wrote, "When you are philosophising you must descend into primeval chaos and feel at home there" (Simon Critchley 2017).

Socrates (470 to 399 BCE) remains relevant to our understanding of philosophy. The "Socratic method": the method of questioning, dialogue, and cross examination forms one of the basic principles of our thinking. Plato and Aristotle occupy a unique position. Much discussion on western philosophy begins with their work during the period that is called 'classical'. This was followed by the Hellenistic period dominated by the Stoics, Epicureanism, Cynicism and Scepticism.

Much Indian philosophy is also non-theistic in its nature. The exposition of these is called 'darshans' or 'sight' or 'views' rather than the word 'philosophy.' The written text 'Astika darshans' accept the authority of Vedas and are 'orthodox.' The 'heterodox' do not accept the Vedas. Buddhism or Jainism and Charvak Lokayat belong to the latter group. Buddhism asserts that there is no Atman, no Brahman, no absolute reality; there is not only no self but no permanence of any kind. The postulation of a permanent self is the very source of suffering itself.

Wittgenstein argued that philosophical problems are matters of linguistic expression: 'There is no 'pure sensory perceptions uncoloured by thinking (in language) nor is meaning ever unequivocal because language is pluri-valent. Analytic philosophy curves its path through this intertwined jungle of sensory process and language.'

"The order of nature is ordered by the human brain. Just as colours are produced not by nature, but by our eyes and our optic nerves, so the human mind creates an order and imposes it on nature. Thus, Man has a perceptive and cognitive capability to structure the world. The understanding does not draw its (*a priori*) laws from nature but prescribes them on it" (Kant 1783/1977).

Seneca (4 BC to 65 AD) suggested: 'Life divides into three periods; that which has been, that which is and that which is to be. Of these, the time we spend is short, that we will spend, doubtful, that we have spent, fixed.' Present time is very short, so short indeed that some people think there is none.

EXISTENTIALISM

Concerns about non-existence must have been part of life ever since we existed. When humans became capable of asking complex questions beyond those involving immediate survival, they would have wondered about: Who am I? Where do I come from? Where do I go from here? We have described religion as essentially an immortality project.

Existentialism has a long tradition, extending as far back as Socrates. It was about becoming a certain kind of person. Kierkegaard saw it as finding 'a truth which is true for me, to find an idea for which I can live and die.' The first to propound a philosophy of *Existenz* was Karl Jaspers. Heidegger believed that only humans ponder why they exist at all. And this raised the characteristically existentialist issue of our contingent existence. (The term Existentialism was first explicitly used by Paul Sartre).

"Existence precedes Essence" was Sartre's signature slogan. Sartre and de Beauvoir were the only philosophers who admitted to being existentialists. Sartre's public lecture delivered on 29 October 1945 titled: 'Is Existentialism a Humanism?' became the manifesto of the existentialist movement. It is probably his most widely read work, though the only piece that he later openly regretted having published and perhaps was coloured by his proximity to the France of World War II.

Existentialism has come to be identified with a cultural movement which flourished in Europe through the 1940s and 1950s following the two world wars where rationalism and empiricism seemed to have become redundant. It was as much a literary phenomenon as a philosophical one. Though considered by some to be a cultural movement of a bygone era rather than an identifiable philosophical tradition, it is still relevant now that waning religious certainties leave an increasing sense of loneliness to accompany our search for meaning.

To "exist" is always to be confronted with the question of meaning. Most theistic beliefs also have existence as their central concern but resolve them through two unverifiable mechanisms, eternal life informed by an omniscient creator. In theism essence precedes existence. Existentialism opposes the idea of predetermination by some absolute power but stands on two central tenets: (1) Existence precedes essence. (2) A further set of categories, governed by the norms of authenticity and freedom are necessary to human existence.

The formal school of existential philosophy had it's beginning in 1834 and SÖren Kierkegaard is generally regarded as its founder. His work, however, was not translated until after the World War 1 when it was taken up by Martin Heidegger and Karl Jaspers. Both pursued the psychiatric implications of his ideas. The existential psychiatry tradition was developed through the interpretation of Heidegger's work by the Swiss psychiatrist, Ludwig Binswanger. Karl Jaspers, who entered philosophy through psychiatry, remains a very influential figure in existential psychiatry. The phenomenological approach championed by Jaspers is quite central to our current understanding of mental disorders.

Kierkegaard attacked the three most potent forces of conformity: the popular press, the State Church and the reigning philosophy of Hegel. In his view, the popular press did the thinking for the people, the Church its believing for them and Hegelianism their choosing for them. He believed that Christianity promoted complacency, greed and tokenism towards the poor and their suffering while profiting from its identification with the political and economic power of the day. The popular press was a demoralising institution undermining the search for truth by advocating opinions which many will not oppose because it may risk their possible exclusion by the majority.

Kierkegaard talked about "the single individual" in which the singularity of existence becomes known from the conflict between ethics and religious faith. In contrast to "the singularity of an individual" stands "the crowd" or more specifically "the crowd of untruth." The crowd is public opinion in the widest sense: the ideas that a given age takes for granted; the ordinary and accepted ways of doing things; -the complacent attitude coming from the conformity necessary for social life - and what condemns it to "untruth" (Crowell 2020). This relieves the person from the burden of being himself. However, to "exist" is always to be confronted with the question of meaning. When confronted with tricky situations raising existential concerns, the search for meaning acquires greater significance.

Fredrich Nietzsche is also considered to be one of the pioneers in the field. He worked on his thesis of the death of God. He sought to see it as the collapse of any theistic support for morality. Both Nietzsche and Kierkegaard saw "the crowd as untruth," and believed that the so-called autonomous, self legislating individual is just a herd animal trained by itself to docility and unfreedom through conforming to the "universal" standard of morality.

Nietzsche's thoughts were influenced by the cultural situation in nineteenth century Europe in which religious beliefs were eroding in favour of the natural sciences in general and Darwinism in particular. To him, the consequence of the death of God meant getting rid of any theistic support of morality. He saw a complicity between morality and the Christian God as perpetuating a life denying a nihilistic stance.

We are born biological beings but must become existential individuals by accepting responsibility for our actions. This was what Nietzsche meant by, "become what you are." The Judeo-Christian moral order arose as an expression of the resentment of the weak against the power exercised over them by the strong. Eventually that power became internalised in the form of conscience which created a "sick" animal whose will is at war with his own internal instincts. In this way, a herd animal was created and trained to confirm to the universal standards of morality leading to a life of docility after losing a sense of autonomy, self-regulation and freedom.

Martin Heidegger (1927) in his book *Being and Time* made an inquiry into the "being that we ourselves are" which he termed 'Dassin.' He outlined the tension between the individual and the public or crowd. He introduced "authenticity" as the norm for understanding self-identity and tied the project of self-definition through freedom, choice and commitment. He saw the "I" as "an entity whose (essence) is precisely 'to be' and nothing else than 'to be.' Who I am depends on what I make of my properties."

The central idea in Heidegger's ontology is that humans have their existence by being-in-the-world, and the world has its existence because there is a Being to disclose it (Heidegger, Macquarrie, & Robinson, 1962). He observed that, having been thrown into the world at a point in history beyond our control, we must fashion the best life we can from this contingency.

Heidegger believed in two fundamental ways of existing in the world: (1) A state of forgetfulness of being. One lives in the world of things and immerses oneself in the everyday diversions of life. One is "levelled down," absorbed in "idle chatter," lost in the "they" and (2) A sense of mindfulness of being, often referred as the "ontological mode" (Greek word '*ontos*' meaning existence). One marvels not about the way things are but that they are. To exist in this mode means to be continually aware of being. One remains mindful of being, not only mindful of the fragility of being but mindful, too, of one's responsibility for one's own being. Ordinarily, one lives in the first state. Its only when entering the second mode of being (mindfulness of being) that one exists authentically.

Heidegger emphasised the dual nature of human existence. The individual is there but also constituting what is there. The ego is two in one: an empirical ego (an object of the world) and a transcendental ego (which constitutes itself and the world). Nothing in the world has significance except by virtue of one's own creation.

Existentialism concerns itself with the conflict flowing from the individual's confrontation with the 'givens' of existence (certain ultimate concerns, certain intrinsic properties that are a part of the human being's existence in the world). Existential concerns have been recognized and discussed since the beginning of written thought. Their importance has been uniformly recognized by people from various backgrounds including philosophers, theologians, writers, poets, social scientists and clinicians involved in the caring profession.

Sartre believed each one of us must forge our meaning from an inherently meaningless world. "Man is what he does" or "The only reality is in action." He exhorted others to embrace their freedom and thus realize themselves as true human beings. "Man is nothing other than his own project. He exists only to the extent that he realizes himself, therefore he is nothing more than the sum of his actions, nothing more than his life."

Sartre's equation also held that freedom is self-determination which itself is good. The world acquired significance only through the way the human being constitutes it, 'for-itself.' There is no meaning in the world outside of or independent of the for-itself. Jean-Paul Sartre, Simone Beauvoir and Maurice Merleau-Ponty were fellow students in the 1920s. Their philosophical influences and interests were very closely aligned during the subsequent two decades and are seen as 'a phenomenological trio' developing their ideas through collective discussion (Howell 2011). Sartre and Beauvoir focused primarily on an individual's motivations, while Merleau-Ponte concentrated more on the individual's understanding of the world.

Sartre's initial form of existentialism ignored the influence of others over an individual's essence. It lead to a conflict between one's self-image and the image of oneself that other people express. This precipitated his belief that authenticity was rare and bad faith widespread.

Merleau-Ponty (1945) believed that one's freedom is constrained by the surrounding material and social situation. "The world around me is already filled with objective languages, customs, opportunities and limitations inscribed there by generations of people. All this exists in an economic situation dependent on the activities of the people I live alongside."

The idea of projects was central to Beauvoir's existentialism. She saw it as temporal. They were not determined by innate nature but developed through one's circumstances. She developed an alternative theory of freedom by recognising that metaphysical freedom could become weighed down by the social structures constraining the individual's life. This effect is mediated through the sedimentation of freely chosen projects.

For her, the slogan 'existence precedes essence' was not a fixed essence, since the idea of sedimentation entailed its continuing development and, in principle, any sedimentation project could be weakened or removed over time. Beauvoir recognized that the values and social meaning in the projects can become so firmly embedded in the individual's outlook and behaviour that they may find it difficult to overcome them and may even be unlikely to want to do so.

Sartre (1952) wrote *Saint Genet* and had by this time given up on his idea of radical freedom in favour of sedimentation. He came to accept freedom as inherently engaged in its social context through the sedimentation that gave projects their 'temporal thickness.' Once he had accepted the idea of sedimentation, he could describe Genet as imbued with the morality of the people who raised him without attributing it to him having any prior project of bad faith (Webber 2019).

Both Sartre and Beauvoir agreed there was no human nature, no fixed set of qualities explaining human behaviour in general, and no such fixed qualities of any group of people, such as gender or race. No individual has a fixed personality. Their behaviour is explained by their projects and the values they pursue.

West and King (1987) coined the term "ontogenetic niche" to emphasize that development unfolds in an ecological and social setting. It is a legacy structuring development, a crucial link between parents and offspring in an envelope of life chances. All children inherit their parents, as well as their peers, and the places they inhabit. They are also products of their times and the prevailing social structures.

Webber (2018) sees existentialism as more than a theory of the nature of human existence, but a theory that all value is grounded in the structure of what it is to be human. Crowell (2020) believes that the fundamental contribution of existential thought lies in the idea that one's identity is constituted neither by nature nor by culture, since to "exist" is precisely to constitute such an identity. It is in this light that key existential notions such as facticity, transcendence (project), alienation and authenticity must be understood.

FACTICITY denotes the '*givens*' of our situation such as our race and nationality, our talents and limitations, the others with whom we deal as well as our previous choices. From an existential viewpoint, the kind of person that I am cannot be defined in factual or third person terms. It is the first-person account of the person. 'The kind of being I am,' is also defined by the stance I take towards my facticity.

TRANSCENDENCE refers to an ability for a person to take a stance towards their own characteristics and their practical engagement in the world. Transcendence denotes the '*takens*' of our situation, namely how we face up to facticity. Through transcendence a person acquires an agent's perspective with the ability to make choices and decisions. Existentialists describe the perspective of engaged agency in terms of "choice." However, the meaning of the choice may not always be transparent to the individual making the choice.

Existence is co-constituted by facticity and transcendence and hence it is the embodied being-in-the-world, a self-making situation.

ALIENATION: This refers to the estrangement of the self both from the world and from oneself. While it is through 'my projects' that the world takes meaning, the world itself is not brought into being through my projects. The self-understanding or project through which the world is there for me in a meaningful way, already belongs to that world, and derives from the traditions of the society. My very engagement in the world alienates me from my authentic possibility. We yearn for autonomy but recoil from autonomy's inevitable consequence – isolation. Kaiser (1965) called this paradox "mankind's congenital Achilles heel."

AUTHENTICITY refers to the attitude with which I engage in my projects as my own. I do something authentically when I do it because I choose this action as my own, something to which I commit myself. I do not do so because that is what I am supposed to do for moral or any other reason. It reflects my choice of myself, a commitment I make to be a person of this sort. The norm of authenticity is a kind of transparency regarding my situation, a recognition that I am a being responsible for who I am.

The measure of an authentic life lies in the integrity of a narrative, that to be a self is to constitute a story in which a kind of wholeness prevails, to the author as a unique individual (Nehamas 1998, Ricoeur 1992). It defines a condition of self-making, a way of being autonomous. It is a mark of my freedom. At the same time, no account of authenticity can neglect the social, historical and political aspects of existence. The 'situation' under consideration stems from the very character of existence itself. An authentic choice strives to respond to the claim history makes on people with whom one belongs to seize its destiny.

FREEDOM is the ethical theory placing freedom at the core of human existence. It is not only valuable, but also the very foundation of all other values. It tries to foster an authentic stance towards values based on engagement and commitment. Freedom in existential terms is seen as choice and transcendence. Freedom is not simply a matter of the ability to pursue one's projects but includes the freedom not to pursue these projects.

According to Sartre, the patterns in a person's deliberations, decisions and actions result from the reason they find in their situations. These, in turn, are determined by the projects they are pursuing, the goals and values they are oriented towards, whether or not they are explicitly aware of this. When we describe people in terms of character traits, we are referring, whether we know it or not, to the projects they are pursuing whether they know it or not (Webber 2009).

ENGAGEMENT: Values acquires significance only if I am at some level engaged. Freedom cannot be exercised, and choice made to live an authentic life, unless one is earnestly engaged in projects governed by these beliefs.

BAD FAITH is one of the fundamental beliefs of Sartre's existentialism. Our usual inclination is to deny responsibility for our situation, that is, to be in bad faith. It is seen as a form of self-deception that is quite well spread. Exploitative and oppressive societies rampantly foster self-deception leading to existential anguish (Angst). This denotes our implicit awareness of our freedom as the sheer possibility of possibility. All forms of bad faith adhere to a falsehood about the human condition.

One version of bad faith comes from trying to collapse transcendence (our possibility) into our facticity (our attendant condition). We try to claim: 'That's the way I am.' This relieves us from the anguish of our freedom by denying we are free in the creative and existentialist sense. This type of bad faith resigns us to the life-pattern laid out for us, over which we take no control, and thus frees us from any responsibility.

Another form of bad faith allows a person to determine the 'identity' to which we can conform. Sartre termed it as 'being-for-others.' In this way, one becomes an image expected by others. Bad faith dismisses any other kind of behaviour as conceivable. Pre-reflectively, one can be aware of what is going on but reflectively they keep following the role and exclude other possibilities.

One other form of Bad faith is that of the dreamer who discounts our antecedent condition by sheer wilfulness, as if there's pure possibility with no actuality. The dreamer lives entirely in the future, unencumbered by any past.

Crowell (2020) sees existentialism to be a useful broad term of intellectual history illuminating the work of philosophers and several others who rejected the label. There is a core of philosophical content in existential thought grounded in the phenomenological approach giving philosophical shape to the basic existential insight that thinking about human existence requires new categories not found in the conceptual repertoire of ancient or modern thought.

The powerful and reciprocal dependency of thoughts and feelings explain why so many people are so predictably unpredictable. There are so many good ideas and intentions available and yet we fail to enact them.

In summary Steven Crowell (2020) says that, as a cultural movement, existentialism belongs to the past, however "As a philosophical inquiry that introduced a new norm of authenticity, for understanding what it means to be human - a norm tied to in-the-world-existentialism has continued to play an important role in contemporary thought in both the continental and analytic tradition." Other theories of human behaviour can be classified as forms of existentialism only if, or only to the extent that, they agree that our existence precedes our essence, that human individuals have no fixed nature, and their motivations are rooted in their chosen projects.

ENACTIVISM: AN APPLIED EXISTENTIALISM

Varela, Thompson and Rosch (1991) introduced *the enactive approach* in their book *The Embodied Mind* out of dissatisfaction with the cognitive view of the mind. They were unhappy with the prevailing view of the human mind being likened to a computer. To them the mind was being seen as the software running on the hardware of the brain. Varela and colleagues viewed cognition as an 'embodied action' highlighting two important points: (1) that cognition depends upon the kind of experiences that come from having a body with various sensorimotor capacities and, (2) that these individual sensorimotor capacities are themselves embodied in a more encompassing physiological, psychological, and cultural context.

They brought to focus four main characteristics of cognition: (1) embodied (2) embedded, (3) a form of action, and (4) intertwined action and perception. So, we cannot understand cognition in isolation from the bodily being doing the cognising, nor from the environment at which it is directed.

They saw the organism and the world as dynamically coupled. All living beings were self-organising unities which actively maintained their own boundaries by interacting with their environment. To remain alive, living beings need to eat and breathe and defecate. In an environment consisting of many other living beings whose needs may be detrimental to their own, organisms need to find their way and adapt to the dynamics of their environment.

The mind is not a separate faculty, nor something inner, it is not hidden in the brain where it is causing actions; the notion of 'mind' instead refers to a type of interaction with the environment (de Haan 2020). "Sensemaking" can be defined as an organism's evaluative interaction with its environment. Living beings rely on making sense of their environment for survival. In its basic form it is about distinguishing (perceiving) what is supportive of one's existence and what entails threats. This is inherent to all living beings. It is in this sense that life, cognition and mind are continuous.

There are three dimensions of sense-making including: (1) Basic sensemaking of the here and now. It involves the relevant aspects of the present environment, recognizing food, mates, danger etc. (2) Evaluative sensemaking signifies the desire not just for survival but for living a good life. The meaningfulness of our worlds and the values that guide our actions surpass the functional or the life-maintaining. (3) With stance-taking a different type of values emerges: 'existential values' such as respect, honour, dignity, friendship and love. This existential dimension can even transform our basic needs.

The interaction between the organism and the environment is a constant back and forth, acting and reacting, mutually adapting and changing. It is not just the present relation that counts but also the history of couplings which shaped the present interaction. The proper unit of analysis is the person in interaction with her world. An estimation of someone's current situation also requires that the history of these interactions be also considered.

The capacity for sense-making depends on there being a body needing to be sustained and requires interaction with its environment to do so. The brain is an indispensable organ for thinking but remains an organ and, as such, depends upon the whole body for its functioning. The environment we make sense of is a social and cultural world. Our existential sense-making capacities are also, to a considerable extent, learned in and through social and cultural interactions.

Our environment is primarily a social one not only because most of our interactions are with people, but also because our material world and objects in it are mostly human-made. "Even if I stay in my apartment and don't see anyone, sociality still permeates everything from the fact that I live in a building, to the newspaper I read, the music I listen to, and the food that I eat, all is shaped by the specific community I am part of, with the specific sociocultural practices. The sociocultural practices reflect histories of coupling. They are continuously being shaped and reshaped by the actions of the participants" (de Haan 2020).

Taylor (1985) described persons as 'self-interpreting' animals. Stance-taking is unavoidable. Once you can take a stance, you cannot refrain from doing so. Once you have become conscious of yourself as being visible to others, of the fact that others can see you and have a perspective on you and can evaluate you, there is no going back to oblivion. Once you realise that what you say and do says something about you, that you express yourself, this cannot be undone.

Even our basic biological needs are transformed and acquire an existentially meaningful dimension. Eating, for instance, is much more than just filling your stomach with nutrients. What one chooses to eat is meaningful, as it with whom, and where.

The existential dimension is about our stance-taking which shapes the way we interact with our world. It also shapes our everyday life. We reveal our stances through our behaviour but, at the same time, our stances are constituted by the behaviour. Our stance-taking capacities form the very precondition for the development of psychiatric disorders (Fuchs 2011). Only an organism capable of stance-staking, of being self-conscious, of relating to past and future, of evaluating themselves and others, of making moral judgements, of living a good life are also vulnerable to mental disorders.

Our stance-taking position adds depth, not just to the meanings we encounter in the world, but also to our sufferings. Our capacity to reflect gives rise to the emergence of guilt and shame. The more we relate to others the more we worry about such emotions.

PART III

STORIES WE LIVE

Autobiographical memories are the bedrock of life. When we are born, we are only a part actor in our lives. So much of what we think, believe, and do is determined by the significant others in our lives who, in turn, have been shaped by the generation(s) before them. One of the basic tasks of growth as an individual is separation/individuation. To do so we must gradually become the actor, script writer, director and editor of the movie called 'my life.' How well one can assume these roles varies markedly from person to person. The outcome of individual efforts may not entirely be up to themselves.

We live a life-script which is slowly encrypted and elaborated with our emerging sense of self. These are not rigid scripts followed in letter and spirit. They are always subject to change with what we encounter along our journey through life. Our life-scripts are determined by a variety of factors ranging from our senses to the individual neurons and the complex process of physical health, emotions, cognitions, behaviour and sense-making. Of course, there are also social and cultural factors.

UNDERSTANDING OUR PHYSIOLOGY & THE PHYSICAL ENVIRONMENT

The fundamental and basic unit of existence is our body (anatomy), and every living body must be functional (physiology). The key to physiology is the metabolism (the process of exchange of matter with the environment through which the organism can maintain itself) and homeostasis (the ability to maintain the functional operations of the body continually and automatically, chemically, and physiologically, within a range of values compatible with survival).

"Our physical existence cannot be adequately explored as if it were merely a matter of anatomical structure and physiological function, arbitrarily located in space. It must be regarded as a living engagement with the world around it, whereby it achieves form and reality through constant adaptation to stimuli, which it receives in part and in part creates" (Jaspers 1959).

Our body is a complex but very finely tuned machine. The various systems are interdependent and delicately coordinated. For the sake of convenience, we divide our physiology into various systems though they are quite interlinked. Given the complexities of our physiology (as well as anatomy) the surprising thing is not why it sometimes breaks down, but how effectively and for how long it continues to work. A lot is going in our body at any given time, yet we address it piecemeal, targeting one problem or system at a time.

If our body were an orchestra, the symphony is the hypothalamic adrenal axis (HPA), and the hypothalamus is the conductor. It is just a small structure located deep in our brain (the location may signify its importance to us and hence the need to protect it as deeply as possible within the bony cranium). It acts as the coordinating centre of the body, keeping it in a stable state through homeostasis. It does that by directly influencing our autonomic nervous system and by managing hormones. It plays a crucial role in many essential functions, including releasing hormones, maintaining daily physiological cycles, controlling appetite, managing sexual behaviour, regulating emotional responses and body temperature.

The Catechol-o-methyl transferase (COMT) gene serves as an example illustrating the complexity of our physiology. This gene provides instructions for making an enzyme called catechol-O-methyltransferase which is critical in the metabolic degradation of dopamine, a neurotransmitter hypothesized to influence human cognitive function. It may directly affect our stress reactivity, health and well-being. Those with this gene appear to experience both negative and positive emotions more strongly. Those with the COMT gene variation Met/Met tend to be more neurotic and have lower stress resiliency.

An estimated 20-30% of Caucasians of European ancestry have a COMT gene variation which limits the body's ability to remove catecholamines including dopamine, norepinephrine, estrogen by 3-4 times. This "slow" variation of the COMT gene is associated with greater levels of cortisol and it interferes with the body's ability to calm itself and de-stress.

How the body makes sense of bodily changes has a profound effect on life. Pain on the right side of the chest has a potentially dire interpretation which may cause anxiety. On the other hand, anxiety can also cause chest discomfort. The common symptoms of mitral valve prolapse (a generally innocuous condition, only diagnosed through routine examination) includes bursts of rapid heartbeat (palpitations), chest discomfort and fatigue and can be interpreted as panic. A panic attack has implications for life and death and is experienced as a 'fear of dying.'

Some people are known to be 'highly sensitive persons' (Aron 1996). They are extremely perceptive to every subtle change in their body and their environment. It is just the way they are and understanding their presentation in the light of their sensitivity would make greater sense. As Scott Stossel (2014) put it: "My anxiety is a reminder that I am governed by my physiology - that what happened in the body may do more to determine what happens to the mind than the other way around." He goes on to suggest that "the truth is that anxiety is at once a function of biology and philosophy, body and mind, instinct and reason, personality and culture."

Nietzsche believed the body was superior to philosophy. The body knows things we cannot put into words. It knows them directly, without mediation. The mind can deceive us with its thoughts and assumptions. It can make us believe things that are not true or that we do not want to be true. The body, on the other hand, does not lie. It tells us what is happening in the present moment without judgment or bias.

In the words of Aubrey Lewis (1934): 'There is no theory of psychopathology which can neglect the preponderant role of one's body in giving substance to consciousness and relevance to reality. It is not to be supposed that a meaningful change in the body can leave the mind just as it would be if there were no such change.'

In many ways, disordered physiology could and often does determine destiny. Being born with one or more major physical problem (blind, deaf or with cerebral palsy and a variety of severe physical and developmental problems) will have a profound effect on managing life. Having a condition is one thing and making sense of having that condition, and learning to live with them can have even greater significance. Stephen Hawking outlived his life expectancy by almost half a century. He was physically extremely limited yet made an enormous contribution to humanity and is considered amongst the brightest persons to have ever lived.

COMPLEXITY OF THE MIND

The brain is not a piece of hardware with mind as its software. Both interact in an inseparable and complex manner. The brain is the organ of the mind and mind is one of the various functions of the brain.

Robert Burton (2008) in his well-articulated book *On Being Certain* points to some of the complexities of mind. The 'holy grail' of science (and much of the philosophy of mind) is to explain how the brain creates a mind. Scientists do not know how a collection of electric brain signals creates subjective experiences. Seeing each individual neuron as a simple on-and-off "device" is convenient and yet deceptive. The final yes-no decision to fire or not to fire is influenced by complex control mechanisms ranging from the interaction of genes to moment to moment shifts in hormone levels. Once they leave the individual neuron, the scale of interaction becomes exponentially more complex. Individually "mindless" neurons join to mysteriously create the MIND.

The theory of *emergence* has been used to explain our understanding of how consciousness arises out of "mindless neurons." Burton takes the example of the tiny termites who can work in unison to construct huge mounds measuring up to twenty-five feet in height. No termite with their tiny brains has a clue how or why to build a mound. Its brain is not large enough to carry the information. There are no termite engineers, architects or critics. All termites are low-level labourers operating without blueprints, or even a mind's eye notion of a termite mound.

The same process may apply to the human brain. Each neuron is like a termite. It cannot contain a complex memory or hold an intelligent discussion. There are no super-neurons, nor are there any master plans contained within each neuron. Each neuron's DNA provides general instructions for how a cell operates and relates with other cells. It does not provide instructions for logic, reason, or poetry. And yet, out of this mass of cells, comes Shakespeare and Newton.

Consciousness, intentionality, purpose, and meaning all emerge from the interconnections between billions of neurons not containing these elements. Termites are to termite mounds as single neurons are to the mind. Primary modules provide the *bricks and mortar*, the secondary association areas build the *house*, and yet more complex interactions are necessary to call this building *home (*Allen 2013).

Supporting the neurons is a cast of three other varieties of brain cell—microglia, oligodendrocytes and astrocytes—collectively called glial cells. Microglia are gardeners. They prune links between neurons to keep the network in order. These cells prune synapses during brain development, and this process continues into a person's mid-twenties. By hunting down and swallowing rarely used synapses, microglia keep the brain lean and mean, streamlining the computations neurons perform and ensuring the organ remains as efficient as possible. Getting rid of rarely used synapses helps artificial neural networks to encode added information and store memories.

Oligodendrocytes have crucial roles in tweaking axonic signals. Misbehaving glial cells are now implicated in a range of conditions, from autism to multiple sclerosis to obsessive-compulsive disorder. They produce myelin which wraps around axons to improve those fibres' electrical conductivity and fine-tunes the velocity of electric signals in axons. This fine-tuning (achieved by adjusting the diameter of the axon and of the distances between the nodes of the myelin sheath) compensates for any remaining difference which reflects the actual interval between the times of a sound's arrival at each ear. And it is that real difference which the brain uses to locate from whence a sound has come.

Astrocytes are snowflake-shaped cells sporting tendrils, each terminating in an appendage called an "end-foot." Every astrocyte governs a territory of its own, and these tessellate to form a three-dimensional mosaic across the brain. End-feet hunt down and envelop synapses, allowing astrocytes to eavesdrop on the chatter between neurons and then, by strengthening or weakening particular synapses, exert control over the computation done within networks of neurons. Consequently, they play a crucial role in memory formation, especially in the hippocampus, which consolidates relevant short-term memories into long-term ones. Astrocytes regulate between 50% and 90% of human-brain synapses in this way. They also seem able to perform computations of their own.

Misfiring microglia in those with autism may fail to prune synapses thoroughly enough during brain development, resulting in overconnected brains with heightened sensitivity to stimuli, both sensory and emotional.

Dysfunctional oligodendrocytes have been thought to be a cause of psychosis in conditions like multiple sclerosis, bipolar disorder and schizophrenia. Such dysfunction disturbs the myelin on axons, disrupting the timing of their signals. The hypothesis is that this results in the hallucinations - imaginary sights and sounds - the defining feature of psychosis.

There is also compelling evidence that misfunctioning astrocytes play a role in mood disorders such as depression and anxiety and in neurodegenerative diseases like Alzheimer's. Most strikingly, in 2021 Liam O'Leary at McGill University in Montreal reported that the brains of depressed suicide victims had markedly reduced densities of astrocytes, compared with healthy brains, in parts of the prefrontal cortex (the brain's executive), the caudate nucleus (which helps control goal-directed behaviour) and the thalamus (which passes sensory information to the cortex).

We should not see our knowledge of physiology as closed either. The gut is receiving increasing attention as "the second brain." The enteric nervous system relies on the same type of neurons and neurotransmitters that are found in the central nervous system. This second brain in our gut, in communication with the first brain in our head, is thought to play a key role in certain diseases in our bodies and in our overall mental health. Research suggests that the gut microbiota differs significantly between patients with major depression and healthy individuals. Modifying this with a probiotic diet has been shown in several small studies to improve stress and depression scores.

Studies are afoot to explore why sound can ease pain. A recent study on mice showed that relative sound intensity might play a role in helping reduce pain. Low intensity sound can inactivate the audio-somatosensory pathway and thus the activation of the somatosensory thalamus. A noise played at low volume appears to blunt activity in parts of the brain responsible for signalling pain (Yuanyuan et al 2022). Sound induces analgesia through corticothalamic circuits. The ideal volume was 5-decibel, but the type of sound played made no difference. There is quite obviously a long way to translating these findings in mice to the human context. Whether this would have implications for psychic pain (for example different forms of depression) only time will tell.

OUR PHYSICAL ENVIRONMENT

"The organic even in its lowest forms pre-figures mind, and.... mind even on its highest reaches remains part of the organic" (Jonas 1966/2001). The fundamental characteristic of life is that all organisms have metabolism, whereas no non-living thing has it. The organism is structurally coupled to its environment. The environment affects how the organism acts and how the organism acts in turn affects the environment.

Our body is made of various elements of our physical world. We need oxygen for survival and nutrition for the functioning of our systems. Water constitutes 80% of our body and is essential for the maintenance of homeostasis. Nutrients include adequate quantities of carbohydrate, protein, fat, vitamins, minerals (Iron, Sodium, Potassium, Iodine, and a range of trace elements).

There was a time when food was in short supply and the percentage of the world population suffering from under- or mal- nutrition was quite high. Thanks to automation, better irrigation, genetic engineering and better food preservation we can now produce enough food for all humans. Animal farming has also helped overcome protein deficiency. However, the distribution of food is still asymmetrical. Overabundance of food has created its own set of problems including the dramatically high incidence of obesity and diabetes. Techniques used for increased production and preservation often deliver unwanted, unanticipated, and harmful effects.

Scarcity of drinking water is a major problem in certain parts of the world and is likely to worsen. As a result of increasing population density, overuse of water and unpredictable weather patterns, the underground water tables are being depleted. It is feared that the next great war may be driven by the need for countries to control water resources.

IRON is an important mineral essential for the formation of haemoglobin in our red blood cells. Haemoglobin enables oxygen to be carried from the lungs to various parts of the body. Deficiency of iron in the body can result for a variety of reasons ranging from dietary deficiency, inability to absorb food from the gut, and the loss of blood due to many causes. Iron deficiency leads to anaemia and that has been associated with many physical symptoms as well as depression and anxiety.

IODINE is a trace element available in many food items. It is essential for synthesis of the thyroid hormone. Hypothyroidism is associated with many physical symptoms as well as anxiety and depression. The same is true for hyperthyroidism.

LITHIUM has existed since the dawn of universe as one of the three elements (along with helium and hydrogen) believed to have come into existence because of the big bang about 13.7 billion years ago. Lithium is found across the earth in rocks, water, plants and animals. It was first identified in the early 1800s. It was shown to be useful for treatment and prevention of relapse in manic depressive illness (bipolar disorder) in 1949, predating most other psychotropic drugs in current day use.

The amount of lithium available in drinking water varies from place to place. The first evidence that trace amounts of lithium in tap water might affect mental health appeared in 1972, when Dawson et al reported that psychiatric hospital admissions and homicide rates were lower in Texas counties with higher lithium levels in the water supply. In 1990 Schrauzer & Shrestha published a study on lithium levels in water in Texas and concluded that lithium at levels encountered in public water supplies may have a moderating effect on suicidal and violent criminal behaviour.

VITAMIN D is made by the body from sunlight. In recent times, major interest has been shown to evaluation of Vitamin D in our body and it has been touted to be necessary for the prevention of several physical and mental disorders. Sales of vitamin D have skyrocketed recently.

Agus (2011) pointed to the complexities surrounding the massive recent interest in the story of Vitamin D. People who are dark skinned evolved in this fashion so they would be exposed to enough sunlight to maintain adequate levels of Vitamin D, as they are often from regions with limited light exposure. Conversely, those who live closer to the equator have many opportunities to make Vitamin D and thus evolved to have darker, more impenetrable skin.

The ability to tan is a trait that evolved several times throughout evolution. We had to learn to survive not only in various regions of the globe, but we further had to develop ways to offset wild fluctuations in the sun's intensity from season to season.

LIGHT is a major factor in how our body and our lives operate. The individual cellular clocks run on a cycle that is close to 24 hours - the circadian rhythm. The clocks of individual cells can drift apart from each other during the earth's day-night cycle. To keep these clocks coordinated there is a master clock located in the brain, the suprachiasmatic nucleus (SCN) located in the hypothalamus which regulates many basic body functions. The SCN is composed of about 20,000 closely networked cells whose rhythms are coordinated so that the firing rate of the cells varies together in a near-24-hour rhythm. The firing of SCN cells is then transmitted directly and indirectly to many other regions of the brain which then pass on this clock signal to the rest of the body by neurochemical and hormonal means.

Two of the best characterized rhythms driven by this clock signal are the body temperature cycle and the production of the hormone melatonin. The SCN regulates body temperature via connections to other areas of the hypothalamus. Body temperature varies in a wave-like pattern, reaching a maximum during the day and a minimum during the night. Among the most important of the body rhythms controlled by the SCN is that of the sleep wake cycle.

The pineal gland is a small, pea-shaped gland just above the suprachiasmatic nucleus. The SCN projects to the pineal gland to affect melatonin secretion. Light suppresses the secretion of melatonin. Descartes regarded it as 'the principal seat of the soul' and the place in which all our thoughts are formed.

While the concept of soul may be disputed, the importance accorded to pineal gland and melatonin is interesting.

For most human history, our sleep-wakefulness cycle was dependent on the amount of natural light available to us. The circadian rhythm dictated our lives, and we slept longer hours in winter as the light period was short. Conversely, we slept less in summer due to the longer light periods. The other rhythms (such as cortisol secretion) followed the sleep-wakefulness cycle.

We slowly developed the ability to lengthen our day by burning wood, oil, kerosene lamps etc. However, the light produced was dim and not very cost effective. A major change took place with the invention of the incandescent light bulb and the generation and distribution of electricity throughout most of the world.

With the invention and further innovation of television, internet and smart phones, we have further shrunk our night. We live in times when a large segment of the population is sleep deprived. Many scientists believe that the increase in the prevalence of depression in recent decades is due to the disruption in the circadian rhythm allowing for disruption of other body.

POPULATION EXPLOSION

The population of the world is multiplying exponentially. Ironically, the population explosion started most dramatically in the 1960s when the pill became widely available. Despite a recent decline, the world's overpopulation has major implications for the way we live including our housing, food requirements, water needs, consumption of fossil fuels and other resources.

CLIMATE CHANGE

Our environmental circumstances have a major influence on three most important existential requirements: breathing, drinking and eating. They are the basic preconditions for our existence. Concerns have been raised by widespread air pollution due to rising levels of fossil fuel consumption and rising population density. There are major uncertainties regarding the adequacy of water supply and food production.

Adverse psychiatric outcomes are well documented in the aftermath of (natural) disaster and includes post-traumatic stress disorder, major depression and somatoform disorders. There is reason to believe that people with mental illness are particularly vulnerable to heat-related death.

Indirect consequences of climate change, such as migration and economic collapse, are potential drivers of adverse health outcomes. Low-lying coastal areas will become uninhabitable as coastlines disappear. This is particularly concerning as thirteen of the world's largest twenty cities are situated on the coast as well as all the small island nations of the world. Coastal areas in poor countries will be the worst affected.

In 2009, a Lancet Commission on Climate Change asserted: "climate change is the biggest global health threat of the 21st century." Climate change is expected to impact mental health via a range of direct and indirect pathways. Direct pathways include exposure to traumatic events, such as bushfires and other severe weather-related events. Indirect pathways operate through a range of social, political, and economic determinants of mental health such as poverty, unemployment, and housing.

Charlson et al (2021) did a scoping review to explore the existing original research literature investigating climate change and mental health using WHO's global research priorities as a framework. They identified 120 original studies published between 2001 and 2020 specifically referencing climate change impacts, adaptation, mitigation, and other interventions relevant to mental health. Most studies were quantitative, used a cross sectional design, were conducted in high-income countries, and were concerned with assessing the mental health risks associated with climate change-related exposures. While interpretation is therefore difficult, the existing evidence overwhelmingly points to a negative association between climate change and mental health.

UNDERSTANDING OUR EMOTIONS

The paradox of emotion is that on face value they are self-evident and obvious. However, when examined introspectively, they are not so easy to define. Attempts to reach a consensus definition has repeatedly failed.

Antonio Damasio (2003) described emotions as the "continuous musical line of our minds, the unstoppable humming." According to many, emotional experiences are a consequence, and not cause, of the various responses that are evoked by a particular stimulus (Anderson and Adoloph 2014). They argue that emotions in effect constitute an internal, central state, which is triggered by specific stimuli (extrinsic or intrinsic to the organism). This state is encoded by the activity of particular neural circuits that give rise to externally observable behaviours and the associated cognitive, somatic, and physiological responses.

PSYCHOLOGICAL THEORIES OF EMOTION

Psychological theories of emotions have emphasised the multi-component nature of emotions. It includes subjective experiences, neuropsychological processes, as well as somatic and endocrine ones. Appraisal theories propose the idea that an organism continuously evaluates a stimulus within a context. This theory stresses that emotions involve highly coordinated and often synchronised effects in behaviour, body, and brain. Darwin had proposed that phylogenetically distant, invertebrate organisms have primitive emotion states that are expressed by externally observable behaviours. However, these primitive emotion states are not necessarily homologous to the specific psychological categories that characterize human emotions (fear, anger, happiness etc.). These states have certain properties which are shared across emotions and across phylogeny, even if the species-typical behaviour that express them are not.

Much of the literature on emotion, regarding the relationship between emotion state and observable behaviour is confusing. There is disagreement about the causal direction in which behaviour is related to emotion. A common lay intuition is that the state causes the expression: "I cry because I am sad." The predominant psychological view typically makes the behaviour a part – and even a cause – of the emotion. Some theories argue that emotion states are so dynamic that it becomes impossible to say whether the behaviour is cause or consequences (Salzman and Fusi 2010).

Colloquial usage of the word "emotion" refers to "feelings" which is our subjective perception of emotion states and their accompanying somatic response. Recent theories have been more careful to make a clear distinction between emotion and feelings (Damasio 2003). The existence of "feelings" can only be assessed by verbal report – and therefore is currently uniquely accessible to study in humans alone.

There are certain features that can be considered as the evolutionary "building blocks" that describe central emotional states. These features are common to different emotions, in different animal species:

1. Scalability: Emotional states have often been classified according to their valance (positive or negative) and their intensity (Russell 1980). One can be annoyed, angry, furious, or enraged: sad, despondent or

grief stricken. Graduations in emotional intensity are also associated with qualitative shifts in the behaviour associated with the states.

2. Valence: In our daily life, we infer the existence of a particular emotion in others through its behavioural expression. According to the "Principle of Antithesis" (the second of the three principles enunciated by Darwin), emotions come in pairs of opposites (e.g., joy and anger, happiness, or sadness) which are expressed in physically opposite and complementary behaviours.

   In psychological theories of emotion, valence (antithesis) and arousal (intensity) are taken to be essential features of all emotions, and one that defines what is referred to as "core affect" (Russell 2003, Barrett et al 2007). There may be instances of antithesis that do not seem to fall on opposite ends of a positive versus negative dimensions.

   Susskind et al (2008) have shown that fear and disgust expression in humans have opposite effects on increasing or decreasing the intake of sensory information, respectively (fear widens the eyes and nostrils to acquire cues about a potential danger; disgust squints the eyes and nostrils to shut out aversive taste and odours).

   Valence and intensity can be the two defining aspects of emotion that distinguish emotions from all other kinds of mental states (Russell 2003, Salzman and Fusi 2010). In humans, many studies have argued for a small set of so-called "basic" emotions, including happiness, fear, anger, disgust, sadness, which are thought to be culturally universal, especially in their facial expressions (Ekman 1992).

3. Persistence: A key feature that distinguishes emotional behaviour is that they often outlast the stimuli that elicit them. In humans anxiety and depression can continue for prolonged periods of time, with a

sustained and pervasive effect on experience, cognition, and behaviours.

4. Generalization: One consequence of persistence is that an emotional state induced by one stimulus can generalize to a different context and thereby influence subsequent responses to different stimuli. In this way, emotions bias cognitions and behaviour. This accounts for "transsituationality."

UNIQUELY HUMAN FEATURES OF EMOTION

There may be emotional states unique to humans or primates, or mammals. The likely candidates are some of the "social" and "moral" emotions (Tangney et al 2007). The emotions of pride, embarrassment, and awe are likely to be uniquely human. All the features that apply to emotions more generally may also apply to these emotion states.

The three important ways in which human emotions may be unique are:

A. Volitional Control: Control over one's emotions is a feature of adult human emotions that is not typically observed in nonhuman animals nor in human infants and children. The prefrontal cortex is one of the latest regions in development to become myelinated. Its protracted developmental timeline may account for the metacognition (aspects of attention, and volitional control over behaviour, thought and emotion) required for the voluntary control of emotions in adults. (Thompson et al 2000)

   A major mechanism for psychopathology in humans is thought to be impaired ability to regulate one's emotions and may account for psychiatric disorders ranging from PTSD to phobias. CBT may be effective by utilizing various strategies to re-establishing cognitive control over emotions. Alternatively, humans can achieve this through active suppression of emotional reactions (Gross 2002).

B. Subjective Report: Psychological investigations in humans are based not on behavioural observation but on verbal reports. We can usually readily observe our own emotions. However, we are more likely to be able to identify emotional states of other people or animals through behavioural observation. Parts of the orbitofrontal cortex and the nucleus accumbens may be particularly important for the subjective experience of emotions.

   Based on their concept of emotions as a central state, Anderson and Adalphs (2014), believe that neither behaviour nor feeling are themselves part of the emotional state. They should instead be viewed as consequences of it.

C. Stimulus-decoupling: A given emotion state may not only be caused by a large set of eliciting stimuli in humans. It can also be caused by no direct stimulus at all. Most of such emotional states may occur through the anticipation or recollection of these stimuli.

The increased metacognitive abilities of humans also make it possible to elucidate emotion states through thoughts and imaginations. They include all kinds of situations that one has never experienced such as one's own mortality. These are unlikely to be found in other animals.

Guilt is supposed to have evolved to: (a) dissuade individuals from harming beneficial relationships and/or (b) motivate them to repair damages done to relationships. Even though the existence of cognitive biases should favour the ability to surreptitiously cheat, yet guilt motivates reparation even when the transgression is undiscovered. This raises the possibility that guilt while premised on emotions such as regret and sympathy, may be the product of cultural rather than biological evolution. This is believed to account for the absence of universal facial or postural expressions of guilt.

Shame and pride motivate an assessment of prevailing norms and awareness of the presence of observers and conformity to pervasive expectations under observation. Consequently, contempt and moral outrage motivate publicizing the actions of nonconformists, excluding them from cooperative endeavours and inflicting cost upon them.

EMOTIONAL INTELLIGENCE

Philosophical considerations on the relations between thoughts and emotions has continued for centuries. We now recognise three distinct kinds of intelligence: verbal intelligence, spatial intelligence and social intelligence.

Emotional intelligence (EI) belongs to the social intelligence category. The two are interrelated and denote the capacity to understand and use emotional information. EI attempts to see thoughts and emotions as adaptively and intelligently intertwined and reflects the emotion system's capacity to enhance intelligence.

The original approach defined EI as noncognitive competencies with five categories: Intrapersonal, including such qualities as self-actualization, independence and emotional self-awareness; Interpersonal, empathy and social responsibility; Adaptability, problem solving and reality checking; Stress management, impulse control and stress tolerance; General mood, which includes happiness and optimism (Salovey and Mayer 1989/1990).

The concept of EI proposed by Daniel Goleman (1995) captured popular imagination. Their conceptualization also included of five characteristics which included: self-awareness, self-regulation, motivation; empathy and social skills.

EI may determine the adaptive ability of the person to find a balance between life events and life outcomes. The general expectation is that people with low EI will adapt less well to stressful life events with increased possibility to experience depression, hopelessness, and other negative outcomes. Those with high EI should show better adaptive response to negative life outcomes and could arrange their lives so to experience fewer negative life events while being more skilled in dealing with high quality relationships.

Many of our everyday choices are made based on expected emotional reactions to probable future events. Daniel Gilbert coined the term ***"mis wanting"*** to describe the common mistake of wanting things that will not make us as happy as we hope and avoiding things that will not be as bad as we fear (Gilbert and Wilson 2000). We can go wrong because we often focus on the wrong details, when imagining a future event and then misunderstand and misread our own reactions. Negative events may often be less traumatic than we expect because of having many spontaneous and subconscious strategies for coping with problems. Therefore, we may suffer more from the anticipation of a negative event that never occurred.

Affect plays a key role in how our memories about the world are organized and activated. This link drives 'affect infusion' into thinking and behaviour. When we are in a good mood, we are significantly more likely to access and recall positive information first encountered in a previous happy mood state. Gordon Bower (1981) developed the "*associative network model*" according to which affective states are intricately linked to any information we store and recall. We can only interpret complex events by calling on our memories of prior experiences.

The most fundamental influence that affective states have is on our memory. Becoming aware of the subtle memory effect is a vital component of EI. These are most likely to occur when people think in an open constructive way. Mood effect can then be eliminated and even reversed. Affect can also impact on real social judgement about people. Judgements involve the tendency to focus on mood-consistent rather than mood-inconsistent information.

Clinical research suggests that people with depression may be more realistic in how they see the world and themselves, whereas "normal" people tend to distort reality in a positive direction. There is also some experimental evidence suggesting negative moods may help avoid certain mistakes in judgement, such as the "*fundamental attribution error*" (FAE). This occurs because people mistakenly believe that most actions are internally caused and ignore external influences on behaviour.

Stephanie Moylan (2000) showed that positive mood tends to increase and negative mood tends to decrease the incidence of a variety of errors and distortions in performance assessment judgements. To be emotionally intelligent means both knowing about these effects and how to avoid and correct them. People hold overly favourable views of their abilities in many social and intellectual domains. This is partly because people who are unskilled in these domains reach erroneous conclusions and make unfortunate choices. Their incompetence robs them of the metacognitive ability to realize it.

In an interesting study Kruger and Dunning (1999) found participants scoring in the bottom quartile on tests of humour, grammar and logic grossly overestimated their test performance and ability. Although their test performance put them in the 12th percentile, they estimated themselves in the 62nd. Several analyses linked this miscalibration to deficits in metacognitive skill, or the capacity to distinguish accuracy from error. Paradoxically, improving the skill of participants, and thus increasing their metacognitive competence, helped them recognize the limitations of their abilities.

In certain individuals, extreme stress and anxiety can produce a dangerous "*neurotic cascade*" of reverberating negative affect and negative thinking (Suls

2001). In such a state, even minor problems are magnified out of all proportion. "Awfulization" refers to the tendency to overdramatize negative outcome. "Overgeneralization" another faulty thought pattern, is often found in this negative state. People in such states sometimes set unrealistic goals for themselves, show decreased flexibility in adjusting their goals, and so inadvertently produce more negative experiences.

ALEXITHYMIA

Alexithymia is a multifaceted personality construct, introduced by Nemiah and Sifneos in the early 1970s encompassing a cluster of cognitive and affective characteristics associated with various medical and psychiatric disorders. These were first observed among patients with classic psychosomatic diseases and later also among patients with substance abuse, posttraumatic stress and eating disorders. Alexithymia is attributed to an arrest in affect development during early childhood. It may also predict mortality from all causes over five years in middle-aged men, independently of other risk factors.

The term alexithymia encompasses four key features: (a) difficulty identifying feelings and distinguishing between feelings and the bodily sensations of emotional arousal; (b) difficulty describing feelings to others; (c) a poor fantasy life; (d) a literal cognitive style focusing on the minute details of external events.

The concepts of alexithymia and low EI overlap closely. Howard Gardner (1983) pointed to the existence of several intelligences, including two forms of personal intelligence, which he labelled: (1) Intrapersonal intelligence, the ability to access one's own feeling-life, and (2) Interpersonal intelligence, the ability to read the feeling and emotion of others, usually referred as empathy. Both are part of the definition of EI.

High alexithymia rates for psychiatric patients ranged between 33% and 42%, in contrast to rates ranging between 4% and 16% in diverse groups of healthy individuals. Men tend to be more alexithymic than women (Taylor 1997, 2000). When under stress, those with low EI are thought to be frequently overwhelmed and act out in unhealthy ways or become mentally and physically unwell. Those who are highly alexithymic usually have a tough time controlling their emotions and impulses to act and in coping positively with stressful situations (Parker et al 1998, 2001). EI is a better indicator of self-actualization than cognitive intelligence.

Those with high alexithymia scores use poor methods to regulate emotions and apply immature defence an adaptive style. They can be more prone to panic attacks characterizing panic and post-traumatic stress disorder. Some clinicians regard panic disorder as overwhelming floods of undifferentiated emotions not contained by neuronal representations but expressed as profound autonomic disturbances. Studies of patients with panic disorders report rates of 47% and 67% of high alexithymia, compared to 12.5% in patients with simple phobia and 13% in patients with obsessive-compulsive disorder.

People with Borderline personality disorder is well known for their difficulties in regulating emotions, especially anxiety and anger, their impulsive self-destructive behaviour, their lack of empathy and their excessive use of maladaptive ego defence mechanisms. These are all suggestive of low EI. Bar on (2001) found that if one scored low on EQ-I, then they would probably score high on a borderline personality feature scale. People high in alexithymia tend to have an insecure attachment style (Taylor 2000).

HAPPINESS DEFICIT DISORDER?

Happiness is an emotional state characterized by feelings of joy, satisfaction, contentment, and fulfillment. The two key components of happiness (or subjective well-being) are: (1) The balance of emotions between positive and negative emotions, feelings, and moods. Happiness is generally linked to experiencing more positive feelings than negative ones. (2) Life satisfaction which relates to how satisfied one feels with different areas of their life including their relationships, work, achievements, and other things that they consider important.

People appear to value happiness more than material possessions. Being happy is associated with better health, higher earnings, a longer life, a stable family upbringing, stable financial situation, employment, good health, freedom, and personal values. Happiness matters as does the pursuit of happiness which refers to pleasure and joy.

Never in the history of human existence have there been so many opportunities for personal development. Never have we had so many possibilities to set, pursue, and achieve our personal goals and life dreams "Everything is amazing, and no one is happy." Muller (1999) observed that "people seem simply to have taken the remarkable economic progress in stride and have deftly found new concerns to get upset about in an important sense, then, things never get better (Pinker 1998).

Pinker drew attention to 'the Easterlin paradox' which postulates that: "Though in comparison within a country richer people are happier, in comparison across countries the richer ones appeared to be no happier than poor ones. And in comparison, over time, people did not get happier as their countries got richer." This was explained by two theories: 1. The hedonic treadmill: People adapt to changes in their fortunes, like eyes adapting to light or darkness and quickly returns to a genetically determined baseline. 2. The theory of social comparison (or reference groups, status anxiety or relative deprivation): People's happiness is determined by how well they think they are doing relative to their compatriots.

Happiness has two sides: an experiential emotional side and an evaluative cognitive side. Happy people live in the present. Those with meaningful lives have a narrative about their past and a plan for the future (Pinker 2018). It is possible that human beings may not just be built for satisfaction. When things improve, expectations balloon and consequently even dramatic improvements in objective conditions can still leave us unsatisfied. In modern times, our expectations of ease and pleasure and our intolerance of inconvenience and discomfort have increased to such an extent that we still suffer from pain more than our ancestors ever did. We have a large variety of tranquillizers and pain killers available to us and yet they fail to make us happy.

The dominant beliefs of the time and our surroundings shape our desires and expectations. Mass media and the advertising industry may be depleting our reservoir of contentment. We are constantly measuring ourselves against the movie stars, athletes, super models or even friends and colleagues (who may have posted their photos when feeling at their best). These are hard to keep up with and likely to leave us with a sense of feeling worse off. However, we are unlikely to find out what may have happened in their real life, or how lousy they may have felt just minutes, hours, or the day after the post. People are unlikely to share photos or feelings that show them in poor light.

The most common reaction to achievement is not satisfaction but a craving for more. Human beings are always looking for better, bigger, and tastier (Harari 2015). Pain and suffering are inevitable, inescapable, and essential to life. Nothing but the mere form in which it manifests itself depends on chance and that our present suffering fills a place, which without it, would be occupied by some other suffering. (Yalom 1980). Happy families are all alike, every unhappy family is unhappy in its own way (Tolstoy: Anna Karenina). We seek easy answers to explain success, though it can be better explained by avoiding many probable causes for failure.

The US Declaration of Independence (1776) included "the right to the pursuit of happiness" as one of the three unalienable human rights along with the right to life and the right to liberty. Time is what life is made of and one matrix of progress is a reduction in the time people must spend in keeping themselves alive at the expense of the other, more enjoyable things in life. (Pinker 2018). The more one seeks happiness, the more elusive it is. This observation (termed the "hedonistic paradox" by many professional philosophers) led Frankl to say, "Happiness ensues; it cannot be pursued." Unhappiness is soaring around the world, he lamented.

The analytics firm "Gallup" first began tracking global unhappiness in 2006. Each year Gallup asks roughly 150,000 people in over 140 countries about the emotions they experience. Jon Clifton, the head of Gallup reported negative emotions—the aggregate of stress, sadness, anger, worry and physical pain—to have reached a record high in 2021 (The Economist 18 June 2022).

The poll attributed five main causes for the rise of global unhappiness: poverty, broken communities, hunger, loneliness, and the scarcity of decent work. Today, 17% of people find it "very difficult" to get by on their present income—one of the highest shares we have recorded. Two billion people were so unhappy with where they live that they would not recommend their community to anyone they know. The contribution of poverty to global suffering remains well known, despite great strides to tackle it in recent decades. A rise in hunger around the world was making matters worse. According to the United Nations Food and Agriculture Organisation "the decades-long decline in hunger in the world [has] unfortunately ended." In 2014, nearly 23% of people globally were moderately or extremely food insecure. Now the share is over 30%.

Gallup found that 330 million adults go at least two weeks without talking to a single friend or family member. Although they had not captured loneliness data globally since the pandemic, other studies suggest it is worsening. The Survey Centre on American Life, a think-tank project, found that 10% of women reported having no close friends in 2021, up from 2% in 1990. And it was worse for men: 15% reported having no close friends in 2021, up from 3% in 1990. Just because someone has friends, it does not mean they have good friends. One-fifth of adults do not have anyone they can count on for help. Loneliness can increase blood pressure and decrease life expectancy. According to a recent meta-analysis, loneliness takes a toll that is physically equivalent to smoking a pack of cigarettes per day.

Global unhappiness is also increasing because of the daily grind of work. Despite a regular pay cheque, someone who is unhappy at work is statistically more likely to experience negative emotions, such as anger, stress, and physical pain, than someone who is unemployed. Some 19% of workers are completely miserable in their jobs. But even among those that enjoy their work, unhappiness is rising. Stress and worry have risen among workers around the world consistently since 2009.

Bregman (2017) pointed out: "Productivity is at record levels, innovations have never been faster, and yet at the same time, we have a falling median income, and we have fewer jobs." He quotes David Graeber's (2013) analysis which showed that innumerable people spend their entire working lives doing job that they consider pointless. They are the jobs that even the people doing them admit are superfluous. Graeber called them "Bullshit jobs." In a poll Dahlgreen (2015) found that 37% of British workers thought they had a 'bullshit' job. He also sites a survey of 12,000 professionals by a Harvard Business Review (Schwartz and Poratz 2014) wherein half said that their job had 'no meaning or significance', and an equal number were unable to relate to their company mission.

In the Gallup poll 2006 (before the widespread use of social media) 3.4% of people had rated their lives a 10 (the best possible life) and only 1.6% rated their lives a zero (the worst possible life). Fifteen years later the share of people with the best feasible lives has more than doubled (to 7.4%), and the share of people with the worst possible lives has more than quadrupled (to 7.6%). The inequality is even more evident if you group the world into wellbeing quintiles. In 2006, the top quintile for life ratings averaged 8.3; the lowest quintile averaged 2.5. Now, look at 2021: the top quintile averaged 8.9, and the lowest quintile averaged 1.2. The gap in the two life ratings is now 7.7 points—the highest in Gallup's history of tracking.

This wellbeing inequality is as serious as income inequality. It reflects a growing divide in emotions rather than possessions. And this type of inequality is plainly evident when you ask people to rate how their lives are going. Life could hardly be better for one fifth of the world, and for another fifth it could hardly be worse. It may be that the people at the top appreciate what they have more than ever before. For the most unhappy, they are more aware of what they lack than ever before. Social media partly explain why. Through online platforms users can see that their misery is not always shared.

Comparison is said to be "the thief of joy, and social media enables comparison like nothing else. They bring people all over the world into each other's homes through handheld devices and more people have smartphones than ever before. Seneca (4 BC to 65 AD) observed that "Nature has made nothing difficult for a man which she has not made necessary for him. But if he desires purple cloth steeped in rich dye, threaded with gold, and tricked out with patterns and colours of various kinds, then it is their own fault, not Nature's, if he is poor. It is the mind that makes us rich.'

Our society while obsessed with success and appearances, it is also drawn to images of damage and destruction. Literature, films, and music are full of stories of the damaged and the despairing. We are all drawn to these images, and narratives of lives that are similarly affected. People want stories about people like themselves or preferably people even worse off than themselves (Whitwell 2005).

A large segment of the population may now be commitment phobic. In the past most of the relationships resulted from living and getting to know a limited number of people from which to choose a life partner. Getting introduced to one another by friends and family was common. These well-established social processes have now taken a backseat. The social media sites may offer infinite possibility of finding someone out there who may be better or more suited. We may be fishing for a relationship in a sea rather than a pond. Another potential cause may be the exceedingly high incidence of breakdown in relationships and its financial implications. The prevalent culture of discarding all that is old and going for the new may be spilling over to relationships as well. Relationships require sustained work and patience. Factors that may be contributing towards greater loneliness a need to work towards more financial independence and resentment regarding need to stay at home for pregnancy and parenting.

The ready availability of news was once seen as a major advancement for our ability to disseminate information of various kinds including 'gossip.' The overabundance of news may have now turned into a curse. De Botton (2014) pointed out that the news is committed to laying before us whatever is supposed to be most unusual and important in the world. We put our lives on hold expecting to receive yet another dose of critical information about all the most significant achievements, catastrophes, crimes, epidemics and romantic complications to have befallen humankind anywhere around the planet since we last looked.

If all the world's information storage capacity were apportioned equally to everyone on earth, in 1986 each person would not have even gotten a full CD-ROMs worth of storage. By 2007 they had 61 CD-ROMs worth each and in

2022 we have each the equivalent of more than 19,000 per person. It has grown by 58% per year on average (Ed Coper 2022).

We had always been a networked society. But, in this internet and smartphone age, for the first time we are a globally connected network society. We are living in 'the information age.' The availability of so much information was predicted to break down barriers but, instead, we may have entered the age of disinformation. Cognitive scientists tell us humans are now much less rational than we previously thought. There is concern about the disintegration of our traditional media landscape and the rise of cheap infotainment in its place. What we know about the world we have been told by others and we are hardwired to believe and trust this while being, unfortunately, incompetent lie detectors. Gradually our news has become dominated by junk information, cheaper and easier to produce in great volume than the real thing.

The more familiar a piece of disinformation, the more likely it is to be taken as true, even if you originally thought it was false or they did not align with your beliefs. We are much better at remembering a claim we have heard than remembering the circumstances about where we heard it.

We humans may not be so well equipped to handle information overload. Too much information from too many sources in all forms of media may be causing an overwhelming emotional overload.. The need to respond quickly on social media may also be adding to the everyday stresses of our life.

THE MENTAL ILLNESS STORY

The word 'mental' simply denotes 'of or relating to the mind.' The mind is a flow of subjective experiences such as pain, pleasure, anger, and love. These mental experiences are made of interlinked sensations, emotions and thoughts that flash for a moment and immediately disappear. Then other experiences flicker and vanish, arising and fading away in variable periods of time. When reflecting on it, we often try to sort out these experiences into distinct categories of sensation, emotions, and thoughts, but they are inevitably all mingled together and can best be termed as experiential.

As life became more predictable, worries about the future took a more vital role in the theatre of the human mind. Medical professionals deal scientifically with 'illnesses' and much less with life processes. "What it means to be ill" in general depends less on the judgement of the doctor than on the judgement of the patient and on the dominant views in any given cultural circle (Karl Jaspers). A person must first experience one or more symptoms. He then must determine the symptoms are cause for concern. Even after that, he must decide that the symptom is of sufficient concern to warrant seeing a medical professional. There are further barriers to consultation, for example the availability of the professional and a time fitting into the other priorities of the person with the symptoms. David Goldberg (1979) did some pioneering work on the various barriers to psychiatric treatment.

Mental health professionals, and the culture at large, have lowered the bar for what counts as mental illness. Robin Rosenthal (2013) observed: "Abnormal is the new normal." The latest version of DSM could diagnose half the American population with mental disorder over the course of their lifetime (Frances 2013). Psychiatric labels can be shattering, particularly those involving children. The labels often stick and may turn out to be "wish fulfilling prophecies."

For the biomedically inclined, psychiatric conditions can best be isolated by studying underlying biological processes, while research-oriented clinical psychologists think they can be identified statistically. Conceptualizing psychiatric disorders as bounded entities in nature is inconsistent both with medicine's understanding of disease, and evolutionary biology is understanding of species (Zachar 2001). According to Kendell (1975): "In terms of the familiar aphorism that classification is the art of carving nature at the joints, it should indeed imply that there is a joint there, that one is not sawing through bone." There are equally good reasons for claiming that psychometric methods for discovering psychological dimensions do not carve nature at the joints either.

The slippery slope of psychiatric diagnoses even by using criteria set laid by DSM is exemplified well by the findings of Widiger and Francis (1994). They calculated there were ninety-three different ways to meet criteria for being diagnosed with borderline personality disorder in the DSM IIIR and 848 different ways to meet criteria for antisocial personality disorder. This may not be dissimilar to the variations in which the criteria for any other disorder can be met.

THE STORY OF THE TWO MAJOR CLASSIFICATION SYSTEMS IN PSYCHIATRY

Until the advent of the nineteenth century only one form of mental disorder was recognised. "Insanity" was the term used to label patients who had lost touch with reality. Neuroses were recognised to an extent but were at the fringes of psychiatry. Evolution of psychiatric categorisation has been a slow process and still leaves a lot to be desired. Most categories of disorder are based on the consensus of experts rather than being empirically validated entities. Here is a brief account of the development of the two major classification systems currently in use.

The international classification of diseases (ICD) has taken a slow and circuitous route. The WHO took the Bertillon Classification of Causes of Death (1890) and its six revisions to represent The International Classification of disease (ICD) I to VI.

The International Conference for the Seventh Revision was held in Paris under the auspices of WHO in 1955. Mental disorders were included in this revision for the first time. Descriptive psychiatry, which had reached its peak with Kraepelin, was mainly concerned with the psychoses. It was based on institutional psychiatry in which a small number of doctors were dealing with large numbers of patients.

The systematic study of neuroses and personality disorders was an even more recent development. Many doctors concerning themselves with these conditions did not enter psychiatry through the mental hospital but via the out-patient clinic and consulting room where psychoses were comparatively rare. They were investigating and treating a few patients, in marked contrast to their colleagues working in mental hospitals. The differences in the types of observational material from which psychiatrists drew their experience and developed their theoretical orientation became an important source of divergence.

Although all Member States of the World Health Organization had recommended this classification for use, it was adopted by only a few countries: Finland, New Zealand, Peru, Thailand, and the United Kingdom. In some it was used only by their Bureau of Statistics.

Section V was the only part of the ICD solely concerned with psychiatric conditions but did not contain all of them. Many mental disorders were listed under the heading: Section V: "Mental, Psychoneurotic and Personality Disorder." Unfortunately, here "mental disorder" just meant "psychosis". A committee was formed to find the causes for the low acceptability of ICD. They found two potential reasons: (a) Every Professor worth his salt wanted a classification of his own and (b) The WHO was like a caravan, the speed of which was determined by its slowest member.

The next International Classification of Diseases (ICD 9) used a descriptive format that included a brief description of each category of diagnosis. ICD 10 and ICD 11 have further extended clearer guidelines towards diagnosis of individual disorders. The current editions of the two major classification systems (ICD 11 and DSM 5) are much closer in their framework than before.

THE DIAGNOSTIC AND STATISTICAL MANUAL (DSM)

In The United States the Association of Superintendents of American Institutions of the Insane was formed in 1844 thus marking the recognition of psychiatry as a medical speciality. It was later renamed The American Psychiatric Association (APA) in 1921. The first American initiative to develop standardized diagnostic criteria was undertaken for the 1920 census to estimate the prevalence of mental disorder. This manual outlined twenty-one disorders, nineteen of which were psychotic disorders. Most psychiatrists ignored the manual. All American Institutions were using their own diagnostic systems. In the 1940s to 1960s American psychiatry was dominated by psychoanalytic theory.

DSM-I was published in 1952 and DSM-II in 1968. Diagnostic reliability and validity of these categories remained poor. A paper by the philosopher of science, Carl Hempel, delivered at a psychiatric conference in New York in 1959 served as a major formative influence in steering psychiatric diagnostic manuals to a more observational descriptions of symptoms, without implicit causal or other theoretical implications. He argued that the early descriptive phase of in a science should use terms that are as observational and as theory neutral as possible.

In 1970, the classic US-UK cross-national study illustrated the importance of having a unified diagnostic system to determine the rates of psychiatric illnesses. A large discrepancy was found between US and UK statistics on the proportions of adults with hospital diagnosis of schizophrenia and manic-depressive illness. Many patients diagnosed with schizophrenia in New York would have been diagnosed with manic-depressive illness in London. The discovery of psychotropic medications paved the way for the need for research and a move away from psychoanalysis.

A small group of researchers led by Eli Robins and Samuel Guze pioneered the goal of developing operationalized diagnostic criteria for reliable and valid diagnosis to pave the way for credible research and provision of quality care. The Research and Diagnostic criteria (RDC) were published in 1972. *The Feighner Criteria* addressed diagnoses of fourteen psychiatric illnesses including: primary affective disorder (depression and mania), secondary affective disorder (depression only), schizophrenia, anxiety neurosis, obsessive compulsive neurosis, phobic neurosis, hysteria, antisocial personality disorder, alcoholism, drug dependence, intellectual disability and anorexia nervosa.

They used the five phases of diagnostic validation: (1) clinical characteristics of the syndrome and of the patients who develop it (including core symptoms, demographic characteristics, and precipitating factors), (2) exclusion criteria differentiating the syndrome from other known disorders, (3) family studies, (4) laboratory data, and (5) follow-up studies (for diagnostic stability, course, and treatment response).

Kendler and colleagues (2010) identified three major contributions made by Robins and Guze: (1) systematic application of operationalized criteria for psychiatric diagnosis, (2) a basis for empirical data rather than clinical opinion to operationalize diagnostic criteria, and (3) emphasis on the course and outcome as a critical defining feature of psychiatric illness.

Robert Spitzer headed the revision of the American diagnostic criteria for **D**iagnostic and **S**tatistical **M**anual III. Based on the Feigner and **R**esearch and **D**iagnostic **C**riteria (RDC) he introduced the formal operationalization of psychiatric diagnosis with established reliability and validity and provided a new hierarchical, multi-axial system of diagnosis utilizing exclusion criteria.

As a concession to psychoanalytically oriented practitioners, the term 'neurosis' was retained in the nomenclature but only as a parenthetical note. It was subsequently removed from later revisions of DSM. When Spitzer's *DSM-III* was published in 1980, it came into universal use, not only by psychiatrists, but by insurance companies, hospitals, courts, prisons, schools, researchers, government agencies and the rest of the medical profession.

All the editions of DSM simply reflect the opinions of its writers. In the case of the *DSM-III*, it reflected the opinion of Spitzer himself, perhaps one of the most influential psychiatrists of the twentieth century. In his own words, he "picked everybody that [he] was comfortable with" to serve with him on the fifteen-member task force, and there were complaints he called too few meetings and ran the process in a haphazard and highhanded manner. Spitzer said in a 1989 interview, "I could just get my way by sweet talking and whatnot."

In a 1984 article entitled *The Disadvantages of DSM-III Outweigh Its Advantages*, George Vaillant, a professor of psychiatry at Harvard Medical School, wrote that the *DSM-III* represented "a bold series of choices based on guess, taste, prejudice and hope," which seems to be a fair description (Angell 2011). Not only did the *DSM* III become the bible of psychiatry but, like the real Bible, it depended on something akin to revelation. There were no citations of scientific studies to support its decisions.

DSM-IIIR in 1987 and DSM IV in 1994 were published with minor changes. The most significant change in DSM IV was the systematic addition of "clinically significant distress and impairment" across the diagnostic criteria. DSM IV TR was released in 2000 to update the research literature between 1992 and 1998.

The number of diagnoses has continued to climb through successive editions of DSM: from 106 in DSM-I, to 182 in DSM-II, 265 in DSM-III, 292 in

DSMIII-R, 297 in DSM-IV and DSM-IVR and 298 in DSM-5. The growth in numbers of diagnoses was also reflected in the manual's volume, which began with 130 pages in DSM-I to 992 pages in DSM-5.

Field trials were conducted with each successive version of the DSM beginning with DSM-III. The DSM-III and DSM-IV field trials focused on reliability of the proposed criteria. DSM-IV trials included an additional focus on clinical utility and comparison of diagnostic prevalence based on criteria from DSM-III onwards. The DSM 5 field trials focused on the feasibility and clinical utility of diagnoses. It emphasised biological research not confined to diagnostic boundaries as conceptualised. A criticism of the DSM 5 trials was the low reliability obtained for its proposed diagnoses.

The increasing dissatisfaction with validity of the criteria become apparent with complaints about it not sufficiently differentiating disorders leading to high rates of diagnostic comorbidity. Diagnoses lacked specificity for selection of treatment, genetics failed to distinguish psychiatric disorders and many observed syndromes did not fit any diagnostic definitions (Kihilstrom and Klein 1997).

The DSM-IV codified mental disorders, not only for patients, families and clinicians, but also for insurance companies, regulatory agencies, the justice systems and others (Hyman 2011). The entrenchment of the DSM system had the unintended consequence of suppressing important avenues of scientific investigations. Researchers and clinicians have rarely asked questions about symptoms going beyond the DSM constructs.

Regrettably, the shared diagnostic language led to a growing body of evidence demonstrating it did a poor job capturing both clinical and biological realities. The frequency of comorbidity was remarkably high. Co-occurring diagnoses tended to form steady clusters across patient populations, suggesting to some that the DSM system had drawn many unnatural boundaries within broader psychopathological states (Robert Kruger 2006). Genetic findings suggested that the DSM IV handling of each disorder as discrete, discontinuous from other categories of disorder and from health, was palpably wrong (Hyman 2011).

Financial conflicts of interest are known to impair objectivity and integrity in medicine. Concern was expressed to the APA about conflict of interest. As many as 57% for DSM-IV and nearly 70% of DSM-5 task force members had financial relationships with pharmaceutical companies. Eighty-three percent of contributors to the psychotic disorders section and everyone responsible for the sleep disorders section were linked to the pharmaceutical industry. These overwhelming numbers raised significant ethical concerns regarding the enormous influence that pharmaceutical companies may hold on to diagnostic system itself.

The expansion of diagnostic categories and new diagnoses (and thus market!) in every DSM is said to be a virtual 'bonanza for the pharmaceutical industry' (Frances 2009). On the other hand, the DSM is a boon for the APA, which sold over a million copies of the DSM IV. Twenty percent of APA funding is said to come from pharmaceutical industries.

Allen Frances (2013) pointed to the excessive ambition of DSM 5: (1) the unrealistic goal of transforming psychiatric diagnosis by somehow basing it on the exciting findings of neuroscience (a bridge too far), (2) to expand the boundary of clinical psychiatry by pursuing the brave new world of early identification and preventive treatment (Trying to copy some medical specialities now discredited), (3) making psychiatric diagnosis supposedly more precise by quantifying disorders with numbers, rather than merely naming them, resulted in unnecessarily complex dimensional ratings which were clinically dubious.

Trying to be great prevented it from being good enough. Evidence of diagnostic inflation is evidenced by four explosive epidemics of mental disorders in the past 15 years: (a) Childhood Bipolar Disorder increased 40fold (b) Autism 20-fold (c) ADHD tripled (d) Adult Bipolar Disorder doubled. Fads in psychiatric diagnosis come and go. People do not change much but labels do. Fads depend on the combination of plausible idea and our copy-cat, follow-the leader herd instinct.

Allen Frances made some scathing remarks in his book *Saving Normal* and dubbed it as an insider's revolt against out-of-control psychiatric diagnosis, DSM-5, big pharma and the medicalization of ordinary life. This was particularly relevant by being the observation of one who was part of the team framing DSM-III and also the chairperson of DSM IV. He lamented envisioning DSM IV as a guidebook, not a bible. He regretted ".... they had failed to predict that even our conservative manual could provide such easy fodder for advertising gold. Within a few years, it was clear the drug companies had won, and they had lost. Big pharma was simply too big, too rich and too politically powerful."

Over the last 30 years a frightening vicious cycle developed. Diagnostic inflation caused an explosive growth in the use of psychotropic drugs. The consequent huge profits gave the pharmaceutical industry the means and motive to blow up the diagnostic bubble into an ever-expanding balloon. The boundary between mental disorder and normality was so blurred it led to confusing people who needed help with others who did not need help.

After the publication of DSM 5, the APA shifted the model of revision. Now the model is one of ongoing, iterative revision, as warranted by advances in the field of a particular diagnosis. Anybody who believes they have data to support a change can submit a proposal for review by the steering committee. If passed, one of five review committees undertakes a more detailed review and makes the recommendation for approval or disapproval. It goes back and forth between the steering and review committee till being made available for public input. It is then sent for the approval process via the APA assembly and, finally, the APA board.

Research Domain Criteria (RDoC) is now being used to explore categories of research interest. There is also a push towards categorisation being taken out of the hand of the APA and given to a scientific organization, such as the Karolinska Institute or the NIMH.

LIMITATIONS OF DIAGNOSTIC CONCEPTS & CATEGORIES

Diagnosis is undoubtedly an important necessary first step to everything done in clinical medicine. It is critical for applying effective and appropriate treatment and informing prognosis. It enables communication among clinicians and scientists and is of unquestionable importance in medical education and research. However, it is also true that diagnoses are often a shortcut concealing more than they reveal.

Robert Kendell provided an insight into some of the challenges. "The fact that any definition of disease boiling down to 'What people complain of,' or 'What doctors treat' or some combination of the two, is almost worse than no definition at all. It is free to expand or contract with changes in social attitudes and therapeutic optimism and is at the mercy of idiosyncratic decisions of doctors or patients. If one wished to compare the incidence of disease in two diverse cultures, or in a single population at two separate times, whose criteria of suffering and therapeutic concern would we use? And if the incidence of disease turned out to be different in two, would this be because one was healthier than the other, or simply because their attitudes to Illness were different."

Irvin Yalom (1980) lamented that he often found official diagnostic categories problematic. At case conferences, many consultants disagreed on the proper diagnosis of the patient presented. He eventually grasped those disagreements ensued, not from practitioners' errors, but from intrinsic problems in the diagnostic enterprise. In inpatient settings, clinicians relied on diagnosis to inform decisions about effective pharmacological treatment. But in psychotherapy practice with less seriously disturbed patients, he found the diagnostic process largely irrelevant. He believed that the contortions psychotherapists must go through to meet the demands of insurance companies for precise diagnoses are detrimental to both therapist and patient. "Making a formal diagnosis is more than a simple nuisance. It may in fact impede work by obscuring, even negating, the full-bodied, multidimensional individual facing us in our office" (Yalom 2015).

We are trained to use DSM code numbers pinning a patient like a specimen to an admission workup or an insurance form. There is substantial evidence of diagnostic labels impeding or distorting listening. Too often, diagnostic categorization is a stimulating intellectual exercise whose sole function is to provide the clinician with a sense of order and mastery. The major task of a maturing therapist is to learn to tolerate uncertainty (Yalom 1980).

Karl Jaspers founded the idea of *Method Based Psychiatry*. He taught that "the truth is not to be found in one place, but dispersed in all places, not just in the august halls of our old universities, but next to the old lady at the bakery, and the child on the playground, and by the mosquito in the swamp and the flower in the valley. The truth is prosaic, not pompous. Seek it everywhere."

Jaspers discerned that the nature of science is that all knowledge is partial, no scientific theory can have validity outside the chosen scope. This is the method-based intuition, one lying at the heart of any notion of science: our methods determine our results. Jaspers called it methodological consciousness. One must pay attention to one's method in science, in medicine and in psychiatry. The question is not "What is the right theory," but “What is the right method?” Different methods had to be devised, for different settings, conditions and purposes.

Jaspers laid special emphasis on **meaningful understanding (Verstehen)**, which is mostly subjective and especially relevant to psychiatry. Mental states occur in the private world of our feelings and desires and much of the work of psychiatry involves getting to know them.

Modern psychiatry has its roots in medicine but has also developed within the broadly psychological thought-space and the manuals for psychiatric diagnosis of mental disorders especially and inevitably operate with normative terms such as ‘rational,’ ‘reasonable,’ ‘meaningful,’ ‘appropriate’, ‘proportionate’ and their ‘opposites’ (Bolton 2008). Psychological dysfunction is a breakdown of meaningful connection in psychic life, between perception and reality, between beliefs and evidence, between an emotion and its object (Its cause), between reasons and actions and so forth.

The question needing to be addressed is: ‘what is the nature and validity of the distinction between mental order and mental disorder?’ There are two main approaches to this question: (a) mental disorder involves a breakdown of meaning at some point in the relations among mental states and between mental states and experience or behaviour and (b) mental disorder is a matter of functioning below the level of an appropriate ‘normal’ group.

The medical model has been vigorously defended by some psychiatrists and philosophers and vigorously criticized by others. Its sociological critics say the medical model mistakes social norms for medical norms. Psychological critics, on the other hand, argue that the medical model pathologizes the meaningful and the normal. While the description of symptoms may be made increasingly observational, they often contain reference to norms of psychological and behavioural functioning. However, normative concepts are not typically observational. It is the status of the norms invoked in demarcating mental disorders that has been controversial.

The judgement of abnormality is based on a comparison with an average reference group. It is unclear exactly which normal reference group is being involved, and why deviance from it should be considered as a dysfunction rather than just difference. A categorical cut-off between mental disorders and mental normality may turn out to be an impossibility.

Psychiatric diagnosis is now based on the limited criteria accessible at clinical interview with no commitment about the possible cause. The causal stories are complex and involve broad factors such as genetics, neurobiology, early experience, social context, the person's attitude, current life circumstances and events. The diagnosis is supposed to be associated with 'significant distress or impairment.' However, what constitutes 'significant' may be subject to large variations.

Dissatisfaction with the current conceptualization of diagnostic criteria has led to calls for a fresh look. Kendler and First (2010) identified two strategies that could be followed in future efforts to revise psychiatric nosology: (1) an "iterative model" involving small incremental changes to the existing model, and (2) a "paradigm shift model" that discards the underlying paradigm to adopt a fundamental new approach to diagnosis. They, however, believe psychiatry is still available for a paradigm shift. According to Hyman (2011), the current progress in neurobiology is not sufficient for it to make a useful contribution to diagnostic classification.

Tinkering around the concept of organic mental disorder illustrates some dilemmas posed by frequent revisions of diagnostic classification. DSM-III introduced the category of 'organic affective syndromes' for organic mental disorders. DSM-IIIR redesignated the category as 'organic mood syndromes.'

Following the introduction of DSM-III there was great interest in the fact that the category and number of conditions thought to cause mood disorder had further expanded. I recognized and published a few case reports on secondary manic syndromes related to tuberous sclerosis (Khanna and Borde 1989) and electrical injury (Khanna et al 1991) and then a study on thirty cases with the condition. However, the 'specificity' of any known organic factors is yet to be proven. No one has provided good evidence that most individuals develop mania following exposure to even one of the organic factors implicated so far in the causation of mania" (Das and Khanna 1993). Association does not easily translate into causation.

A proposal was made to drop the organic mental disorder category from DSM-IV. The category was however retained and placed alongside the diagnostic categories with which they shared phenomenology. The new term used is depression or mania 'due to another medical condition' and remains in DSM 5. The designation "due to" has important implications that may be hard to resolve.

Kahneman (2011) suggested: "Learning medicine consists in part of learning the language of medicine. Systematic errors are known as biases, and they record predictably in particular circumstances. Most impressions and thoughts arise in your conscious experience without your knowing how they got there. The mental work that produces impressions, intuitions, and many decisions go on in silence in your mind. We are often confident even when we are wrong, and an objective observer is more likely to detect our errors than we are."

Unfortunately, too much psychology and psychiatry has been aimed at "Disease-ifying" (that is medicalizing) everyone and everything in sight. Some people may benefit from Plato, just as others may benefit from Prozac. Some may need Prozac first, then Plato, or Prozac and Plato together (Marinoff 1999). If disease is seen to signify just dis-ease (one who is not at ease), then it could merely be a substitute for symptoms causing discomfort. But, in real life, it is almost tantamount to illness. All psychiatric disorders are at best 'syndromes,' and the distinction of them from 'problems of living' are often ill-defined and even contentious.

THE RISE AND FALL OF DIAGNOSTIC MODELS

Several diagnostic models have found favour from time to time and later been dumped. The proponents were so convinced about their relevance and utility they gained some currency despite the reservations of many. These changes make accurate generalisation from previous studies difficult to ascertain. We need diagnostic models but too frequent changes without adequate evidence to support them poses a problem.

THE HIERARCHICAL SYSTEM OF DIAGNOSIS

ICD 9 and DSM II followed the hierarchical system of diagnosis suggesting a gradient of certainty regarding diagnosis. Organic psychoses (dementia and delirium) were followed by schizophrenia, bipolar disorder and then depression. Psychosomatic disorders, personality disorders and paraphilias were lower order diagnoses because of the uncertainty regarding their biological underpinning. Once a diagnosis of a higher order was made, the symptoms associated with lower order diagnoses were less relevant and could be subsumed under the same diagnosis.

This limited research, particularly biological studies, to an extent and was replaced in DSM III with the multiaxial system of diagnosis. Some degree of hierarchy still existed as personality disorder and developmental disorder were put under Axis II signifying that their position as a psychiatric diagnosis was of lower certainty. Multiple diagnoses on Axis I was not only possible but encouraged.

There has always been some favouring a dimensional approach to diagnosis while others, particularly psychologists and social workers, thought a circumplex model to be more appropriate (Russell 1980).

THE MULTI-AXIAL CLASSIFICATION SYSTEM

The basic concept for a multiaxial system was the evaluation of an individual in terms of several different domains of information assumed to be of high clinical value (Williams 1985).

The multi-axial system of DSM III (1980) included six axes of:

- **Axis I**: information about clinical disorders. Any mental health conditions, other than personality disorders or intellectual disability, was included here.

- **Axis II**: information about personality disorders and mental retardation.

- **Axis III**: information about any present medical conditions which might impact the patient's mental disorder or its management.

- **Axis IV**: to describe psychosocial and environmental factors affecting the person. Factors which might have been included here were:

    - Problems with a primary support group
    - Problems related to the social environment.
    - Educational problems
    - Occupational problems
    - Housing problems
    - Economic problems
    - Problems with access to health care services
    - Problems related to interaction with the legal system/crime.
    - Other psychosocial and environmental problems

- **Axis V** was a rating scale called the Global Assessment of Functioning; the GAF went from 0 to 100 and provided a method summarizing in a single number just how well the person was functioning overall.

The decision to separate Axis I and II was to ensure consideration was given to the possible presence of disorders frequently overlooked when attention is directed to the usually more florid Axis I disorders. It recognized that personality disorders may co-exist with, predispose to, or result from Axis I psychiatric disorders and importantly influence their presentation, course management and response to treatment. Mental retardation was at first included under Axis I, but in DSM IIIR included under Axis II.

Axis III aroused its own concerns. Kendell (1980) preferred this Axis to be used for all etiological factors, both proven and suspected, thus allowing the first two axes to be purged of all etiological implications and assumptions. Roth (1983) pointed to the difficulties of deciding what is relevant to record in Axis III.

The severity of the stressors recorded on Axis IV was supposed to be rated according to how stressful they would be to an "average person" in similar circumstances and similar sociocultural values to the patient. This was the subject of most criticism. Controversies surround the use of an 'average person,' inability to distinguish between chronic and acute stressors, lack of specificity in the aspects of stressors being rated to represent an etiological formulation in an allegedly "atheoretical" manual. Rutter and Shaffer (1980) resented the DSM III model of Axis IV assumption that all stressors act through the same mechanism. Research findings showed that this was most unlikely.

Kendell (1980) and Rutter and Shaffer (1980) suggested the rating on Axis V would be meaningless across patients with mental disorders lasting longer than one year.

The multiaxial system was rarely used to its full potential and lacked clinical utility. In 2004, APA first entertained a motion to explore elimination of the multiaxial system unless there was evidence indicating that the system enhanced patient care (First 2010 Paradigm shifts and the development of the diagnostic and statistical manual of mental disorders: Past experiences and future aspirations).

Upon reviewing the literature, a 2005 committee recommended maintaining the system in the next iteration of the *DSM* and suggested APA provide resources to support more widespread and consistent use. Nearly eight years later, the APA discontinued use of the multiaxial system without much public discussion or comment. APA included just three paragraphs regarding this shift in the *DSM 5*, noting that "despite widespread use and its adoption by certain insurance and governmental agencies, the multiaxial system in DSM IV was not required to make a mental disorder diagnosis" (APA 2013).

The main priorities for DSM 5 were to incorporate etiological and neurobiological research into definitions of psychiatric disorders and to improve clinical utility of the criteria. DSM 5 combined the first three axes into one. It was released in 2013. Rationale for this was based on: (1) the unclear boundaries between medical and psychiatric diagnoses (Axis III), (2) inconsistent use of Axis IV by clinicians and researchers (psychosocial and environmental problems), and (3) poor psychometric and clinical validity of Axis V (Global assessment of functioning)

THE BIOPSYCHOSOCIAL MODEL

Ghaemi (2010) held the view that present day psychiatry had become too eclectic, verging on anarchic. "What passed for a conceptual schema for the field – the biopsychosocial model (BPS)– rose from the ashes of psychoanalysis and is dying on the shoals of neurobiology." The story of psychiatry was a battle between two dogmas: those seeing mental illness as simply a brain disease and those viewing psychoanalysis as the ultimate solution.

George Engel (an Internist and a trained Psychoanalyst) received credit for his articulation of the BPS model in his classic 1977 paper. He complained about medicine becoming too biological, but his impact was strongest in psychiatry. His psychoanalytic friends saw the BPS model as a defence against biological psychiatry. Ghaemi pointed to the irony that one of the central tenets of psychiatry was based on an article in which the key example was of a patient with a heart attack, not depression or psychosis. Engel had emphasised the psychological aspects of an individual's reactions to illness and the social aspects of his relationships to his medical team.

Such a linear causality was often appropriate when considering ways of improving population health (Davey Smith 2005). The perspective of complexity tends to be more prominent when we have less, not more, understanding of a disease. For example, peptic ulcer was once considered as a classic psychosomatic illness which now has Helicobacter Pylori infection as a key etiological factor. The first hypothesis of bacterial association was put forward as far back as 1875. Antibiotic treatment for peptic ulcer had been advocated by several researchers since as early as 1948, and an antibiotic was patented for such treatment in 1961. H. Pylori was found to cause peptic ulcer much later in 1983. It serves as a good example of situations where remedy may occur much before a causal link was found.

Ghaemi (2010) noted that the world of psychiatry in the 1970s was like a civil war. On one side stood psychoanalysis with the Old Guards and on the other, the biological renegades with the Young Turks. What was at stake was not only our understanding of mental illness but also power. Patronage of academic jobs, control over training, access to university resources and government funds were contested by both factions of the medically qualified psychiatric profession which had the almost exclusive right to issue prescriptions legally.

Klerman, Robins and Guze joined Kety of the National Institute of Mental Health (NIMH) to challenge the psychanalytic dogmas of the time and dared to study the brain in relation to mental illness. John Cade in Melbourne discovered Lithium. The psychopharmacology revolution appeared to validate and make practical, the Kraepelinian paradigm, with Lithium for bipolar, imipramine for unipolar depression and chlorpromazine for schizophrenia.

The BPS model has been criticised for its over inclusiveness and poor boundaries. It failed to provide psychiatry with a rational ground for the practise of psychopharmacology. The irony was that the acceptance of the biopsychosocial approach partly grew out of the rebellion of psychologists and social workers against psychiatrists (mostly psychoanalysts), but now psychiatrists (mostly psychoanalysts) were using it to assert privilege among mental health professionals. Later non-psychiatrist professionals, especially psychologists and nurses, embraced the BPS model in their battle to gain prescribing rights. It legitimised a search for power, riches and prestige.

David Healy (1998, 2006) argued that a "corporate psychiatry' had developed, heavily influenced by the pharmaceutical industry. Moncrieff (2006) saw modern psychiatry as becoming a handmaiden to conservative political commitments. Treating the unhappiness of the masses, deriving from poverty, racism and other socio-political causes, as if they were biological entities, not only diverted the masses from the real cause of discontent but directly enriched capitalist entities (like pharmaceutical industries and insurance companies).

The pharmacological industry has huge financial resources and exerts enormous social and political power influencing medical and scientific processes. As psychiatry became a drug-intensive specialty, the pharmaceutical industry quickly saw the advantages of forming an alliance with it. Drug companies lavished attention and largesse on psychiatrists, both individually and collectively, directly and indirectly. They showered gifts and free samples on practising psychiatrists, hired them as consultants and speakers, bought them meals, helped pay for them to attend conferences and supplied them with "educational" materials The psychiatric profession receives more money from the pharmaceutical industry than any other medical speciality (Angell 2011).

APA introduced the Conflict-of-Interest Policy (COI). This policy limited the amount panel members can receive from drug companies annually (US$10,000 in cash and $50,000 in company stock holdings). It, however, allowed unrestricted research grants. Participation in lucrative speakers' bureaus (designed to influence communities of prescribers) is permitted and required to be reported as honoraria.

Disclosure may be better than non-disclosure, but it has severe limitations as a strategy for mitigating bias. Cosgrove and Krimsy (2012) identified two reasons how disclosure merely shifts 'secret bias to open bias': (1) it sometimes involves so much information about ties to the industry that the reader is blinded by the sheer 'signal to noise ratio'; and (2) disclosure may be perceived as absolving a person from their responsibility for managing their conflict.

George Loewenstein and colleagues (2012) argued that disclosure led doctors to give biased advice, either through strategic exaggeration (whereby more extremely biased advice is provided to counteract anticipated discounting) or 'moral licencing' such that advice is legitimatized because advisees 'have been warned' (that is, *caveat emptor* or 'buyer beware'). Their experiments have shown that bias is considerably greater when conflict of interest is disclosed. Thus, attempts to stem the conflict problem through disclosure policies may be worsening it (PLoS 2012).

In addition to the money spent on the psychiatric profession directly, drug companies heavily support many related patient advocacy groups and educational organizations. These groups ostensibly exist to raise public awareness of psychiatric disorders, but also have the effect of promoting the use of psychoactive drugs and influencing insurers to cover them.

Whitaker (2010) summarized the growth of industry influence after the publication of the *DSM-III* as follows: "In short, a powerful quartet of voices came together during the 1980s eager to inform the public that mental disorders were brain diseases. Pharmaceutical companies provided the financial muscle. The APA and psychiatrists at top medical schools conferred intellectual legitimacy upon the enterprise. The NIMH [National Institute of Mental Health] put the government's stamp of approval on the story. NAMI (National Alliance on Mental Illness) provided a moral authority."

A PILL WHEN ILL AND A PILL FOR EVERY ILL(NESS)

We have always held the idea of 'a pill when ill.' These pills were provided by Shamans, traditional healers and others anointed by each group/society as possessing the power to heal. When none existed, the old woman of the village took on the role of a healer. Traditional healers usually had nothing other than their 'experience' to guide them or that acquired from the older generation. Often one formula was used for many ills. The concept of illness and cure was based on simpler concepts. We may also be striving to have 'a pill for every ill(ness).'

Ayurveda, meaning to deal with the fundamental knowledge of life, originated in India around 3,500 years ago. This form of medicine focuses on three factors in the body which we refer to as 'tri-doshas' (fault): Vat (wind), Pit (bile) and Kaph (phlegm). Treatment focuses on natural healing to prevent the disease and provide immunity. Ancient Greeks believed the body was made up of four main components or the Four Humours. These needed to remain balanced for people to remain healthy. The Four Humours were liquids within the body: blood, phlegm, yellow bile and black bile. Traditional Chinese medicine also evolved over thousands of years. It uses various psychological and/or physical approaches (such as acupuncture and tai chi) as well as herbal products to address health problems. Other cultures had their own systems of ancient medicine which are rooted in beliefs of the times.

Homeopathy originated in Germany in the 18th century. It is a system of complementary medicine in which ailments are treated by minute doses of natural substances which, in larger amounts, are presumed to produce symptoms of the ailment. Allopathy (comes from the Greek "*allos*" meaning "opposite" and "*pathos*" meaning "to suffer") had its origins in the 1800s. It represents the method of treatment of disease by currently conventional means, which is with drugs having effects opposite to the symptoms. It became the dominant mode of scientific medicine following the recognition of pathogens leading to the 'germ theory' of illness and the discovery of antibiotics providing a cure.

All the ancient systems of medicine appear to have followed a holistic concept of illness and their remedies. Lifestyle was seen as an essential factor in finding a cure. Later systems appear to have lost that focus. The "germ theory" may have played a significant role in this change. There appears to be a dichotomy in our approach. On the one hand, medicine is going back to the 'chronic disease model' for many medical conditions (including psychiatric disorders) and incorporating a broader concept of illnesses and their management. On the other hand, there is a tendency to medicalise many variations from the norm as true disorders and use pills as the remedy.

Human life is full of suffering which cannot be captured under the rubric of psychiatric diagnosis and may not even be amenable to a pill. While the religious texts and stoics may have overplayed the 'life is suffering' card, we must equally be careful not to see all suffering as disorder. There is not a lot of dignity in pain and suffering. Truth, as always, may be somewhere in the middle. Where possible, we must try to alleviate suffering and many pills we have are not disease specific but can be used judiciously to relieve targeted symptoms.

Agus (2011) suggested: it is quite possible that we already have all the drugs we need to treat most diseases. We just do not know how to use them (method), how much to use (dosage), and when (schedule). Aspirin is a good example, a cheap and most used affordable drug. We are currently celebrating the 125th of Anniversary of Aspirin. Initially synthesised for treatment of arthritis, many new indications have been found over the years. These include treatment of migraine and tension headaches. In the 1930s a dentist observed that people taking Aspirin bled more when their teeth were extracted. It was not until 1980 that it was approved as an antiplatelet agent for the prevention of myocardial infarction. Aspirin is now also used for the prevention of transient ischemic attacks and stroke. In keeping with an inflammatory hypothesis for depression, a recent trial studied its potential role in treatment of depression. The results were negative but indicated the ongoing interest in potential usage of the medication.

Propranolol (along with other Beta Blockers) is another drug for which many new indications have been found over the years. Initially marketed as an antihypertensive, it is now used for arrhythmias, treatment of akathisia, tardive dyskinesia, and migraine prophylaxis.

The effectiveness of any medication depends on the compliance of the patient to the prescribed treatment and this, in turn, at least partly depends on nonmedication factors such as the attitude and expectation of the patient as well as the relationship between the patient and the doctor.

THE STORY BEHIND THE FIRST FEW PSYCHOTROPIC MEDICATIONS

"*My Age of Anxiety*" is a biographical account of Scott Stossel (2014) who suffered from severe anxiety since childhood. He was prescribed every psychotropic medication that was ever marketed through his lifelong journey with the condition. At the same time, he was among the lucky few to be in therapy of diverse types throughout that time. Despite limited benefit from treatment, he continued to be productive. He provided a fascinating story of the discovery of some of the first psychotropic medications.

Stossel recounts how every one of the most commercially significant classes of antianxiety and antidepressant drugs of the last sixty years were discovered by accident or was originally developed for something completely unrelated to anxiety or depression such as to treat tuberculosis, surgical shock, allergies, to use as an insecticide, a penicillin preservative, an industrial dye, a disinfectant, rocket fuel. This is a summary which demonstrates how serendipity rather than research has played a significant role in treatment available to treat mental illnesses.

Before 1906 people were ingesting alcohol, marijuana, and opium to deal with mental symptoms. **Heroin** was manufactured by Bayer in 1897. It was widely used on the battlefields as a painkiller and cough suppressant. Till 1904 it was available over the counter in America.

In 1864, a German chemist combined urea (found in animal waste) with diethyl malonate (derived from the acid in apples) to synthesize barbituric acid. In 1903, researchers at Bauer gave barbituric acid to dogs and they fell asleep. Within months Bayer was manufacturing Barbital, the first commercially available **Barbiturate** to consumers. In 1911, the company released the longer acting barbiturate, Phenobarbital. By the 1930s, barbiturates had completely replaced chloral hydrate, bromides, and opium as the treatment of choice for "nerve troubles". By 1947, there were thirty different barbiturates being sold under different names. They had two big disadvantages. They were highly addictive and were often lethal in overdoses.

By 1941, penicillin was proven to be an effective treatment for bacterial infection, but the mould proved rather temperamental. Frank Berger was successful in developing a method for preserving the mould for long enough to allow for better extraction and purification to help distribute it more widely. One of the penicillin preservatives Berger tested was ***mephenesin***, which he had synthesized by modifying a commercially available disinfectant. When he injected mice with mephenesin to test for toxicity, he found it had a quieting effect on the animals. A similar effect was later seen on humans. Berger, by accident, had discovered the first of a revolutionary class of drugs. But mephenesin was not very potent in the pill form. He and his team went about trying to find similar compounds.

Eventually they found **meprobamate** which they patented in 1950. It was longer lasting and less toxic than mephenesin. Meprobamate was marketed in May 1955. It was advertised as being effective for "anxiety, tension, and mental stress." In 1956, the drug became a cultural phenomenon. The new tranquilizer was praised by movie stars. Magazines wrote about "happy pills" and "peace of mind drugs" and "happiness by prescription." Aldous Huxley hailed meprobamate as "more important, more genuinely revolutionary, than the recent discoveries in the field of nuclear physics."

In 1952, Henri Laborit, a surgeon in Paris, decided to experiment with a compound called **Chlorpromazine**. It was a product of the German textile industry developed by chemical companies. In 1950, French researchers synthesised chlorpromazine from phenothiazines, intending to create a more powerful antihistamine. It failed to provide any advantage over the existing antihistamines. Laborit was hoping that chlorpromazine would help mitigate surgical shock by reducing inflammation and suppressing the body's autoimmune response to the trauma of surgery. To his surprise, the drug not only achieved his goals but also sedated the patients, relaxing them to the point where they were indifferent toward the major surgical procedures they were about to have.

Word got around the hospital, and one of Labroit's surgical colleagues told this to his brother-in-law, the psychiatrist Pierre Deniker, who administered it to his most psychotic patients in the back-wards of a Parisian mental hospital. The results were amazing. Violently agitated patients calmed down. Patients who were unresponsive for years emerged from his stupor. Smith, Kline, and French Laboratories licensed Chlorpromazine in 1954. Its arrival transformed mental health care. In 1955, for the first time in a generation, the number of hospitalized mentally ill in US declined.

MAOIs have their origin in the later years of second world war. Germans were bombarding English cities with V-2 rockets. They ran low on conventional fuel and had to use hydrazine as fuel. Hydrazine is poisonous and explosive, but scientist had found that they could modify it in ways that might be medically useful. After the end of the war, drug companies bought left over hydrazine supplies at a steep discount. In 1951, scientists discovered that the two modified hydrazine compounds, **isoniazid and iproniazid** inhibited the growth of tuberculosis. By 1952, both were on the market for treatment of tuberculosis.

After being treated with these "antibiotics," some patients were observed to be "mildly euphoric." In a 1956 study in New York, depressed patients were found to have markedly improved on Iproniazid. Nathan Kline observed their "psychic energizing" effect and subsequently reported that some of his patients had a complete remission of all symptoms. In 1957, Hoffmann-La Roche began marketing iproniazid.

Reserpine, an alkaloid of Rauwolfia Serpentina had been used in India for a variety of ailments including "insanity." After seeing the striking results of chlorpromazine, executives at Squibb provided funding to Nathan Kline to test the compound on a group of his patients. Several of them improved dramatically. In 1955, Paul Hoch, the commissioner of mental hygiene for New York, arranged with Governor W. Averell Harriman for $1.5 billion in funding to give Reserpine to every single one of the ninety-four thousand patients in all of State's psychiatric hospitals. It worked for some, but not as well as chlorpromazine.

In 1954, Geigy, a Swiss pharmaceutical company had tweaked chlorpromazine's chemical structure to create a compound G22355, which it called **Imipramine**, the first tricyclic. Roland Kuhn, a Swiss psychiatrist was trying to develop a better sleeping pill. He tried Imipramine to some of his patients. Rather than putting patients to sleep, imipramine energized them and elevated their mood. In 1957, Kuhn presented the results on his five hundred patients treated with imipramine at the International Congress of Psychiatry in Zurich. Imipramine was released in US in September 1959. The New York Times published an article headlined "Drugs and Depression." The times called Iproniazid and Imipramine "antidepressants" – the first use of the term in the press or in popular culture.

THE LIMITATIONS OF BIOLOGICAL STUDIES

Biological psychiatry attempts to discover biological correlates of psychiatric disorders with the aim of establishing aetiology, treatment, and prognosis. These attempts have been proven to be difficult due the enormous complexity of our brain. Some believe that each passing year makes neuroscience more complicated and less useful.

The human brain contains an estimated eighty-six billion neurons. Those billions of brain cells communicate by passing chemical messages at the synapse using neurotransmitters and neuromodulators, using a process called neurotransmission. Neurotransmitters (small-molecule transmitters) like dopamine and glutamate, act directly on neighbouring cells. Scientists have identified more than sixty distinct types of neurotransmitters in the human brain, and most experts say there are more left to discover. These powerful neurochemicals are at the centre of neurotransmission and are seen as critical to human cognition and behaviour. Neuromodulators (like insulin and oxytocin) work more subtly, adjusting, how cells communicate at the synapse.

Often, neurotransmitters are talked about as if they have a single role or function. Dopamine is a "pleasure chemical" and GABA is a "learning" neurotransmitter and so on. But these are likely to be gross simplification. Neuroscientists are discovering they are multi-faceted and complex, working with and against each other to facilitate neural signalling across the cortex.

In 1986, Leon Eisenberg (one of the first psychiatrists to study the effects of stimulants on attention deficit disorder in children) observed that American psychiatry in the late twentieth century moved from a state of "brainlessness" to one of "mindlessness." Before the introduction of psychoactive drugs, the profession had little interest in neurotransmitters or any other aspect of the physical brain. Instead, it subscribed to the Freudian view that mental illness had its roots in unconscious conflicts, usually originating in childhood, which affected the mind as though it were separate from the brain.

But with the introduction of psychoactive drugs in the 1950s, and even more sharply in the 1980s, the focus shifted to the brain. Psychiatrists began to refer to themselves as 'psychopharmacologists,' and they had less and less interest in exploring the life stories of their patients. Their main concern was to eliminate or reduce symptoms by treating sufferers with drugs that would alter brain function. An early advocate of the biological model of mental illness, Eisenberg in his later years had become an outspoken critic of what he saw as the indiscriminate use of psychoactive drugs, driven largely by the machinations of the pharmaceutical industry.

Alvin Pam (1990) in a provocative article: "*A critique of the scientific status of biological psychiatry*" outlined how each of the four basic modes of investigation used in biological studies were flawed in procedure and inference such that the bulk of existing findings must be called into question. He observed that:

1. Pedigree studies are ruined by selective adoption. These are marred using 'throw away kids' to demonstrate genetic effect, lack of case history data, and lapses in 'blind' diagnosis.

2. Pharmacological response studies are marred by a spurious assumption that drugs which work must be correcting a biochemical imbalance that caused the condition. Aspirin relieves headache but no one contends that headache is brought about by 'aspirin deficiency.'

3. Neuropsychological – Neurophysiological studies are 'heuristic' fishing expeditions to find a presumed abnormality to account for the psychopathology, without doing the prospective longitudinal study to validate such theory.

4. Biochemical correlates of emotions are treated as if each emotion must have a distinctive neuronal substrate rather than representing a general visceral arousal where cognition defines the feeling.

Impressive progress is being reported, but all may not be as rosy as might appear at first sight. Substandard work goes unchallenged and even gets accepted as empirical evidence. He systematically reviewed many strands of studies and concluded that biological psychiatry is often more reductionist than acknowledged. He saw search for organic causes of psychopathology as a 'fishing expedition' that generates massive research and a literature without discovering the constitutional basis for any functional disorder thus far. The history of biological psychiatry can be depicted as a tale of promising leads, rush to print on slender evidence, hyperbole as initial reception to new work, and unproductive results. With each failure, the faith remains undaunted, simply shifting direction in its quest by optimistic lurches from one idea to another.

A decade later while revisiting the issue of brainlessness and mindlessness in psychiatry, Eisenberg (2000) gave credit to psychiatry for making "a virtue of the failure of its biomedical science by remaining the one medical speciality with a persistent interest in the patient as a person in an era increasingly dominated by organ-based medical speciality." He believed that psychiatrists found it useful to emphasise their medical identity for purely economic reasons. Prescribing drugs and monitoring drug therapy required medical license, whereas psychologists, social workers, and counsellors could compete for psychotherapy.

With the advent of psychopharmacology, psychiatry had changed, and that change brought it back into the mainstream of academic medicine. (Kandel 1998). There were three components of this progress: (1) It now had effective treatments for two of the three most devastating illnesses, depression, and manic-depressive illness. (2) It had new clinically validated and objective criteria established for diagnosing mental illnesses. (3) There was a renewed interest in the biology of mental illness and specially in the genetics of schizophrenia and depression. In addition, since the 1980s there were major developments in brain sciences.

Kandel put forth a new intellectual framework for psychiatry which he summarized in five principles that constitute the current thinking about relationship between mind and brain:

1. All Functions of mind reflect functions of brain. All mental processes, even the most complex psychological processes, derive from operations of the brain. The actions of the brain underlie from simple motor behaviour like walking to all complex cognitive actions, conscious and unconscious, such as thinking, speaking, creating works of art and music.

   Behavioural disorders that characterize psychiatric illness are disturbance of brain function. Although this principle is generally accepted, how precisely the brain gives rise to various mental processes is understood poorly. Similarly, even though there are critical underpinnings to all social actions, a biological analysis of many aspects of individual and group behaviour may not prove to be the optimal level or even informative level of analysis.

2. Genes contribute importantly to mental function and can contribute to mental illness.

3. Behaviour itself can also modify gene expression.

4. Maintenance of learned gene expression by structural alteration in neural circuits of the brain.

5. Psychotherapy and pharmacotherapy may induce similar alterations in gene expression and structural changes in the brain.

We must not forget how extreme biological approaches have been championed in the past that has led to disastrous results (Ghaemi 2010):

1. *The focal toxin theory* of mental illness was developed and championed by Henry Cotton. It postulated that mental illness was caused by toxins released by bacteria in the body particularly from the colon and rotted teeth. In the 1920s and 1930s tens of thousands of

colectomies and full mouth teeth extractions were conducted by doctors on patients with mental illness. This practise continued until Cotton died and other physicians lost faith in the treatment.

2. *Psychosurgery*: the idea that mental illness reflected abnormal functions of the frontal lobe. With frontal lobotomy, the belief was that the disconnection of the brain will lead to diminished mental symptoms, if not outright cure. Hundreds of thousands of persons received frontal lobotomies. Initially it was used as a treatment of last resort for schizophrenia but later for the mildest mental conditions. Walter Freeman promoted it in US and himself conducted 2400 lobotomies. The ineffective and harmful treatment did not die until its founder died, and the rise of antipsychotic medications.

It is also worth keeping in mind a few other lessons from our not-so-distant past. Penicillin cured neurosyphilis and emptied a large part of inpatient beds which until then were occupied by those diagnosed as suffering from the "General Paralysis of the Insane." Malaria therapy won its proponent, Wagner-Jauregg, the Nobel prize but was dumped for ever. Insulin Coma Therapy was used and discarded for good. Electro convulsive therapy was first used under the wrong notion that those with Epilepsy did not suffer from schizophrenia. It was used indiscriminately for decades before finding its main use for treatment of severe depression failing to respond to other treatments.

We have not yet found ways of translating basic science into clinical psychiatry. None of the promising biological findings has ever qualified as a diagnostic test. The brain has provided us no low-hanging fruit. Billions of research dollars have failed to produce convincing evidence that any mental disorder is a discrete disease entity with a unitary cause (Allan Frances 2013). Mental disorders are too heterogeneous in presentation and in causality to be considered simple diseases. All the disorders that we treat, and as currently defined, may eventually turn out to be many different diseases.

As Roger Sperry (1981) in his Nobel Prize in Medicine acceptance speech very eloquently put it: "The more we learn, the more we recognize the unique complexity of any one individual intellect, the stronger the conclusion becomes that the individuality inherent in our brain networks makes that of fingerprints and facial features gross and simple by comparison."

Perhaps psychiatry is especially vulnerable to manipulation of the normal/disease boundary because it lacks biological tests and relies on subjective judgements easily influenced by clever marketing. "It is not the tiger's fault it is a carnivore, but it is our collective fault for allowing the drug companies free rein to prey on our weakness."

Robert Burton (2013) reminds us about one of the basic limitations of scientific inquiry: "It is our mind that dreams up the questions and seeks out the answers." Mind is both a measure of the man and the tool whereby we make the measurement. With powerful new imaging techniques such as fMRI scan, cognitive science has become the de facto mode of explanation of behaviour, rushing into the vacuum created by the failure of previous psychological and philosophical theories to fulfill their initial promise.

Philosophers commonly cite neurological case studies as evidence for their theories. Such advances may be seductive to the academic community and the public. What was privately acknowledged among neurologists as metaphysical musings are increasingly being offered and seen as scientifically based facts. Like a child handed a new toy, the scientific community is not likely to proceed with caution.

In the late nineteenth century, Santiago Ramon y Cajal, a Spanish neuroscientist and Nobel Laureate, developed elegant staining techniques that allowed detailed observation of our neurons and their interconnections. He is considered by many as the father of neuroscience. His work led to the so-called **Neuron Doctrine**: the generally accepted view that the neurons make thoughts, while glial cells are the supporting cells that make the star neurons flourish.

Despite accounting for half the volume of the adult mammalian brain and being at least as plentiful as the neuron, glial cells received scant study. But this view may be undergoing dramatic revision. It was not until the 1960s, that the astrocyte was also shown to have action potentials. Then it was found that both neurons and astrocytes responded to and released neurotransmitters. More recently it was found that astrocytes can also create calcium waves that extend to an area a hundred times larger than the responsible astrocyte. Their role in cognition is still undecided. In the 1960s, it was estimated that glial cells accounted for nearly 90% of the brain cells. Knob cites this as the origin of the popular myth that we use only 10% of our brains. Surprisingly, even the estimate of cell counts of the total neurons in the brain vary dramatically, ranging from ten billion to one trillion neurons. Different techniques bring different results.

In summary, Robert Burton asks all concerned to be constantly aware of the essential paradox that drives all investigations of the mind. The mind exists in two different dimensions – as a 'felt experience' and as an 'abstract concept.' A constellation of involuntary mental sensations plays a critical role in how we think about what mind "is" and "does." No neuroscientist, philosopher, or observer of humankind has the final answer. Each of us are weaving stories, not covering absolute truths. The mind is and will always be a mystery.

Neuroscientists are quickly becoming the prominent narrators of the modern story of the mind. They have the tools, language, and experience to tell us informed, engaging, and important stories. Neuroscientists, however, must see their conclusions about the mind as one interpretation among several or many. Humility, reverence, and respect for the unknowable should be the default mind-set.

Functional MRI uses indirect parameters. It does not measure neuronal activity directly but measures the blood flow and blood oxygen level in the brain. These parameters cannot discriminate between inhibition and activation of neurons: an increase in the BOLD (blood oxygen level dependence) signal can be caused by either 'firing' or 'inhibition of firing' of neurons. fMRI requires complex statistical programming to filter out the relevant information from the 'noise.' 'Masking' entails removing 'uninteresting' data and analysing only the data from those parts of the brain that one expects to be interesting. 'Subtracting' means that the activation of the brain in 'default mode' is subtracted from the activation pattern that shows up during exposure to the stimuli.

Different scanners provide different results. To achieve comparable results, one should preferably use the very same scanner or at least a scanner of the same brand and tesla-force, otherwise results are likely to vary. Each individual brain is different in the same way as all faces are different. fMRI takes place in a highly unnatural situation. We have at best found a neural signature or neural narrative, but not conclusive evidence. Correlation does not imply causality.

It is much easier to do research using modern technology underpinning the biological nature of the disorder while retaining faith in psychiatry being a medical speciality. Subjects are chosen using diagnostic categories having their own limitations but necessary for research to proceed. Given these limitations, there is bound to be confusion about what the results mean and how they would advance our understanding of mental disorders and their treatment.

As far back as 1865, the French physiologist Claude Bernard warned that the use of group averages in medicine leads necessarily to error. The greatest obstacle to applying calculations to physiological phenomena is still, at bottom, the excessive complexity which prevents their being definite and comparable to one with another. Averages must be rejected because they confuse while aiming to unify and distort while aiming to simplify. This applies most prominently to psychiatry where the great diversity of symptoms contained within our psychiatric syndromes means that the average case is even more of a mythical beast than the so called 'classic cases' of other branches of medicine. Bernard said, we 'thus have a description that will never be matched in nature.' The actual individual subject is lost in the average.

One of the key limitations in all biological research may be that it is conducted using subjects who have been diagnosed with conditions which themselves have limited validity. The researcher needs to identify his cases before he can count them and should be able to define and classify what he identifies. The nature of psychiatric disorders remains rather loosely defined and the meaning of the findings, given the tools we use, also give rise to uncertainties. van Praag (1993) noted that the "biology" uncovered in mental disorders appear to be devoid of diagnostic specificity. As most disease entities are on the whole "pseudoidentities," it would be little less than a miracle if a single marker would be found identifying such an 'entity.'

Groopman (2007) in his book: *How Doctors Think* quoted Renee Fox and Jay Katz to highlight the uncertainties of the expert. Fox had identified three basic types of uncertainties: (1) an incomplete or imperfect mastery over available knowledge, (2) Limitations in the current medical knowledge itself, and (3) The difficulty in distinguishing between personal ignorance or ineptitude and the limitations of present medical knowledge.

Katz lumped all the three categories under the rubric of "disregard of uncertainties." Katz thought that the greater burden is "the obligation to keep these uncertainties in mind and acknowledge them to patients." He further adds: "The denial of uncertainty is one of the most remarkable human psychological traits. It is both adaptive and maladaptive, and therefore both guides and misguides."

Physicians' denial of awareness of uncertainties serves the important purpose of making matters seem clearer, more understandable and more certain than they really are thus making action possible. Another defence against uncertainty is the culture of conformity and orthodoxy beginning in medical school. Groopman pointed to other related phenomenon: "Confirmation bias" (the attention to data that support the presumed diagnosis and minimisation of data that contradict it) and "Diagnosis Momentum" (once an authoritarian senior physician has fixed a label to the problem, it usually stays firmly attached, under the assumption that the specialist is usually right.

PART IV

WHEN STORIES GO HAYWIRE

The mind is seen as a collection of stories. We look for explanations of our behaviour and of the behaviour of others and try to make sense of them. When talking about a series of events occurring over a period, we look for overall patterns rather than attempting to relate to every event that ever happened. We look for generalizations that our listeners can understand. We do not store the particular words that compromise the story itself, but the index of the story is what is held in the memory (Schank and Abelson 1995).

While recalling the story, we transform the index into a story in a way suitable for the person(s) listening. We can tell the same story in diverse ways to satisfy different goals. The memory is distilled through two processes: (1) The process of memory which allows an index of the stories to be constructed. The events themselves may be lost as an easily retrievable entity, while the index is available to use. (2) The translation process which expresses this index in a natural language. The index keeps evolving over time. Details can be added by further experiences, by reconstruction of existing ones, and/or by adaptation. People also talk to themselves to analyse experiences and form a story that is coherent.

The fact of a 'personal world' is both a subjective and objective phenomenon. Just as feelings give rise to thoughts, which clarify the feelings and increase them by acting back on them, so the subjects total frame of reference grows up into a world, which manifests itself subjectively in emotional atmospheres, feelings, states of minds and, objectively, in opinions, mental content, ideas, and symbols (Jaspers 1959)

This section elaborates on the theme that many mental disorders can be understood as the story of the person and/or his perception of what he observes about himself and the world around going haywire/erratic/out of control. To start with, certain relevant issues regarding some common mental disorders are discussed. A later section deals with the centrality of the person and their personality making them construct a story about themselves and their world in a certain way. Subsequent stories are constructed on this substrate.

There appears to be a continuum of psychopathology and that reflects in how many of the treatment modalities can be used across different diagnostic domains.

A revised model of existentially informed formulation is presented that could form the basis for clinical work in psychiatry. A broad framework of an existentially informed treatment paradigm is proposed. Pharmacological treatment forms a part of the framework including physical treatments and various forms of therapy.

AFFECTIVE DISORDERS (DEPRESSION & ANXIETY)

Anxiety and depression are two of the most prevalent psychiatric disorders in the community. They were traditionally considered to be part of the spectrum of affective disorders. These two disorders are highly comorbid, their symptoms overlap and the two are frequently inseparable. There were factors other than clinical that led to Depression and anxiety being separated into two distinct categories.

Bipolar disorder (Manic Depressive illness) also falls under the broad category of affective disorders. Every person classified as having depressive disorder has the potential to turn out to have bipolar disorder. The switch can happen at any stage in the course of the illness. Besides genetics/familial factors, an early onset, a relapsing course of illness and use of antidepressants have all been associated with increase in chance of developing a bipolar disorder. People with bipolar disorder spend a much larger proportion of their illness in depression rather than in hypomania or mania. Anxiety disorders are the most frequent condition associated with bipolar disorder. The current discussion is however limited to the more frequently occurring conditions of anxiety and depression.

A world-wide survey showed that 45.7% of individuals with lifetime major depressive disorder had a lifetime history of one or more anxiety disorder (Kessler et al 2015). As many as 41.6% of individuals with 12-month major depression also had one or more anxiety disorder over the same 12-month period. From the perspective of anxiety disorders, the lifetime comorbidity of depression ranges from 20 to 70% for social anxiety disorder (Dunner 2001), 48% with PTSD (Kesler et al 1995), 43% with generalised anxiety disorder (Brawman-Mitzer et al 1993). In the STAR* D study 53% of patients with major depression had significant anxiety and were considered as anxious depression (Fava et al 2004).

Depression has been described over several millennia of human history. It is the most easily recognisable psychological disorder and has been described throughout history. From the ancient Greek medical writing to the early 20th century depressive disorder was referred to as melancholia. Writings in the fifth century B.C., Hippocrates (460-377 B.C.) provided the first known definition of melancholia as a distinct disorder.

Poet W. H. Auden termed the period after World War II as the "age of anxiety." The intense anxiety of that era was a normal response to the extraordinary circumstances, such as the devastation of modern warfare, the development and the first use of a nuclear weapon, the horrors of the concentration camps, and the tensions of the cold war between the two major world powers. In the same vein, the era at the turn of the twenty-first century can be termed as the "age of depression," or perhaps and more appropriately the "age of affective disorders." While the age of anxiety was viewed as a natural response to social circumstances, the current phase can be viewed more as an extension of the age of anxiety to include depression rather than being replaced by the age of depression, as the 'epidemic' of anxiety continues unabated.

There is a widespread perception that depressive disorder is growing at an alarming pace. WHO recognizes depression as a common illness worldwide with 3.8% of the population affected, including 5.0% among adults and 5.7% among adults older than 60 years. Approximately 280 million people in the world have depression. The overall percentage of the US population in treatment for depression in a particular year grew from 2.1% in the early 1980s to 3.7% in the early 2000s, an increase of 7.6% in just 20 years. The current "epidemic" of depression may partly be the result of a range of social factors. The changes in psychiatric definition of depressive disorder have also contributed by at times classifying sadness as disease.

Depression has been dichotomised in many ways: endogenous vs reactive; agitated vs retarded; melancholic vs non-melancholic, unipolar vs bipolar; and vegetative vs non-vegetative. If one clubs all these dichotomies together then saying depression is the commonest mental disorder is like saying 'fever' is the commonest disorder or 'headache' is the commonest 'disorder' for which people consult a doctor all over the world. Fever and headache are the symptoms that underlie many disorders and is not a disorder in themselves.

Out of all the dichotomies of depression, perhaps the most significant is the one between those with or without vegetative symptoms that are sufficiently severe to impair most areas of a person's functioning. The international classification of disorder tries to capture this but then manages to obliterate its boundaries. The goal of this quest is to find a disorder that is distinctly biological in nature and where biologically based therapies are most likely to be effective. Depression with melancholic symptoms is considered by some to represent such a disorder but is used only as one of the specifiers of major depressive disorder in DSM 5.

It should be easy to distinguish these from 'happiness deficit disorders' (described earlier), dysthymia, adjustment disorder with depressive disorder, and all conditions where non-biological factors may play a key role. In the real world of psychiatry, this may be a lot more complicated. Language (idioms of distress) used by people seeking help plays a significant role in the evaluative process. The stoics tend to minimise their symptoms while those high on neuroticism may exaggerate their symptoms and overstate their distress. For some pain always means ten out ten if not 'out of the chart.'

Certain idioms of distress turn out to be 'pivotal' symptom and sways diagnosis in a certain way. For example, any patient presenting with only a limited number of symptoms of depression who also talks about suicidal ideas or plans is much more likely to be seen as suffering from a major depressive disorder and be prescribed antidepressant.

It has been pointed out that one of the basic flaws in the DSM definition of major depressive disorder is that it fails to consider the context of the symptoms and thus fails to exclude from the disorder category intense sadness other than in reaction to a loved one, that arises from the way human beings naturally respond to major losses. While pathologizing normal condition may cause harm, the avoidance of such pathologizing may decrease such harm.

Distinguishing disordered and normal sadness could help with more accurate diagnosis, allow appropriate epidemiological studies, allow more accurate research, and allocation of funds and appropriate treatment. DSM 5 does go into some detail in trying to explain the need to differentiate between major depressive disorder and other disorders with low mood. But lot of these distinctions are not as easy to use in clinical practice. The world of clinical psychiatry is different to the world of research and academics.

Negative emotions such as sadness, anger, and fear response to certain situations are results of natural selection. Such emotional responses are likely to reflect learned socially constructed scripts (stories). Allan Horwitz and Jerome Wakefield (2007) in their book "The Loss of Sadness" outlined three lines of evidence to support this position:

1. Nonhuman primates also show a clear resemblance to humans in the way they respond to loss - that is their observable features of expression, behaviour and, and brain functioning. Darwin had noted the similarities in facial expressions of apes and humans in situations associated with sadness including elevated eyebrows, drooping eyelids, horizontal wrinkles across the forehead and outward extension and drawing down of the lips. They also include decreased locomotor activity, agitation, slouched or foetal posture, cessation of play behaviour, and social withdrawal.

The loss situations that commonly lead to depressive responses are similar in primates and humans. Primate studies show that symptoms of depression that develops after separation rapidly disappear when the situation of loss is resolved, such as when an infant monkey is reunited with its mother. Such transient sadness response to separation is part of innate coping mechanism among many species. However, prolonged separations and separations marked by profound isolation can produce significant neuroanatomical changes that permanently affects nonhuman primate brain functioning, analogous to the triggering of genuine depressive disorder in humans.

Michael McGuire and colleagues (1983) had studied Vervet monkeys, who possess strong and enduring hierarchical status relationships with one dominant male in each group. The highest-ranking males have serotonin levels that are twice as high as those of other males in the group. When they were removed from the group their serotonin levels fell and they refused food, showed diminished activity, and appeared to human observers as depressed. Conversely, the serotonin levels of previously dependent monkeys who gained high status after the removal of the previously dominant male rose to values that characterize dominant males. Studies of wild baboons living freely shows the same tend (Sapolsky 2017). Jordan Peterson (2018) quoted similar findings in Lobsters.

John Price (1994) views depression as part of an 'Involuntary Subordinate Strategy' (ISS). Animals develop ISS response when they judge themselves to be weaker than the competitors. Many of the symptoms of ISS involve behaviour that communicate that the loser will not confront the winner, will not attempt to gain dominance, and will give up the struggle.

2. The human tendency to become sad in certain contexts appear early in infancy. John Bowlby demonstrated how attachment losses led to depressive reactions among infants. Healthy infants who were separated from their mothers initially reacted by crying and displaying other expressions of despair. When separation was prolonged, the infants withdrew and became inactive and apathetic, like the symptoms of an intense adult loss response.

   The capacity for intense sadness response to loss appears to be a universal feature found in all human groups. Charles Darwin noted the universality of sadness response. He provided a description of grief among Indigenous Australians that was comparable to the expression of this emotion among Europeans. The constriction of the muscles at the corner of the mouth is recognized across cultures as representing grief.

   Paul Ekman (1976) researched facial expressions as they were less susceptible to cultural influences. Results indicated an overwhelming agreement among persons in different countries about the emotion each photograph expresses. These findings lead to the belief that there are some innate features of the expression of sadness, and they are present in all cultures. They may have stemmed from the evolution of humans as a species.

Culture may have evolutionarily shaped the loss responses in a variety of ways:

1. Cultural meaning influence humiliation and entrapment, which count as losses. These meanings also influence contextual factors, such as humiliation and entrapment, which determines the severity of loss.

2. All cultures display norms or "scripts" that guide people towards overt expression of emotions. Cultural norms also affect what is viewed as the appropriate duration of loss response.

3. George Brown's cross-cultural studies found rates of depressive responses to vary tenfold across societies. These variations were to a considerable extent due to varying exposure to the kinds of loss events that naturally cause depression. There was a nearly perfect correlation between the number of severe loss events that befall members of different societies and resulting rates of depressive symptoms. Strong interpersonal ties and networks of social support, as well as powerful collective religious rituals and belief systems help make people less vulnerable to loss.

Allen Frances (2013) summed up by iterating: 'Major depression is not always that major.' A lot of what passes for MDD is not really "major," is not really "depressive," and is not really "disorder." Loose diagnosis has created a false epidemic of MDD. Mild major depression is a peculiar contradiction in terms. Sadness should not be synonymous with sickness. There is no diagnosis for every disappointment or a pill for every problem. We are usually resilient, lick our wounds, mobilize our resources and our friends, and get on with it. Our capacity to feel emotional pain has great adaptive function equivalent in its purpose to physical pain. The DSMs have made it too easy to get a diagnosis of MDD. Doctors bought the story line that all depression results from a chemical imbalance in the brain and therefore requires a chemical fix – the prescription of an antidepressant medication.

DISTINGUISHING GRIEF FROM DEPRESSION

At the behavioural level grief is associated with sadness, lack of pleasure, decreased initiative, and tendency to withdraw from life. It must have had some adaptive advantage at some stage in a way like acute pain that results from an injury. It makes one to stop, take stock of the situation, and thereby avoid further damage to the tissues. Chronic pain unrelated to any physiological damage on the other hand would be harmful in the way that depressive disorder is certainly harmful.

A central premise of evolutionary science is that forces in our distant past helped make us who we are today. The environment of evolutionary adaptedness (EEA) refers to a group of selection pressures occurring during an adaptation's period of evolution responsible for producing the adaptation (Tooby and Cosmides 1992). This occurred when humans lived in hunter-gatherer societies. It shaped the many genetic traits that humans still have. Sadness was designed to cope with contexts that arose in those ancestral conditions but that may be less apparent in current environment.

Another explanation of the adaptive function of depressive feelings is the communication of these to other people and thus attract social support after attachment losses. Sir Aubrey Lewis proposed that depressive reactions could function as a "cry for help." The culturally defined period of mourning following the death of a loved one is a good example of eliciting care and compassion for others in the kinship and society. In the past dress codes and forms of behaviour were proscribed and adhered to. In the Indian culture a shaved head was the clearest indication that a man has lost someone close. The erosion of such practises as well as living in much larger communities has taken away these adaptive measures to deal with grief.

Severe depression is associated with more marked and sustained states of low mood without sufficient situational cause. These states are more likely to alienate others and diminish social support leading to isolation and rejection, and fitness disadvantage. Thus, reactive states of depression may be easier not just because of the lower severity of symptoms, but also because of its increased ability to elicit caring response from others relative to those with endogenous depression.

Ethological studies indicate that the capacity to become depressed, as indicated by lower testosterone, elevated cortisol, and retardation of behaviour, is deeply rooted in the reptilian brain and is present in most vertebrates and all mammals (Price 1994). Such depressive response might have arisen widely as signals of defeat in status contests that are ubiquitous in the animal world. SSRIs work on both the disordered and the non-disordered depression (Knutson et al 1998). Grieving people who are not disordered report fewer symptoms after treatment with antidepressants (Zisook et al 2001).

Throughout our life we go through a series of attachments and losses. One day we grieve for those we lose and when we die others will grieve for us. Mistaking grief as depression may have unfortunate consequences. It runs the risk of reducing the dignity of the pain, the existential processing of the loss, wasting the many well-established cultural rituals that not only help with grieving but may also help making or reinforcing other bonds.

DSM 5 considers the importance of grief and reactions to losses. It does encourage to identify the simultaneous occurrence of major depressive disorder. This is a useful approach, but it is by no means an effortless process as many of the symptoms of grief and depression overlap. It finally boils down to the clinical judgement of the professional and a truly collaborative decision-making process with 'the one who suffers.'

DSM 5 has created a category of Persistent Complex Bereavement Disorder under the group of conditions for further research. It may be easier to produce the proposed criteria, but further research is likely to face many roadblocks.

DISTINGUISHING OTHER FORMS OF DEPRESSION FROM MAJOR DEPRESSION

It is important to distinguish between major depressive disorder from dysthymia (persistent low mood associated with low self-esteem, low self-confidence, and self-loathing) and reactive depression (crises in life that cause distress). Dysthymia can go unrecognised in some or mislabelled as Major Depression depending on whether help is sought or not and the idioms and phrases used while seeking help. The same may be true with people presenting with an adjustment disorder with affective (depressive and/or anxiety) symptoms. The distinction is of importance as dysthymia and adjustment disorder with depressive and/or anxiety symptoms are less likely to need or benefit from antidepressants. If misdiagnosed and inappropriately prescribed antidepressants, they may be taking an unnecessary medication for a long time and suffer unwanted side effects too.

The new category of persistent mood disorder amalgamates dysthymia with chronic persistent major depressive disorder. This would be seen as an indication for antidepressants for dysthymia as well. The utility of antidepressants in dysthymia is less certain.

The analogy from other branches of medicine may be quite appropriate. "It was only after Sydenham had demonstrated that "the pox" was in fact two distinct syndromes: Chicken pox and Smallpox, that it was possible to predict with any accuracy who would certainly recover and who would remain scarred for life and was in danger of dying. And only when physicians had learned to distinguish between the renal and cardiac forms of dropsy was it possible to predict which patients were likely to benefit from digitalis (Kendell 1998).

Some medication can be used in case of adjustment disorder with significant physiological symptoms that is interfering with everyday functioning.

Without a diagnosis of major depressive disorder medication may be used in a targeted way and for a much shorter period and therapy would be seen as likely to be more helpful in ameliorating grief. Making sense of loss and addressing the other adaptive needs is a basic existential project. Each loss may pose different issues and having dealt with them once does not make a person a master at this dilemma. As Yalom put it, 'psychotherapy is often cyclo-therapy.'

For mental health clinicians and researchers' symptoms-based measures of depression is a necessity. They are easy to use, reduce the cost and complexity of research studies, allow for higher research productivity, and confers enhanced scientific respectability. Psychiatrists like all other professionals seek prominence and distinguishing ourselves through research and publication plays a key role in achieving these goals. However, inappropriately diagnosing grief, dysthymia, or adjustment disorder as major depression muddies the waters in any research undertaking.

THE SEARCH FOR CAUSES OF PSYCHIATRIC ILLNESS:

Kenneth Kendler (2019) in a classic paper explored the search for causes of psychiatric illness "From many to One to many." He traced this back to Robert Burton who in 1621 in his encyclopaedic book: "The Anatomy of Melancholy" had listed forty-four causes for melancholy which were as diverse as old age, temperament, parents, poverty, over-much alcohol, sorrow, anger, immoderate eating, and envy. In 1786 Thomas Arnold was even more extensive in his list of bodily and mental causes of "insanity." Jean Esquirol (1838) provided the most common causes of "insanity," dividing the causes into two groups: physical and moral (or psychological).

Kendler sought to rigorously assess informal impression by reviewing all studies that addressed the aetiology of psychiatric disorders in the first four 2013 issues of twelve major psychiatry and psychology journals. He was able to identify thirty-seven potential causes of depression distributed across eleven levels of scientific inquiry, almost equal to Burton's number of forty-four in the year 1621. In this article he explored the causal theories in psychiatry, largely in conformity with the rest of medicine, but for a period of time out of step with it.

From many to one: The causal paradigm of medicine shifted dramatically in the second half of the 19th century to the doctrine of specific etiology due largely to the work of Pasteur and Koch. The task was to define a disorder in relation to its one specific underlying cause. Disorders not amenable to such causal clarification were of lower status-syndromes and not real diseases. The monocausal theory derived from bacteria and viruses-soon spread to include parasitic and vitamin-deficiency diseases. Psychiatry sought to participate in the diagnostic revolution. Like the rest of medicine, it sought to turn symptom-based diagnoses into distinct diseases discovered using an iterative clinical research paradigm of signs, symptoms, and course of illness. This quest was aided by the discovery of Treponeme palladium as the cause of the General Paralysis of the insane (GPI) which accounted for up to 45% of urban public mental hospitals.

From one to many: Susser and Susser (1996) described three successive eras of epidemiology: The first focussed on sanitary statistics. The second epidemiological phase, termed infectious disease, has as its paradigm "the germ theory, lasted roughly from 1850 to 1950 and was dominated by monocausal etiological theories in which the relationship between putative etiologic agent and specific disease was one to one (although most investigators recognized such factors as "host resistance").

The third epidemiological phase was termed "chronic disease" began around 1950 and has lasted until recent times. It incorporated multifactorial disease model for what was termed as chronic noncommunicable diseases associated with certain lifestyles (e.g., diabetes, heart disease, certain forms of cancer, and hypertension). The intense debate about and eventual resolution of the causal association between smoking and lung cancer played a key role. The debate led to the proposal and eventual acceptance of the Hill criteria for causation. Smoking became a paradigmatic risk factor that was a worthy cause for lung cancer despite unequivocal evidence that many people who were long-term smokers never developed lung cancer and many individuals with lung cancer never smoked.

Multicausality underlined that most identified causes are neither necessary nor sufficient to produce a disease. Nevertheless, when a component that is neither necessary nor sufficient is blocked, a substantial amount of the disease may be prevented. Kendler points out that the approach in major parts of psychiatry in the second half of the 20th century was out of step with the rest of medicine. The continuing quest for monocausal models has two prominent phases, both fuelled by new scientific developments.

The stage was set in 1957 by Montagu's discovery of dopamine in brain tissue quickly followed, in 1960, by the dramatic finds from Ehringer and Hornkeiewicz of the decreased content of dopamine in the post-mortem brains of patients with Parkinson's disease. Even greater excitement followed the impressive effects obtained from L-dopa (Levodopa) in patients with Parkinson's disease. A major neurological disorder fitted a monocausal neurochemical theory and had a viable treatment predicted by the causal theory.

In the early to mid-1960s, through histo-fluroscence stains the cell bodies and neuronal pathways of the three monoamine neurotransmitters (Dopamine, Norepinephrine, and Serotonin) were identified. These led to the "catecholamine hypothesis of affective disorders," the "dopamine hypothesis of schizophrenia," and the "serotonin hypothesis of depression." The primary support for these theories was reasoning backward from therapeutic mechanism to aetiology. It is now widely accepted that these "chemical imbalance" theories claiming a dominant causal pathway to illness are false although debate continues regarding the dopamine hypothesis.

The second wave of monocausal theories was genetic. The first successful linkage study of Huntington disease in 1983 elicited intense excitement in psychiatric genetics and launched many linkage studies, especially in schizophrenia and bipolar disorder. Psychiatry was deeply committed to establishing its medical legitimacy. However, such an approach fitted better in the world of medicine in the late 19th century than the late 20th century. Psychiatry needed to claim that we treated "real" disorders because they were multicausal, like coronary artery disease, hypertension, rheumatoid arthritis, and type 2 diabetes, not that they were monocausal, such as classic infection or mendelian medical disorders.

The current journals are now filled with evidence for multicausal nature of psychiatric disorders (Paulus and Thompson 2018). The chemical deficiency theory of depression originated with psychiatrist Joseph Schildkraut's 1965 hypothesis that low levels of amines were associated with the development of depressive disorder. The success of drug treatment that raised the levels of amines and alleviates mood symptoms was a major contributor to the theory.

The causal hypotheses that we use is influenced by the prevailing paradigm of the time. "To Ivan Ilyich only one question was important: was his case serious or not? But the doctor ignored this misplaced enquiry. From the doctor's point of view, it was a side issue not under consideration. The real issue was the assessing of probabilities to decide between a floating kidney, chronic catarrh, or appendicitis. It was not a question of Ivan Ilyich's life or death but one between a floating kidney or appendicitis" (*The death of Ivan Ilyich* by Leo Tolstoy 1886).

THE EMPIRE OF DEPRESSION

There are two senses in which depression can be seen as having an empire (Jonathan Sadowsky 2021). First, in Western psychiatry and societies, depression has become a dominant way of interpreting mental distress. Second, this linguistic shift then began to spread globally.

Increasing rates of diagnosis of depression in recent decades is a fact, but its cause and meaning is not obvious. There are three possible reasons: (1) There could really be more depression. (2) We may be catching more of it and (3) the possibility of a diagnostic drift – the relabelling of states that were considered different illness or were not considered illness at all. The history of depression is in part a history of the tug-of-war over where the line should fall. Sorrow is everywhere you turn, but when is sorrow sickness?

Some who argue for a rise in true prevalence of depression point to depressing conditions in the world, rapid changes in social roles and expectations, or increased social isolation (due say, to the internet), or even a worsening human diet. Anxiety is an expectation of danger to come. Depression is a sense of loss already felt.

The growth of outpatient psychiatry led to an increase in the number of people being treated for depressive illness. No longer was treatment reserved for the most severe depressive cases. The growing interest in depression led more people, both professional and lay, to learn to label problems as depression, which was a growing idiom of distress before the advent of antidepressants. That is part of the reason some medications came to be called antidepressants at all. Another reason, as discussed later (When anxiety became a dirty word) was the bad name that was generated by the widespread and improper use of the tranquillisers. The medications provided new incentives for multiple actors – pharmaceutical companies, doctors, patients, and patients families to identify cases of depression.

At least some of the rush to diagnose and treat depression may be related to our fear of death. Suicide is a form of death that elicits the greatest concern. However, suicide is a complex problem. Many of the problems associated with suicide are unlikely to alter using an antidepressant alone. There is a strong association of grief with death that is seen as untimely (younger the person who dies, the more the 'life not lived' and more the misgiving) and preventable (depression was naively thought to be a condition that was easy to diagnose and treat).

Concerted efforts were made for General practitioners, primary care physicians, community nurses and other health professionals to use checklist approach to diagnosis of depression. In contemporary times, most often a diagnosis of depression has already been made and a person so diagnosed is started on antidepressant much before the patient in seen by a psychiatrist. The fear of the coroner and doing what can be done to avoid the possibility of having to face one remains a source of anxiety and nightmare for all professionals.

In recent times there has been a weakening in people's faith in scientific certainties. There is a growing cynicism that knowledge claims reflect power and narrative structures more than objective truths. There is a renewed interest in all kinds of alternative treatment models. Natural therapy (the practice of being in nature to boost growth and healing, especially mental health) and traditional forms of treatment (Ayurvedic, Chinese, and others) and nonchemical therapies (Yoga, Meditation, Tai Chi etc). The market for barely researched and unregulated herbal and other drug is enormous and still growing. We are strangely not as concerned about them.

For depressed patients, the world appears as uninviting and unattractive. How deep and pervasive these thoughts and feelings are may largely depend on the severity of the depression. Depression affects not only how they feel (hopeless, helpless, and worthless), but also what they perceive (the rejecting, disapproving faces of the family and carers, and the seeming uselessness of activities and pursuits people around them appear to be engaged in) and the way they act (underactivity) and interact (avoiding contact with others). Their sense-making is disordered in that it is distorted and biased in a negative direction and it is long lasting. All this creates a vicious cycle that makes it hard to elicit an appropriate nurturing environment for recovery.

The concept of 'emotional intelligence' and 'mis-wanting' may be of considerable importance is understanding depression. These were explored in some detail in the earlier chapter 'understanding our emotions.'

ANXIETY DISORDERS

Anxiety disorders are among the most prevalent mental health conditions, affecting 264 million individuals worldwide in 2017 with large-scale general population estimates suggesting 12-month prevalence rates of 18.1%–22.2%. According to NIMH, some forty million Americans (nearly one in seven) suffer from one or more of the various kinds of anxiety disorder at any given time, accounting for 31% of the expenditure on mental health care in US. As recently as 30 years ago, anxiety per se did not exist as a clinical category, however the new epidemiological data shows the lifetime incidence of anxiety disorder as more than 25%.

The increase in prevalence of anxiety disorders has partly been because of the identification of newer categories. Before 1980, no one had ever been diagnosed with social anxiety disorder. Twenty years later, about ten to twenty million Americans were estimated to be suffering from the illness. NIMH estimates that more than 10% of Americans suffer from social anxiety disorder at some point in their lifetime, about 30% of them in an acute form. Sceptics view this as medicalising shyness and introversion.

Anxiety extends far beyond those who are officially designated as mentally ill. Everyone alive has at some point experienced the torment of anxiety. Anxiety is at once a function of biology and philosophy, body and mind, instinct and reason, personality, and culture. In computer terms, it is both a hardware problem ('I am wired badly') and a software problem ('I am faulty logic program that makes me think anxious thoughts'). There is an underlying consistency of experience across time and culture which speaks of the universality of anxiety as a human trait.

Fear signifies that something in the world is threatening, and one sees oneself as vulnerable. In anxiety one sees oneself as threatened or vulnerable, but unlike fear, in anxiety there is no direct object or situation that is really threatening. Some degree of anxiety is essential for survival. According to what is known as "The Yerkes-Dodson law," performance increases with physiological or mental arousal (stress) but only up to a point. When the level of stress becomes too high, performance decreases.

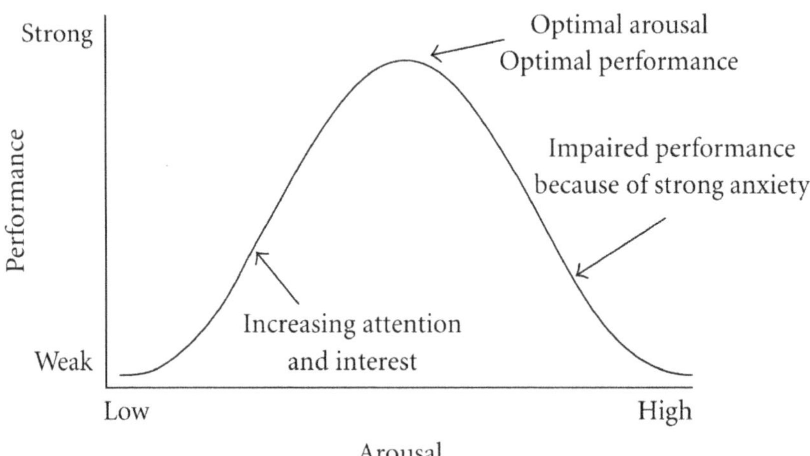

Anxiety is associated with arousal and the level of anxiety that is associated with increased performance is labelled as 'signal anxiety' and levels beyond that associated with decreasing performance is seen as pathological.

Kierkegaard (1884) wrote: "If man were a beast or an angel, he would not be able to be in anxiety. Since he is both beast an angel, he can be in anxiety, and the greater the anxiety, the greater the man." The ability to worry about the future goes hand in hand with the ability to plan for the future-and planning is what gives rise to culture and separates us from other animals. Most of the threat that leads to anxiety lay not in the world around us but rather deep inside us - in our uncertainty about the existential choices we make and in our fear of death.

Kierkegaard added, "Learning to know anxiety, is an adventure which every man has to affront if he would not go to perdition either by not having known anxiety or by sinking under it." "He therefore who has learned rightly to be in anxiety has learned the most important thing."

When anxious, people often perceive their surroundings only partly and take notice only those things which confirms their worries. It elicits a certain type of reactions from others, one that in turn affirms the person's experience. No behaviour, thought, or feeling, is in itself disordered. One cannot assess the appropriateness of sense-making without taking its context into account. Any assessment is shaped by the norms and values of the sociocultural community of which we are a part.

One can see death anxiety to underlie many of the anxiety-based disorders. In panic disorder one of the main symptoms is the fear of having a heart attack and an associated dread of dying. Separation anxiety is associated with the fear of doom for the child or their parents. Most of the specific phobias involve objects, animals or situation that increase possibility of death such as snake, spider, heights, flying, enclosed spaces, and water. The most common symptoms in obsessive-compulsive disorder include germs, washing, cleaning, violence etc. Germs kill and so can violence. Rituals are often directed at avoiding the possibility of the harm that could occur due to the obsessions.

WHEN ANXIETY BECAME A DIRTY WORD

During the 1950s antianxiety drugs like Meprobamate were mistakenly seen as a remedy for distress caused by problems of living. They were able to provide relief from some of the symptoms associated with stress through sedation and muscle relaxation and this was received with lot of optimism and enthusiasm. Demand from these drugs skyrocketed and they were widely misused. By 1956, one in 20 American were taking some sort of tranquillizer (the term in widespread use around that time). In the early 1960s, the benzodiazepine Chlordiazepoxide and diazepam were developed. By 1969, diazepam became the most prescribed medication in US. Women received two of every three prescriptions.

The use of these drugs for everyday stresses of life caused significant concern. They were seen as numbing people's reactions to social problems and allowing many to use them to avoid confronting oppressive interpersonal situations. The director of NIMH expressed unease whether "the chemical deadening of anxiety" was harmful and whether "Western culture (would) be altered by widespread use of tranquillizers." Serious concerns were also expressed about their addictive qualities, adverse side effects, and overdose potential.

Charles Edward, the commissioner of FDA expressed growing concern of his agency that "advertisements have also prompted their use in the treatment of symptoms arising from the stresses of normal living which cannot properly be defined as pathological. In 1971, FDA requested that advertisers of psychotropic drugs refrain from promoting their use in coping with everyday life strains. The popular press also took a strong stand. The craze for antianxiety drugs was tapering off by the time the DSM III was published in 1980.

THE RISE OF ANTIDEPRESSANT DRUG TREATMENT

Horwitz and Wakefield (2007) pointed to the way pharmacological companies were quick to capitalize on the DSM's focus on symptoms, which allowed them to broadly construe states of intense sadness as depressive disorder and thus to vastly increase the potential market for antidepressant medication. The approval of direct-to-consumer advertisements in 1997 may have influenced the increase in the use of the antidepressants as well.

'Ask your doctor' increases the myth of a simple cure for a complex problem. Once the 'client' raises the question the 'care provider' may find it hard to say no. It also takes a longer consultation to explain the reason behind not prescribing compared to dishing out a prescription. SSRI group of drugs accelerated the use of antidepressants as they had fewer side effects and were safer than the earlier antianxiety and antidepressants.

SSRIs could also be used to treat a variety of problems besides depression including anxiety, panic, obsessive-compulsive disorder, post-traumatic stress disorder and, eating disorder. They could have been easily marketed as antianxiety medications but were approved as antidepressants because of the negative associations that had developed around the anti-anxiety medications. By 2001, about two and a half times more people were using SSRIs than antianxiety medications. The "antidepressant" label provided tremendous impetus for marketing depression, rather than anxiety, even though they were being used for a variety of anxiety-based disorders.

The diagnosis of major depression used common symptoms such as sadness, lack of energy or sleeplessness as indicators. It was particularly suited for expanding the market for psychotropic drugs because it inevitably encompassed many patients who formerly might have been thought to be suffering from problems of living.

The overlap between the symptoms of anxiety and depression has always been known. Anxiety was generally viewed as the most common psychic problem resulting from the stresses of daily life. Yet the DSM III attempted to identify a pure depressive syndrome independent of anxiety. The condition which is emphasised depends not only on the diagnostic fashions of the time, the interests of various professional and advocacy groups, but also the economic costs and benefits that accrue from such emphasis. By 1980, the balance of these factors had shifted away from anxiety because of the backlash against the anxiolytics. DSM III and its various revisions have also provided drug companies with a way out of the dilemma they faced in marketing their antianxiety medications.

Reducing health care expenditures has been a significant concern in today's world. General practitioners and primary care physicians have increasingly become the source of prescriptions for antidepressant drugs. These consultations cost less than that that of the specialist.

As a result of cost considerations, visits to office-based psychiatry have become shorter and more often includes a medication prescription.

Medications also involves lower out-of-pocket costs for the patients than psychotherapy. By 1998 two thirds of elderly persons for depression received only an antidepressant, whereas a little more than 10% obtained only psychotherapy. Payment for long term psychotherapy almost disappeared.

It had taken FDA fifteen years from the application (1972) to approval (1987) of Prozac, but when it finally reached the market, it proved to be sensational. Peter Kramer's "Listening to Prozac: A Psychiatrist Explores Antidepressant Drugs, and the Remaking of the Self" helped to galvanize the formulation of life problems as problems of depression and their treatment with antidepressant medications. His use of the term antidepressants to characterize SSRIs and his book's focus on depression helped associate both the drugs and the condition they treated specifically with depression (Peter Kramer 1993). Kramer's book also helped create a mythic status for Prozac, his generic term for SSRIs. By 1994, Prozac (Fluoxetine) had become the second best-selling drug in the world followed closely by its siblings Paxil (Paroxetine) and Zoloft (Sertraline).

It is widely acknowledged that a large proportion of real-world patients fail to participate in industry trials of antidepressants because of exclusionary criteria.

The NIMH sponsored Star*D study was the largest, longest and most ambitious study ever done to evaluate depression treatment in real-world patients at a cost of 35 million US dollars. Over the course of all four levels of treatment, almost 70 percent of those who did not withdraw from the study were claimed to have become symptom-free (Rush et al 2006).

Pigott et al (2019,2023) reanalysed the data and accused Star*D investigators of not using the protocol-stipulated Hamilton Rating Scale for Depression (HRSD) to report cumulative remission and response rates in their summary article and instead used and non-blinded clinician-administered assessment. This inflated their report of outcomes as did their inclusion of ninety-nine patients who scored as remitted on HRSD at study outset, as well as 125 who scored as remitted when initiating their next level treatment. These patients should have been excluded from data analysis. In contrast to the study reported 67% cumulative remission rate after up to four antidepressant treatment trials, the actual rate was 35.0% when using the protocol stipulated HRSD in data analysis.

Evidence indicates that the SSRIs are no more effective than older antidepressants. They are simply better tolerated, their side effects are more benign, and they lack the addictive nature and potential lethality of the antianxiety medications (Mann 2005). A metanalysis by Cipriani et al (2018) looked at the comparative efficacy and acceptability of twenty-one antidepressant drugs for the acute treatment of adults with major depressive disorder. It was well greeted as it apparently showed that all antidepressants were more effective than placebo.

Nassir Ghaemi (2018) in a critique of the study disputed the claim. "The real truth isn't found within the published paper but rather within the busy table on page 142 of the online appendix." "Here we see that the Cohen's standardised mean difference effect sizes range from a low of 0.19 to a high of 0.62 with amitriptyline. Thus, amitriptyline exceeds the clinically meaningful threshold of 0.50 with a traditional meta-analytic method. No other drug does so with the closest second place with being fluvoxamine with the Cohen's d of 0.44. Ten drugs had values of less than 0.30 and four between 0.30 to 0.34. Thus 74% (14/19) of antidepressants clearly had no clinically important benefit in this analysis."

A 2022 study by Joanna Moncrieff and colleagues (including Mark Horwitz) aimed to synthesise and evaluate evidence on whether depression is associated with lowered serotonin concentration or activity in a systematic umbrella review of the principal relevant areas of research. They included seventeen studies: twelve systematic reviews and meta-analyses, one collaborative meta-analysis, one meta-analysis of large cohort studies, one systematic review and narrative synthesis, one genetic association study and one umbrella review.

This comprehensive review of the major strands of research on serotonin showed that there was no convincing evidence that depression is associated with, or caused by, lower serotonin concentrations or activity. Most studies found no evidence of reduced serotonin activity in people with depression compared to people without. Methods to reduce serotonin availability using tryptophan depletion do not consistently lower mood in volunteers.

This resonates well with the assertions made fifteen years ago by Horwitz and Wakefield (2007) who pointed to many problems that beset the monoamine theory of depression:

1. The SSRIs cause immediate changes in levels of serotonin, but the resulting effects on depression typically take several weeks to transpire. Thus, there may be several other processes associated with the change in the amine activities may be playing a role.

2. Some drugs that do not affect either serotonin or norepinephrine (e.g., dopamine) also can alleviate depressive symptoms (Valenstein 1998)

3. The drugs used to treat depression work with at least equal effectiveness on other disorders, including those of anxiety, eating, attention deficit, substance abuse, personality and a host of other conditions that may or may not be comorbid with depression.

4. Measures typically show that only about 25% of depressed patients actually have low levels of serotonin or norepinephrine.

5. The hypothesized deficiencies of serotonin or other chemicals quite possibly may be the consequences rather than causes of depression.

The main issue is not that serotonin deficiency is the cause of major depression, but that depression itself is a heterogenous disorder with a lot of overlap with anxiety and is of multifactorial origin. At the same time, antidepressants do benefit many with depression. The precise way it does so may still elude our full understanding. Nonspecific changes that help with homeostasis may be relevant. The non-specificity of all psychotropic medication is discussed further in the section of treatment.

Johann Hari (2019) in his international best seller, *Lost Connections* asserts: "You are not suffering from a chemical imbalance in your brain. You are suffering from a social and spiritual imbalance in how we live. Much more than you've been told up to now. It's not serotonin; it's the society. It's for sure. But it's not the cause. It's not the driver. It's not the place to look for the main explanation, or the main solution." He lists disconnections from 1. Meaningful work, 2. Other people, 3. Meaningful values, 4. Status and respect, 5. Natural world. 6. A hopeful and secure future and 7. Childhood trauma as the social causes for depression.

Hari does concede that: "It is foolish to deny there is a real biological component to depression and anxiety (and there may be other biological contributions we haven't identified yet) – but it is equally foolish to say they are the only causes.' And this concession makes the chasm between a brainless and mindless psychiatry pertinent and emphasises the need for them to work together. Many of his conclusions about biological or more specifically medications have some validity, but he has overstated the clarity afforded by psycho-social research. They are as hard, if not harder, to conduct and as limited in their ability to find clinically meaningful conclusions.

Human life is complex without doubt and so are their mental disorders. In an existential framework physiology is seen as the starting point on which life experiences and social and cultural factors work.

CULTURAL VARIATIONS

Depression has been called the single most fraught psychiatric diagnosis for cross cultural study. Psychiatry is a cultural system, with a set of beliefs about depressive illness that are not universal but becoming more global in their influence every day.

It is possible to use local categories, or 'idioms of distress' that are used by distinct cultures, instead of supposedly universal diagnoses. A Punjabi idiom "sinking heart" has some overlap with the English word "depression." If one, simply calls it depression they lose aspects of how Punjabis see the problem. Western psychiatry roots emotion more in the brain. Loss of control of the heart is loss of control of the self for Punjabis.

Another idiom of distress found in numerous places translates as "thinking too much." Having 'taken things to heart' is a commonly used expression to denote perturbation because of events beyond one's control. Perhaps many of the languages without a word for depression are calling it "thinking too much." In Indian culture there is a greater emphasis on interpersonal interdependence. To say that 'I am depressed' could mean that someone close may be 'the cause' of me being depressed. So, people may be more likely to present with somatic symptoms rather than emphasising their depressed mood. The low frequency of depression in India was reported in the past, though the rates are showing an increasing trend with changes in the social fabric and lifestyle.

African studies showed a significant increase in the incidence of depression in the times following the end of the colonial rule. Several theories were proposed. One of them was a post-colonial revival in which culturally it seemed like saying, 'I can also have the White Man's disease.'

While talking about culture we must remain vigilant against creating cultural stereotypes. Every culture is made of many individuals, and they are all unique people with differing characteristics.

ARGUMENTS IN FAVOUR OF RECLASSIFICATION:

When both depression and anxiety symptoms occur together, it is generally assumed, that depression should be seen as the primary disorder. This notion can be disputed. There are many more variations in anxiety disorder than depression. Across all disorders, the presence of significant anxiety symptoms predicts worse outcome. In Star*D study those 53% of patients with anxious depression were less likely to remit and had a greater side effect burden. In a recent study, when examining diagnoses without hierarchy, the parent offspring transmission from anxiety disorder (AD) to major depression (MD) and from MD to AD were nearly symmetrical and a result of a similar mixture of genetic and rearing effects, with relatively high genetic and rearing environmental correlation (Kendler et al 2022).

This intergenerational Swedish study comprising over two million families found a modest genetic influence on the transmission of anxiety, depression and the cross transmission of anxiety and depression within families. The proportion of correlations was 70% for the genes and 30% due to the rearing environment and these were remarkably similar for anxiety and depression. It appeared likely that there were some common sets of social determinants that effect of anxiety and depression in both parents and offspring generations.

A reclassification of anxiety and depression under a unified category appears worthwhile:

1. Anxiety and depression are highly comorbid conditions, and their symptoms are frequently inseparable.

2. They cluster within families, often co-occur, and cross predict each other (Rice AJP September 2022)

3. They are both considered to belong to the broader category of internalizing disorder.

4. Both tend to emerge around adolescence.

5. Neuroticism is a personality trait or temperamental characteristic that is associated with the development of both anxiety and depression and the genetic risk for developing neuroticism also appears to be shared with that of internalizing disorders (Hettema et al 2006)

6. Antidepressants are the mainstay of treatment of both anxiety and depressive disorders. The so-called antianxiety medications are useful only for the short-term treatment of anxiety. Besides lack of efficacy in the long term there is the added burden of tolerance and dependence. It has been shown that all the antidepressants work for anxiety disorders.

Our body can respond in three ways in response to stress. The origins of these responses can be traced back to the naked humans living a nomadic life with constant threat of other animals who were often stronger, larger, and faster. The most common response was to fight or flight. When they felt to be in in danger, but they could overpower the threat, they went into the fight mode. Their brain released signals to the body, preparing it for the physical demands of fighting. If they believed they cannot overcome the danger but can avoid it by running away, they went into the flight mode. A surge of hormones, like adrenaline, gave the body the stamina to run from the danger. When faced with insurmountable danger, when they made a judgement that neither fight nor flight was going to be effective, they went into the freeze mode. They laid on the ground very still (pretending to be dead or merge into the ground) to evade the predator. The success of this response depended on every member of the group remaining frozen.

In the stress model of affective disorder, presentation as predominantly anxious may signify being in the fight mode, but not in a very effective way. Presentation as predominantly depressed mode represents being in the flight mode, whereas the mixed anxious and depressed presentation signifies being in both flight and fight mode. Severe depression (with psychomotor retardation) may represent the freeze response. People with severe depression are often at greater risk of suicide in the initial stages of treatment, as they may refreeze without being any decrease in their depression and take the refuse of suicide to run away from their severe depression.

Stengel (1959) had very eloquently put forth the idea that any adequate classification should utilize categories which are "mutually exclusive and jointly exhaustive." In keeping with the idea mood disorder, anxiety disorders, and anxiety-based disorders could form part of the broad category of affective disorders with the following subcategories:

1. Affective disorder with predominantly depressive symptoms (Present day Major Depressive Disorder)

2. Affective disorders with predominantly anxiety symptoms (Present day Generalised Anxiety Disorder)

3. Affective disorders with mood and anxiety symptoms

4. Specific Anxiety based disorders: Panic Disorder, OCD, PTSD

Each of these categories may be further classified according to the severity of symptoms as mild, moderate, severe and severe with mood-congruent and mood-incongruent psychotic symptoms. Other specifiers like persistent symptoms may be used for each category. Those associated with other medical conditions may be mentioned separately.

Anxiety may be hardwired in our brain while depression may be more a problem with our software. The ever present "fear of death' or 'ceasing to exist' made the human brain evolve to be hard-wired to anxiety. It offered an advantage for survival. Increasing concern about the future became a preoccupation as we gave up our nomadic life to live as farmers having greater control over our life circumstances. Depression made a debut in human life later, possibly over the last 15,000 years. We now had a fear of losing other givens of life rather than life itself. Depression could represent a "fear of life," the fear of loss of significant connections with people and possessions dear to them.

These two fears (life fear and death fear) are often present together which may account for the frequent co-occurrence of anxiety and depression. Anxiety is defined as an anticipation of something going wrong while depression signifies sadness and inability to experience pleasure. The two constitute overlapping aspects of the same overarching condition of affective disorder.

THE STORY OF POST-TRAUMATIC STRESS DISORDER

Trauma is usually defined as (1) a serious injury to the body, resulting from physical violence or an accident or (2) the severe emotional or mental distress caused by an experience. The medical profession is inextricably linked to diseases and injuries. Psychiatry as a subspecialty of medicine has a significant role to play in dealing with mental and emotional problems that affect people as they go through the journey of their life, including those secondary to trauma. In its Greek origin the word 'trauma' simply means 'wound'. More than the trauma itself, it is the way we deal with our 'woundedness' is what matters the most.

To Freud and his contemporaries, the primacy of childhood trauma was seen as the basis of future psychopathology. Volumes were written about the traumatic experiences of childhood leaving a person vulnerable to later psychopathology. Trauma experienced in later life was thought to be of lesser importance. Otto Rank (1929) argued that birth is an interruption of blissful uterine life from which people spend the rest of their lives trying to recover. He believed that birth trauma, and the fantasy of returning to the mother's womb, are far more important than any subsequent traumas and fantasies.

A major impetus to study of trauma came from the aftermath of the Vietnam war. Traumatology has since spilled over to all aspects of life and has started a new age in everyday psychology and psychiatry.

THE CULTURAL CONTEXT OF TRAUMA:

At the heart of the concept of trauma is an enduring conflict of interest between the employer and the employee (of various kinds) and has been shaped over many centuries of our contemporary ways of living. While the average worker wants a safe work environment with equitable wage, the employer wants the best output with minimum input that maximizes profit. Injury sustained in 'the line of duty' is more likely to be perceived as trauma.

In the preindustrial world, it was the peasant who did all the hard manual work and led a life of deprivation and disadvantage. They worked long hours in dismal conditions. The king and his men and later the property owners, and moneyed few controlled every aspect of their lives. Following the industrial revolution, a new class of manufacturers acquired power.

Bertrand Russell (1935) observed in his essay, *In Praise of Idleness*: "The conception of duty, speaking historically, has been a means used by the holders of power to induce others to live for the interest of their master's rather than for their own'. He noted: "In England, in the early nineteenth century, fifteen hours was the ordinary day's work for a man." 'It was only after urban working men had acquired the vote, certain public holidays were established, to the great indignation of the upper classes."

The lowly paid workers putting long hours at work were more likely to suffer from injury, see their women die in childbirth and children die in infancy and childhood. They were themselves more likely to die of cold, frost, heat stroke, accidents and injuries. Yet, having no collective voice, they were supposed to suffer in silence.

After the industrial revolution, things changed to some extent. However, the socioeconomic divide continued. The haves and have nots continued to lead different lives. The worker gained limited rights but were still much more likely to face adversity while suffering in relative silence. Larger factories allowed more workers to collaborate with each other and fight for their rights. There was always underlying tension between the landlord and the peasant, the industrialist and the worker. Profit was the main driving force for the landlord and the industrialist and safety and fulfilling the needs of life were the main concern of the peasant and labourer/worker.

There were wars too. The ruler needed an army to defend their territory. People joined the army for a living or were made to do so. Wars were traumatic, both on account of death and injury (physical and emotional). People who went through these traumatic experiences were supposed to have 'shell shock." Individual vulnerability was supposed to be a major factor in these post traumatic experiences.

There were gradual turns in social mores leading to increasing empowerment of the working class. Processes that contributed to increasing empowerment included: the democratic process, the need for the society to be more egalitarian, the socialist movement, the rise of organized labour and the power of the unions. From the fifteen-hours a day, six to seven days a week for the working class, a forty-hour week gradually became the standard in most of the developed world. Now we are striving towards a 30-hour week norm or even less. Work life balance keeps gaining increased impetus.

The prevalent opinion was that anxiety could spread by contagion, so army aggressively sought to contain it. During the civil war, the union army tattooed, or branded soldiers found guilty of cowardice. During World War I, any British soldier who developed 'neurosis' because of the war trauma was declared to be "at best a constitutionally inferior human being, at worst a malingerer and a coward." Medical writers of the time described anxious soldiers as "moral invalids." Until the second world war, the British army punished deserters with death.

That war was the first conflict in which psychiatrists played a significant role, both to screen soldiers before combat and as healers of their psychic wounds afterwards. More than a million US soldiers were admitted to hospitals for psychiatric treatment of battle fatigue. This caused lot of unrest among the army generals. Psychiatrists had to face criticism for their "hypersensitive professional attitude." High ranking officers on both sides of the Atlantic agreed that soldiers diagnosed with "war neurosis" should not be allowed to poison the gene pool with their cowardice.

THE VIETNAM WAR:

People who came back from the Vietnam war faced a hostile world. They were subject to abuse, being labelled as 'baby killer' and 'psychopath'. They were frequently being disowned by even their own families. These ex-army personnel had significant difficulties in adjusting to the life beyond the war. They often made news headlines for all the negative reasons. Most of these war affected soldiers had been conscripted. A major change in thinking was taking place after the deeply unpopular war. The ravages of the war were seen by much wider population on expanding television channels in graphic details and in colour. It had to be stopped because of the growing unease of the society.

The antiwar lobby was very vocal and lent a strong voice to highlight the curse that the war had ravaged on the young soldiers. They lobbied hard for the veterans to receive specialized care. There was a sense of collective guilt in the society for the plight of ex-servicemen who had been thrust into an unpopular war. Government still needed to recruit and maintain armies. Solution and restitution were necessary. Now suddenly and for the first-time war related trauma gained immense currency.

The concept of "Post-Vietnam Syndrome" was formulated by antiwar psychiatrists led by Chaim Shantan and Robert Jay Lifton in the late 1960s. It was thought that these symptoms did not emerge until months or years after the veteran returned home. This led to seeing the Vietnam veteran as a 'walking time bomb', 'living wreckage' or 'rampaging loner.' The introduction of DSM III in 1980 saw the emergence of a new diagnostic category.

THE DIAGNOSTIC LABEL: POST TRAUMATIC STRESS DISORDER

The newly minted diagnosis of PTSD was meant to shift the focus from the details of a soldier's background and psyche to the fundamentally traumatic nature of the war. PTSD legitimized their 'victimhood' and gave them 'moral exculpation' and guaranteed them a disability pension because the diagnosis could be attested by a doctor (Summerfield 2001). DSM III while claiming to take an atheoretical stance in diagnosis, made an exception with PTSD. It pronounced a direct link between a traumatic incident or incidences and the emergence of psychiatric disorder. Past trauma and individual vulnerability were not a deterrent to the diagnosis. Trauma 'generally outside the range of usual human experience' was seen as sufficient for the diagnosis.

The use of this disorder also moved from military to civilian trauma and post traumatic experiences. Rape, combat, torture, and fires were all included. It led to the emergence of a massive new area of study as well as controversy. The diagnosis has been seen as a legacy of the American war in Vietnam. It became one of the most studied conditions and yet remains highly controversial. The definition of the disorder and its diagnostic features have been redefined in successive revisions of DSM and ICD.

THE HISTORICAL PRECEDENTS OF PTSD

Young (1995) argued that the concept of PTSD has been 'constructed' over time. He doubted that the disorder had always existed, waiting to be discovered by psychiatrists at a time when society was ready for it. During the first world war terms like: soldier's heart, Irritable heart, Shell shock, Conversion hysteria and Neurasthenia was used. The prevailing theory was that both the soldier's predisposition to stress and his exposure to hostilities contributed to their breakdown. Young, termed PTSD as "The harmony of Illusions."

Numerous reports in the past described clinical presentations that would now be considered as PTSD. These include traumatic hysteria from railroad injury (Andrews 1891) and rape trauma syndrome (Burgess and Holmstorm 1974). During the second world war, the top five of the nineteen most common symptoms were restlessness, irritability, fatigue on arising, difficulty falling asleep, and anxiety (Grinker and Spiegel 1945). The view had changed to "even the bravest and fittest soldier could endure so much," and "every man has his breaking point." The symptom of intrusion and avoidance which are at the heart of the concept of PTSD figure quite infrequently.

Jones and colleagues (2003) studied the medical files of severely traumatized British war veterans who had received pensions for chronic psychiatric illness: Flashback almost never appeared in the medical files until the Persian Gulf War (36 of the four hundred patients of the Persian Gulf war veterans (9%) mentioned broadly defined flashbacks). Only three out of 640 patients from World War one reported phenomena even remotely suggestive of flashback and only 5 of 367 patients from World War two did so. Thus only eight of the 1007 world war I and II veterans had broadly defined flashbacks and only five of these would qualify for DSM IV criteria for PTSD and none from 428 psychiatric casualties from Victorian campaign or Boer war. Based on these observations, they concluded that PTSD may be a 'contemporary culture bound syndrome."

THE CENTRALITY OF TRAUMA:

While every psychiatric diagnosis is conceptualized as being multifactorial it is only PTSD that other factors are not considered for diagnosis. McFarlane (1990) suggested that the decline of interest in psychoanalysis as an explanatory model has decreased the emphasis on the unconscious conflicts in the causation of psychiatric disorders. This in turn has led to an increasing focus on life events, and in particular traumatic life events, as causative factors.

Studies of those exposed to a range of human-made and natural events have consistently shown that factors before the event account for more of the variance in symptoms of the disorder than do characteristics of the event. These include: (a) tending to respond to life with negative emotions (trait neuroticism) (b) believing that one is helpless in the face of events (c) using an emotion focussed coping style ('how am I feeling?) rather than a problem focussed coping style (what do I need to do?) (d) having a history of psychiatric disorder (e) whether social support is available, (f) whether religious or political commitment is present and (g) the person's level of intelligence (Bowman 1999).

A 2-year prospective follow-up study in firefighters concluded that specific personality traits characterized by high levels of hostility and a low level of self-efficacy at baseline accounted for 42% of the variance in PTSD symptoms. These may constitute markers of vulnerability to the development of PTSD. Early identification of the risk factors may lead to effective prevention and intervention (Heinrichs et al 2005).

THE SIZE OF THE PROBLEM

The 1990 National Vietnam Veterans Readjustment Study (NVVRS) remains the landmark study. Data was collected during 1986 and 1987 revealed that 15.4% of a random sample of 1000 male Vietnam veterans met criteria for PTSD at the time and 31% had suffered at some point since the war.

A group of researchers from Columbia University undertook a reanalysis of the NVVRS (Dohrenwend 2006). They culled the poorly documented cases and found that the rate was 9.1% for current PTSD and lifetime rate of 18%. Richard McNally (2007) took the definition of impairment to at least 'moderate difficulty' in social and occupational functioning to qualify as having PTSD. Then the estimate of diagnosis fell to 5.4% and lifetime prevalence to 11%. Thus, it was one in nine veterans who suffered from PTSD and not one in three as originally reported.

The Walter Reed Army Institute of Research (Thomas et al 2010) assessed over 18,000 army soldiers in infantry brigade from wars in Iraq and Afghanistan: pre deployment, 3 months after deployment and 12 months' post deployment. PTSD rates as defined by symptoms with 'serious impairment' rate was 6.3% higher than pre deployment rate after 3 months and 7.3% higher at 12 months.

THE DELIMITATION OF PTSD TO CIVILIAN LIFE:

PTSD has come to be associated with a growing list of commonplace events such as accidents, mugging, difficult labour (with healthy babies), verbal sexual harassment, or shock of receiving (inaccurate) bad news from a doctor, even when in cases in which the diagnosis has been rescinded shortly afterwards (Summerfield 2001). Increasingly, every workplace is being portrayed as traumatogenic even for those who are just doing their jobs.

The profile of this category has risen spectacularly and has become a means by which people seek victim status – and its associated moral high ground – and pursuit of recognition and compensation. It was rare to find a psychiatric diagnosis that anyone liked to have, but posttraumatic stress disorder was one (Nancy Andreasen 1995). When it comes to certain situations, there is no scope anymore for mere accidents to take place.

If there is an injury, someone other than the injured must take responsibility. It is almost presumed that an unsafe condition must have prevailed that resulted in the accident and hence injury Claim for cost of care for the injury and eventually compensation claims often follow. If the injured is reluctant to pursue that goal, there are many who will covertly or overtly encourage them to pursue it. Suggestions and recommendations can come from friends and family, co-workers, and unions. Billboards and advertisement of legal firms specializing in compensation are hard to miss. One common theme is 'the need to look after oneself.'

THE CONTEXTUAL MEANING OF A VIOLENT INCIDENT

Witnessing the torture and execution of human beings has since antiquity been 'a form of entertainment' throughout the world. The amphitheatres of Rome and similar allocated grounds in palaces and forts are testimony to that. Public hangings and lynching were commonplace. Hunting was and continues to be seen as a game, hobby, or pastime. One maims and kills animals and bring the remains as trophy. The skin and head are often displayed in homes as a mark of bravery and honour. Boxing is considered a sport, even though that may lead to blood spilled on the faces and body of the boxers and thousands witnessing it.

The difference here is essentially that of choice that one has in watching or choosing to stay away. PTSD is more likely to occur in people traumatized while involved in 'roles thrust upon them.' The increasing emphasis on individualism and freedom of choice may play a key role in how one perceives an event and how they react to it. Traumatic stress caused by another person has a greater negative impact than do natural disasters.

We may also be living in a less violent world (Pinker 2011). Birth rate has been exceeding death rates over decades. Infant and maternal mortality rates have been declining steadily. We fight infections better and can treat many life-threatening conditions thereby increasing life expectancy. The life expectancy on an average has increased by 3 years every decade. We can also save ourselves from the ravages of nature so much more effectively. As a result of these changes, the present population may be less exposed to trauma commonplace in earlier centuries. This may have made us less resilient to stress and more inclined to react adversely to trauma. An increasing sense of entitlement may also play a significant role in symptom formation and continuation.

CROSS-NATIONAL PREVALENCE:

Some data suggest that PTSD in the developing world appears to be partly a function of exposure to the Western trauma culture (Yeomans et al 2008). The result of a community survey of 245 randomly selected adults in war torn Freetown Sierra Leone in which PTSD was diagnosed in 99% makes it appear like a pseudo condition. (De Jong et al 2000). Some survivors of the Asian Tsunami in Sri Lanka reported PTSD symptoms, mistakenly believing that affirmative response to questions about PTSD were prerequisites for receiving food, clothing, and other forms of material aid (Watters 2010).

Duckers et al (2016) collected general population studies on lifetime PTSD and trauma exposure, measured using the WHO Composite International Diagnostic Interview (CIDI - DSM IV). A broad collection of data sets was brought together and combined into a vulnerability index, reflecting a variety of social and economic country features (World risk report compiled by UN University and University of Bonn). In the 2013 report, the vulnerability of 173 countries was summarised using twenty-three indicators.

The highest prevalence rate of PTSD was found in Canada, The Netherlands, and Australia, and the least in Nigeria, China, and Romania. Exposure to trauma was the highest in the Netherlands, Columbia, and the USA, and the lowest in Romania, Spain, and Italy. The most vulnerable countries were Nigeria, Iraq, and Columbia, and the least vulnerable were The Netherlands, Germany, and Belgium.

Exposure to trauma was a significant positive predictor for PTSD (accounting for approximately one third of the variance). Country vulnerability was a significant negative predictor, accounting for approximately 25% of the variance. When both variables were included simultaneously they explained 60% of the variance. Together exposure and vulnerability and their interaction explain 75% of the variance in the national prevalence of PTSD. Based on these averages' countries were divided into four groups:

1. Australia, Canada, The Netherlands, and the USA: Higher rates of exposure and lower vulnerability levels. Average lifetime PTSD of 7.34%

2. Eleven countries (including Belgium, Germany, Italy, Japan, and Spain): Average lifetime rate of 1.96%.

3. Five countries with higher exposure and vulnerability: PTSD average of 2.1%

4. Others e.g., Columbia, Israel, Lebanon, Mexico, and South Africa.

The possible explanations include: (a) Less vulnerable countries may be inhabited by more individualistic cultures with a more equal power balance, less uncertainty, a more long-term orientation, higher indulgence, and less restraint and (b) PTSD prevalence may be higher in low vulnerability countries as the relative impact of a traumatic event on long term goals is greater because there is greater expectation of achieving such goals.

THE CHANGING DEFINTION OF PTSD

The term Trauma has undergone a conceptual bracket creep whereby the range of qualifying events continues to expand.

DSM III conceptualized PTSD as arising from a limited set of traumatic stressors such as rape, combat, torture, and natural disaster. According to DSM IV one may not even be present at the scene of the trauma to qualify as a trauma survivor. Someone who feels helpless when learning about threat to other people qualifies as a trauma survivor as much as the recipient of the trauma threat.

Four percent of Americans living far from the terrorist attack of September 11, 2001, apparently developed PTSD by viewing scenes of violence on TV (Schlenger et al 2002). A series of studies suggested that stressors failing short of the current definition of trauma can produce more PTSD symptoms or higher rates of disorder than stressors that do meet the current definition of trauma.

In July 2010, Veterans Affair (VA) in USA announced that: 'The VA would no longer require a veteran to provide documentation of his exposure to combat trauma.' It also established that 'one can sustain an enduring and disabling mental disorder based on anxious anticipation of a traumatic event that never materialized.' Calls are now being made by Paramedics and Police association to introduce legislation that would create a presumption that PTSD diagnosed in frontline workers was caused by their jobs. That would reverse the onus on emergency service workers to prove to the insurer that their jobs made them sick.

DSM 5 removed the previous requirement for a fear-based response to the traumatic event. Very frequently people said they did not have any emotional response. "I was just doing my job." It was the training that kicked in at that time and it ruled out a lot of people. It tightened the scope of qualifying events to reduce bracket creep. For example, losing a child to aggressive cancer was not classifiable. Of the seventeen original DSM IV symptoms, eight underwent significant edits and three symptoms added.

Symptoms were restructured into four clusters based on factor analyses, including new, separate requirements for active avoidance and negative cognition/mood. PTSD moved out of anxiety disorders and into a "Trauma and Stressor Related disorders" chapter of DSM 5. Adjustment disorder has been recommended for subthreshold PTSD.

PTSD is defined in DSM-5 as the presence of at least 6 of 20 symptoms across reexperiencing, avoidance, alternations in mood and cognition, and hyperarousal categories. This definition results in 636 120 potential clinical presentations of PTSD (Galatzer-Levy and Bryant 2013). In a study involving 10,965 participants there were 3511 with a PTSD diagnosis, out of which there were 2181 different pattern of symptoms (Bryant et al 2022).

ICD 11 has the simplest system (6 symptoms and three clusters) for the diagnosis of PTSD. Both DSM 5 and ICD 11 have been parallel processes involving some of the same members). Research is likely to be hampered by such large heterogeneity of the disorder.

The Trauma Trail: A QUADRANGLE

The trauma trial can be seen as quadrangular in its dimension. The four angles are:

1. The trauma victim
2. The Medical Profession: (Treating professional and IMEs)
3. The Purse Holder: (DVA, Workcover, Insurer)
4. The defenders of the rights of the victim (Interest groups, Legal system. Politicians, and the media)

Each of these are significant stakeholders walking alongside each other on the trauma trial. Each has their own dilemmas and conflict between them is rife. Battle lines can be drawn due to differing interests that tie them to a certain viewpoint. Besides the Veterans of war, workers injured in their line of duty, those affected by disability claims are all affected by similar issues and travel along the same trauma trail.

THE TRAUMA VICTIM:

The frequency of exposure to trauma varies with the kind of work one performs. Working in the armed forces of course is associated with greater exposure to death and related issues. Working for the police forces, fire brigade, ambulance services and emergency departments are substantial risk areas.

The trauma victim has an onerous task at hand. On the one hand lies their symptoms and distress and on the other is the task of navigating through the process of seeking help by negotiating complex pathways. There is often suspicion about the extent of suffering and they are often subject to surveillance by certain agencies.

Daniel Kahneman and Amos Tversky (2000) described the peak-end effect that we may be more prone to creating strong memories for the more rewarding aspects of a past scene and obscure the rest. Memories tend to be imperfect. Predictably, the pessimists are less likely to resort to this sort of affectively positive reshaping of remembrances. Moreover, the very concept of trauma precludes any chance of it being a positive experience.

There is more social utility attached to expressions of victim-hood than to survivor-hood. Compensation contingent upon being sick often creates the perverse incentive to remaining sick. There may be a lingering fear of losing financial safety net if someone on disability benefits tries to go to work that ends up proving to be too much. Once it becomes advantageous to frame distress as a psychiatric condition people will choose to present themselves as medicalized victims rather than as feisty survivors (Summerfield 2001).

THE MEDICAL PROFESSION:

The medical profession plays an especially important part in the trauma trail. The claim must be first substantiated by a medical professional and later by an independent medical examiner. The treating psychiatrist is required to always take the health interests and needs of the patient to be paramount in responding to a request for a medicolegal report. An independent medical examination and report is requested by a third party and provided by a psychiatrist not involved in any past or present therapeutic or other interpersonal relationship with the examinee.

A medicolegal report is a written opinion by an expert on a medical matter arising out of legal proceedings before a Court, Tribunal or another decision maker. Although the psychiatrist may be retained by either party to a dispute in a civil matter or the prosecution or defence in a criminal matter, the principle of honesty and objectivity is paramount. There are often significant differences in the opinions expressed by treating psychiatrists and the IMEs which may arise from:

(A) The definitional problem

In DSM IV PTSD is defined as the presence of three symptom clusters that arises in response to life threatening event: re-experiencing (nightmares and flashbacks), avoidance (numbing or withdrawal) and, hyperarousal (irritability, insomnia, aggression, poor concentration). The construction of this definition is suspect. Research shows that memory is spectacularly unreliable and malleable. We routinely add or subtract people, details, settings, and actions to and from memories. We conflate, invent, and edit (David Dobbs 2009).

A 1990s study asked 59 Gulf War veterans about their experiences (19 specific events including witnessing death, losing friends, and seeing people disfigured) one month after return and 2 years later. Seventy percent of them reported at least one event they had not reported initially and 24% reported at least three such events for the first time. Veterans recounting the 'newest' memories also reported the most PTSD symptoms.

J A Bodkin (2007) in an elegant study showed that the PTSD rate had zero relation to the trauma rate. Ninety clinically depressed patients were screened separately for PTSD symptoms and trauma. Although the symptom screens rated seventy of the ninety patients positive for PTSD, the trauma screens found only fifty-four who had suffered from trauma. The PTSD symptoms were equally distributed among the trauma positive and trauma negative groups.

A possible explanation may come from the observations of Schank and Abelson (1995) on the nature of memory. As mentioned earlier, stories change over time because of the process of telling and embellishments added by the teller. The actual events giving rise to the story in the first place have long been forgotten. **McNally** believes "this has nothing to do with gaming or working the system or consciously looking for sympathy. We do all this: we cast our lives in terms of narratives that helps us understand them." With memory unreliable and biological markers elusive, diagnosis depends on clinical symptoms (re-experiencing and avoidance) and eliciting signs (some of the symptoms of hyperarousal).

As Allan Frances (2013) pointed out: "A diagnosis of PTSD may be hard to get right. Paradoxically it is one of the most underdiagnosed and one of the most over-diagnosed conditions" (underdiagnosed when people suffer its symptoms stoically and in silence and over-diagnosed when a trigger for financial gain). The human reaction to trauma is a great equalizer. Without concerns about compensation, for most people the intrusive images gradually become less intrusive, and the triggers become less terrifying.

(B) Distinguishing Trauma Associated Narcissistic Symptoms from PTSD

Robert Simon (2002) introduced the term Trauma Associated Narcissistic Symptoms (TANS) to display a discrete cluster of psychological symptoms arising from narcissistic vulnerability closely mimicking those of PTSD.

TANS usually follows a traumatic stressor (which may be relatively insignificant) overwhelming the grandiose self thereby producing shame, humiliation and rage that drive re-experiencing avoidance and arousal symptoms. Severe traumatic stressors are especially narcissistically wounding e.g., exploitation, harassment, abuse, rape and torture can cause both PTSD and TANS.

In individuals who develop TANS, the traumatic stressor usually contains a strong interpersonal element. The trauma is 'up, close and personal.' The severity of the stressor often is inversely related to the degree of narcissistic pathology exhibited. The individual continually ruminates, licking the wounds of humiliation and plotting revenge. Dreams with scenes of humiliation related to the current and/or earlier narcissistic injuries may emerge.

In a US study, 12% of currently serving personnel and 20% of veterans met criteria of problematic anger (Adler et al 2020). They found problematic anger was most prevalent among service members separating from the service for disciplinary and medical disability reasons including problematic relationships with spouses, partners and children. Anger was associated with a greater likelihood of behavioural and functional health outcomes (e.g., PTSD), relationship health difficulties (e.g., low social support) and economic difficulties (e.g., substantial financial insecurity). In a large Australian study 16% of actively serving personnel and 31% of recent military veterans met criteria for problematic anger (Varker et al 2022).

(C) The challenges faced by the treating psychiatrist.

Psychiatrists involved in treating trauma victims face several challenges. In the usual specialist/client or patient interaction it is a dyad with a person seeking and another providing help. In the context of trauma related consultation, compensation and related issue is always the elephant in the room which alters the dynamics of the interaction.

The vital role of trauma for the diagnosis can become a tricky issue, as the client may be reluctant to address other issues that may also be relevant to the causation and perpetuation of their condition. In an age where there is a significant sense of entitlement getting better may deprive the financial gains that are associated with maintaining disability. This may not be a conscious process with the aim to defraud. The significance of a 'sick role' is well known in medical sociology (Talcott Parsons 1951).

The psychiatrist may be in a dilemma as to the limit to which the defences used by the trauma victim can be challenged without risking further traumatization. It is common to find the trauma victim to need less care once their claims are settled. Were they in need of extra care to help with secondary traumatization emanating from the complex claim process. It may also be possible that, after the lengthy settlement, they realise not much more can be gained by continuing to see the medical professional.

(D) The challenges faced by an Independent Medical Examiners

The independent medical examiner (IME) may be more likely to focus on the vulnerability of the trauma victim, while the treating Doctor may more exclusively focus on trauma as a possible cause of the PTSD.

The IME may similarly put a greater emphasis on the trauma-associated narcissistic symptoms (TANS) where the person exhibits symptoms of both

PTSD and TANS. The brevity of the interview and a perceived conflict of interest by the examined may make it more likely to become apparent. On the other hand, the treating Doctor and patient, having a long-term involvement, may more easily identify and understand those symptoms.

Hoge et al (2014) in a well-controlled head-to-head study showed that 30% of combat soldiers who met DSM IV symptom criteria for PTSD failed to meet DSM 5 criteria. Discordance among those who met either criterion was nearly 50%. ICD II definition offered no clinical advantage and even greater discordance (Hoge et al 2015). One multinational study (Stein et al 2014) scored diagnostic interviews according to DSM IV, DSM 5, ICD 10, and ICD 11 criteria. Concordance across all four definitions was so low that they even suggested using all four definitions for future epidemiological studies.

THE PURSE HOLDER

Insurance companies are mostly independent businesses run for a profit having many shareholders to whom they have primary allegiance subject to the law.

They try to limit costs through various methods. The more claims they settle, the less profit they make. There is an inbuilt inclination then for an insurance company to issue many policies and then minimise the claims made against them, the claimant is usually a novice and commonly unwell and stressed. These large financial institutions have dedicated legal arms and individual trauma victims may be unable to match the financial strength of the institutions. Justice has a price tag.

They may also selectively seek medical opinions from consultants known to have views less favourable towards trauma claims. An insurer dealing with multiple claims every day, always has the upper hand against the novice. An individual trauma victim can hardly ever match the financial strength of the institutions. Justice has a price tag.

In the book, NOISE, Daniel Kahneman and colleagues (2021) discuss a study about the discrepancies seen in insurance companies' assessments. They employ numerous 'Underwriters' who quote premiums for financial risks such as insuring a bank against losses. They also employ "Claims Adjusters" who forecast the cost of future claims and negotiate with the claimants when disputes arise. There is a Goldilocks value from the perspective of the company. The 'noise audit' found the median difference for underwriters was 55% and for claims adjustors, 43%. These were just medians: in half the pairs of cases, the difference between the two judgements was even larger. An adjuster is assigned to the claim – just as the underwriter was assigned, because he or she happens to be available. They use the word 'lottery' to emphasise the role of chance in selection of one underwriter or adjuster and a lottery creates noise.

Similar 'noise' is likely to occur in several aspects relating to workover claims, particularly in relation to PTSD.

THE DEFENDERS OF THE RIGHTS OF THE VICTIM:

Veterans Service Organizations actively help veterans to file for disability. These organizations are driven to funnel largesse to their constituents. They are also extremely suspicious of any proposed reforms of the disability system. Attempted changes are met with accusations of dishonouring veterans, dismissing suffering and discounting the cost of war. In civilian life various unions play a similar role. Thus, the pressure groups and organizations are often working at cross purposes and make any shift in paradigm hard to achieve.

The legal system is also an important part in the trauma trail. Advertisements are openly displayed in social media of legal firms advertising for people dealing with trauma claims to contact them. Some firms also work on a 'no win no fee' terms. Once the legal process is initiated, it creates further difficulties in the recovery process. Governments should play a role protecting workers from exploitation. Entrusted to help their constituents in need, they legislate to defend the rights of people but also regulate various agencies including Work cover, Work safe, veteran's affair and insurance companies.

IMPLICATIONS FOR TREATMENT AND OUTCOME

PTSD is now the fourth most diagnosed psychiatric disorder. The expanded definition has allowed many more to receive subsidised care. A soldier who commits war crimes can share the diagnosis with his own victim as can the journalist who witnessed and/or reported on the atrocity, the descendants of the victims, the historian studying the event years later. All can be victims of 'vicarious trauma.' Novelist Will Self suggests that the biggest beneficiaries of the trauma model are trauma theorists themselves, who are granted a kind of tenure, entrusted with a lifetime's work of 'witnessing' and interpreting. As Bonanno put it: "People don't seem to let go of the idea that everybody's traumatized."

On the one hand, suffering from vicarious trauma is now increasingly recognised while, at the same time, news, novels, television series, social media platforms and movies portray violence in graphic detail. The popularity of movies showing explicit violence belies the sensitivity to trauma in contemporary life. Modern technologies 'supersize' the experiential impact of violence. One main difference is that between choosing to witness violence compared to being forced to experience it, real or imagined.

Surprisingly, PTSD has not been of much interest to drug companies. They shy away from advertising for it because none of the medications are very effective, and they fear bad publicity. Are they uniformly ineffective, because the condition is so complex it is difficult to cage into a purely biological model?

Glass (1954) summarised four 'state of the art' basic principles of military psychiatric treatment near the battle front: treatment should combine simplicity and brevity; psychiatric staff should create a therapeutic atmosphere reflecting positive motivation; and the psychiatrist should identify with the needs of the combat group rather than just the individual. With so few psychiatrists available near the battle front, this goal appears to be a near impossibility. Putting the needs of the group before the individual is a reminder of the sufferers being labelled as cowards, thus undermining the morale of the army.

Reviewing 175 years of progress in PTSD therapeutics, Stein and Rothbaum (2018) found the basic tenets of treatment have remained largely unchanged. A 2008 Institute of Medicine report established that trauma-focussed treatment had more evidence for efficacy in the treatment of PTSD than any other intervention, including two FDA-approved medications (sertraline and paroxetine). However, a review of current guidelines for treatment of both military and non-military PTSD revealed that few treatments are endorsed with great certainty, due mostly to a paucity of clinical trials, particularly of pharmacotherapy.

Since 1974 New Zealand has had a comprehensive no fault accident compensation scheme for those who suffer personal injury. All personal injury victims whether injured on the road, at home, in a hospital, at play, or at work are covered by the one Act. Therefore, a person injured in a motor vehicle accident or at work is compensated in the same way as those injured at home. This has been of limited benefit. Recently there has been an upsurge in damage claims due to: (1) Mental trauma being excluded in the Act from the definition of personal injury meaning that damages for mental trauma can now only be claimed in Court. (2) Exemplary damages claims are now allowed in cases of negligent as well as intentional conduct. (3) The abolition of lump sum compensation by the Act.

FIVE STEPS TO MOVING FORWARD

To say that PTSD maybe more of a social construct, does not in any way diminish the importance of the condition. Human beings are social animals. The idioms, and phrases we use to describe distress are influenced by our contemporary life. As professionals, we must continue to strive towards a greater understanding of the conditions leading to distress including those involving Workcover and Insurance claims. Reducing the antagonism between various aspects of the trauma trail is essential to making a move forward. This can be achieved through several important steps:

(A) NEW WAYS OF DEFINING THE ISSUE

Any news report of natural or humanmade disasters are now always accompanied by discussion about the need for counselling and therapy for the survivors (Bracken 2001). A large industry has grown around PTSD. Bracken believes that postmodernity has caused an undermining of social stability and coherence and a systematic weakening of those cultural institutions which provide meaning and order for individuals. He suggested that the condition that the diagnosis PTSD attempts to capture is in fact something particularly associated with life in contemporary postmodern societies.

Eastmond (1998) compared two groups of Bosnian refugees in Sweden. These refugee families were from the same town and had been detained in the same concentration camp in Bosnia. The group who settled in a location where they were offered temporary jobs fared best. In the other group when offered psychological intervention but no work, most of the adults were on indefinite sick leave one year after arrival.

Sally Satel (PTSD's diagnostic trap 2011) identified two overarching problems requiring remedies: (1) The culture of clinical diagnosis. Some disability evaluators use a detailed interview checklist to gauge the degree to which daily function is impaired, but its implementation is uneven. The distinction between reversible and lasting incapacitation is complex. (2) The inadvertent damage that disability benefits themselves can cause like the award of compensation does confirm that they are indeed beyond recovery, Risk of a 'sick role' depriving them of the estimable value of work (the daily structure, the distraction from depressive ruminations, opportunity for socializing and cultivating friendships). People who take those jobs and have an inherent increased risk for trauma are likely to be at greater risk. Training should include preparation to deal with the aftermath of trauma. They may also need to be equipped to proactively identify and deal with problematic anger.

(B) A BALANCED APPROACH BY PSYCHIATRISTS

Sometimes reading the report from an IME and often the scathing remarks about the claimant and the treating professional makes it appear like a turf war. And yet both the treating and independent examiners are members of the same craft group with similar abilities and competence.

A recent study (De Jong et al 2016) reported an association between doctors enjoying meals costing more than $20 had higher relative prescribing rates of certain medications including antidepressants supplied by their hosting pharmacy company. A position statement for engagement with the pharmaceutical industry has been published by the College of Psychiatrists to minimise the influence of any industry on the conduct of its members (RANZCP June 2016).

The role of specialized units being able to provide superior outcomes is open to debate. It is sobering indeed to note Christopher Fruech who researched and treated PTSD for VA from the early 1990s to 2006 found that Veterans getting PTSD treatment from the VA are no more likely to get better than they would on their own. The reason was the collision of the vagaries of PTSD with the VAs disability system, in which every benefit seems to be structured to discourage recovery.

(C) RECOGNITION OF CONFLICT AS BEING INHERENT TO THE TRAIL:

Workers' compensation has a fraught history. It is socially responsible to provide for a universal system of insurance covering work related injury to recognise the value of workers and the risks of work. It is also economically responsible both to support a return to work and to ensure that premiums neither stifle business nor bankrupt the state.

An investigation by the Ombudsman in the state of Victoria, Australia (Deborah Glass 2016), found Workcover agents cherry-picking evidence to support a decision to reject or terminate a claim – as little as one line in a medical report – while disregarding overwhelming evidence to the contrary. They found Independent Medical Examiners (IMEs) – whose opinions agents use to support their decision-making on compensation – receiving selective, incomplete, or inaccurate information. They also saw evidence that some IMEs were used selectively to advantage the insurers – including those described by agent staff as 'good for terminations.'

She found examples of agents maintaining unreasonable decisions at conciliation, in some cases despite acknowledging that the decision was unreasonable and would be overturned. In effect, the investigation found cases in which agents were working the system to delay and deny seriously injured workers the financial compensation to which they were entitled – and which they would eventually receive if only they had the support, stamina and means to pursue their cases through the dispute process.

The impact of this on vulnerable people cannot be overstated. The cessation of payments – for up to two years before a case is concluded – will inevitably lead to financial hardship and as the cases illustrate, can equally lead to depression and despair. In such cases the system itself compounds the injury – not only to the detriment of the worker, but ultimately to all of us who bear the social and financial cost. They proposed that the system needs a better safety net for the vulnerable.

(D) 'TREATMENT FIRST' MUST BE PROMOTED

Returning from war is a major existential project and so is the case for those trying to come to terms with major traumatic experiences and adjusting to life after that.

In 2008 Senator Richard Burr introduced the Veterans Mental Health First Act. It stipulated that the veteran be eligible for a "wellness stipend" to adhere to an individualized treatment and agree to a pause in claim action for at least a year or until completion of treatment, whichever came first. The bill died in committee.

Standing in the way of reform is conventional wisdom, deep cultural resistance, and the foundational concepts of trauma psychology. "Saving PTSD from itself" will require a shift so that most trauma related stress is assessed not as a disorder but as part of a normal, if painful, healing. The task needs to be seen as re -contextualization by integrating trauma into normal experience. as we do when face to face with other traumas such as death of loved ones, breakup, and loss of jobs.

(E) HANDLING THE PROCESS

Agencies such as Work safe need to be strengthened and empowered to ensure safe working environments. We know that, despite all precautions, accidents will still occur but that does not mean someone must be held responsible or punished.

Any claim for trauma associated conditions vetted by a doctor could receive a provisional acceptance. The claimant may then be appropriately assessed by a medical panel with experienced consultants deciding the legitimacy of the claim. Provisions can be made for assessments to be done in a timely fashion, say within 2 to 6 weeks. The panel may also be able to ascertain the kind of treatment steps warranted as well as an appropriate time for review.

Medical Panels are used where there is a disagreement or uncertainty about aspects of an injury or medical condition. They are convened to answer referred questions and to provide a more conclusive opinion on the medical issue/s in dispute. They can serve the valuable purpose of accelerating, fair, and cost-effective resolution of medical disputes in relation to workers' compensation claims. They must also provide detailed reasoning for the decision reached.

In most university exams, an examinee is assessed by at least two examiners and the result vetted by an examination committee. Why should a single independent medical examination be entrusted to make a judgment likely to have major implications for the injured person? Such an approach could also relieve individual examiners from arbitrating a claim process so complicated as to provoke profound, unhelpful negativity from the patient.

In case of further dispute, a Review Tribunal may be constituted as a specialist quasi-judicial body constituted like the one reviewing involuntary treatment for mental illnesses. Each Tribunal panel may consist of three or more members: a lawyer who chairs the hearing, one or more specialists (depending on the complexity of presentation), and another suitably qualified member. The role of a representative of the community, with a lived experience of trauma may be of help. it is essential that the Tribunal receives the absolute best evidence available when hearing applications and making its decisions. The Tribunal's decisions can involve the consideration of quite complex issues and can impact directly on people's health and lives.

These steps could reduce the antagonism among the different people along the trauma trail. The need for lengthy, expensive, and traumatizing legal battles could be avoided. The insurance premium would be lower and some of the savings can be used to pay for provision of safe work environment.

The balance can be restored between 'victimhood' to age old values of 'Survivor hood.' Stoicism can be once again come to be regarded as a virtue. The much-celebrated writer H. G. Wells pointed out: "We all have our time machines, don't we. Those that take us back are memories… And those that carry us forward, are dreams." Jonas Salk (the inventor of the first vaccine for Polio) famously said: "I have had dreams, and I have had nightmares. I overcame the nightmares because of my dreams."

COVID-19 PANDEMIC RELATED PTSD?

The Covid-19 related stress may emerge as another major challenge over the coming months and years. Health care workers (doctors, nurses, ambulance workers) have had to deal with the lack of resources, the high frequency of death of patients, witnessing patients die in isolation, being stretched to provide care, and having to isolate themselves to protect their own families are some of the stressors that they had to go through day in day out.

Many others in the community may have been affected through death of family, inability to meet family and friends in nursing homes and hospitals, inability to participate in funerals, social isolation, economic fallout due to

Covid-19 are some of the negative experiences. Many were affected by the conflict regarding the safety of rapidly developed vaccines and the need to get vaccinated or risk losing their job.

DSM 5 criteria excludes naturally occurring illnesses, such as a virus as a qualifying trauma for the diagnosis of PTSD. This does not however rule out claims for PTSD directly from the virus but due to the events surrounding the pandemic.

THE STORY OF ATTENTION DEFICIT DISORDERS

Attention plays a vital role in our life. Evolutionarily, good attention allowed animals as well as humans the ability to orient and respond quickly to any threat to survival. Effort is required to maintain in memory several ideas that require separate actions or that may need to be combined according to some rule.

The scientific study of attention is carried out in the fields of psychology, psychiatry, neuroscience and, more recently, machine learning. They all recognise its core quality to be "the flexible control of limited computational resources." It can be enhanced and impaired by a variety of factors.

A disorder characterised by hyperactivity, inattention and impulsivity was recognised in children as early as in 1902. Various terms were used to describe it before being labelled as Hyperkinetic disorder. An overlap between such a condition and learning difficulties, emotional difficulties, and conduct problems was well documented.

DSM-III (1980) transformed the concept of hyperkinetic disorder to attention deficit disorder. The primacy accorded to attentional difficulties as being of critical importance as opposed to hyperactivity opened new avenues that were so far unavailable. Now one could have attention deficit disorder with hyperactivity (like hyperkinetic disorder) but could have no hyperactivity and still be diagnosed with attention deficit disorder without overactivity. It was a significant change in basic assumptions.

Interest in this disorder has expanded exponentially in recent decades. It remains a highly controversial diagnostic category. At first there was wide discrepancy across borders (UK vs USA) and within different states of a country (such as Western Australia compared to rest of Australia). Attention Deficit Disorder has fast become an explain-all for all sorts of performance problem at all ages. There is no reason to think the kids have changed, but much more likely that the labels and diagnostic practices have. Strangely, in US boys born in January have at a seventy percent greater risk than those born in December.

In DSM IV, a few words were changed so that the definition would be more female friendly – considering that girls were more likely to be inattentive, "space cadets" and less likely to be hyperactive. Field testing predicted a 15% increase in rates, but clever drug marketing caused rates to triple. Several newly patented and expensive ADHD medications were marketed around the same time.

THE REMARKABLE INCREASE IN PREVALENCE

In the 1980s, around one in every twenty children in the United States were diagnosed with ADHD, but today that number is one in nine. Between 2003 and 2011 in US the diagnosis of ADHD soared by 43% overall and by 55% among girls. A 123% increase in the number of adults with ADHD between 2007 and 2016. By now it has reached a point wherein 13 percent of adolescents in the US have been given the diagnosis. In many parts of the South in the US, 30 percent of the boys are now diagnosed with ADHD by the time they turn eighteen. The increase has been extraordinary almost everywhere.

Using data from 2016-2019 a national survey of parents estimated that the number of children aged 3–17 years ever diagnosed with ADHD is six million (9.8%). This number includes: 3–5 years: 265,000 (2%), 6–11 years 2.4 million (10%), 12–17 years: 3.3 million (13%). Boys (13%) are more likely to be diagnosed with ADHD than girls (6%). According to a national 2016 parent survey, 6 in 10 children with ADHD had at least one other mental, emotional, or behavioural disorder: About half of the children with ADHD had a behaviour or conduct problem. About 3 in 10 children with ADHD had anxiety.

ONSET AFTER THE AGE OF EIGHTEEN

Initially, it was believed that ADHD began as well as ended in childhood. In the 1990s several prospective studies showed that around 15 to 20% of children continued to show the full syndrome into adulthood, and in a further 50% some of the symptoms persisted into adulthood (Faraone et al 2006). A series of studies have now found out that the syndrome could have its onset in adolescence, or even adulthood (Moffitt et al 2015, Agnew-Blais et al 2016). These have been termed as late-onset ADHD.

Many adults are now being told and now even more frequently have found for themselves that they have attention deficit disorder. Millions have been prescribed stimulants. The market for prescribing stimulants is now worth over $10 billion. It is human nature to point fingers at something else for our own flaws and shortcomings and to avoid any personal culpability. Many point that someone else has been diagnosed with ADD or ADHD to justify that they may have it too due to shared DNA. This could be another red herring. We must remember that DNA tells us about our risks and not destiny. "DNA is simply a list of parts or ingredients rather than a complete manual that explains how those parts work together to generate results" (Agus 2011).

Many are being misdiagnosed whose problem in concentrating is really caused by some other disorder. Any late onset of attentional problems is more likely to be caused by some other condition rather than ADHD. Adult ADD was already too easily diagnosed but DSM 5 by lowering the requirement made it more likely to capture 'many adults who want to be sharper but don't have specific or serious enough problem to qualify for a mental disorder.'

Frances (2013) pleaded to keep DSM as a manual of mental disorders and not a vehicle for performance enhancement.

Sibley et al (2018) studied a group of children initially without ADHD who had served as a comparison group in a well-known Multimodal Study of ADHD. They had repeated, detailed clinical assessment into adulthood. Forty percent of these participants during adolescence and 20% during adulthood screened positive for ADHD on a symptom checklist. The numbers plummeted to 3.3% once three sensible constraints were applied such as (i) Impairment across multiple contexts, (ii) Not better explained by substance misuse or another mental disorder, and (iii) mapping the exact chronology of symptoms. The prevalence fell further to 2% if those with childhood symptoms that fell near the diagnostic threshold were excluded, suggesting that their ADHD was as much late-recognised as late-onset. The study demonstrates the poor predictive power of diagnosis by checklist.

They concluded: "Individuals seeking treatment for late-onset ADHD may be valid cases, however, more commonly symptoms represent non impairing cognitive fluctuations, a comorbid disorder, or the cognitive effect of substance abuse. False positive late-onset cases are common…." They further added that "Without clear exclusionary guidelines for ADHD in adolescents and adults, there is a risk that ADHD may become a catchall diagnosis for executive dysfunction stemming from any source."

Many cases of late-onset ADHD may be illusory and stem from a lack of consideration of impairment, symptom chronology, and mental health history. Philip Shaw (2018) in an editorial piece "Growing Up: Evolving Concepts of Adult Attention Deficit Disorder" pointed to two points arising from the study by Sibley et al (2018) worth a thought. First, there appears to be a nontrivial incidence of late-onset, impairing ADHD that is not better explained by another mental disorder or substance misuse. The minimum current estimate may be 2 to 3%. Secondly, the study had an under sampling of females.

It is possible that quiet, nondisruptive but inattentive girls are being overlooked in childhood, particularly when they have a higher-than-average IQ and can perform well at school. When these women become primary informant after the age of eighteen, they declare their history of attention, which may have become more impairing in less structured adult settings.

In a meta-analysis of six studies published between 1996-2005, Simon et al (2009) estimated that the pooled prevalence of adult ADHD was 2.5%. Wilcutt (2012) based on pooled data from eleven studies published between 1996-2011 estimated the prevalence of ADHD to be 5.0%. Song et al (2021) based on studies published from January 2000 onwards reported the prevalence of persistent adult ADHD (with a childhood onset) and symptomatic adult ADHD (regardless of a childhood onset) both decreased with advancing age. By adjusting for the global demographic structure in 2020, the prevalence of persistent adult ADHD was 2.58% and that of symptomatic adult ADHD was 6.76%, translating to 139.84 million and 366.33 million affected adults in 2020 globally. The heterogeneity of the studies is an obvious problem, but a rising trend from 1996 to 2020 is quite unmistakable.

POINTS OF CONTENTION:

Problems with attention and concentration is a significant part of many mental disorders and is also one of their core symptoms: (a) Impaired attention is a fundamental cognitive deficit in patients with schizophrenia, (b) Diminished ability to think or concentrate, or indecisiveness, every day is one of the core symptoms of Major Depression, (c) Impaired concentration or feeling as though the mind goes blank is one of the major diagnostic criteria of generalized anxiety disorder, (d) In PTSD, trauma-related arousal and reactivity that began or worsened after the trauma includes hypervigilance, heightened startle reaction, difficulty concentrating.

All the above conditions need to be ruled out before an adult is diagnosed with attention deficit disorder if they were never diagnosed when they should have been picked up. The erstwhile concept of hyperkinetic disorder considered it to be a disorder of three Rs: reading, writing, and arithmetic.

Harrison et al (2007) found the increasing use of stimulants as performance enhancers among students. This also led to recreation of a large and illegal market for stimulants. Stimulants may be able to improve performance in the same way as many others such as caffeine or energy drinks, other drugs as also transcranial direct current stimulation. If that is the desired goal that people must follow it does not mean that it should change diagnostic processes or be legitimized by medical professionals.

REASONS FOR SCEPTICISM:

Diagnostic overreach emphasising one diagnosis over the other has repeatedly caused problems in the past. Slavney (1991) pointed out to the concept of a disjunctive category such as citizenship (a person can be a citizen of a country if he is born there or if he lives there for several years or if he marries a native).

Schizophrenia as defined by Eugene Bleuler was a disjunctive category defined by the 4 As (Alogia/Loosening of Association, Autism, Ambivalence, and Affect blunting). These were considered as pathognomonic of schizophrenia. Gradually it was assumed that the subtle presentations of the disorder were much more common than the obvious ones. This led to both a lowering of the diagnostic threshold and proposals for a variety of atypical presentations. Every presentation with a trace of psychosis was seen to represent schizophrenia. This trend in the 1950s and 60s were fuelled by the advent of potent antipsychotic medications and greater optimism about the treatability of schizophrenia.

The US-UK diagnostic project showed that American Psychiatrists diagnosed schizophrenia more often, and affective disorder less often, compared to their British counterparts. Bleulerian criteria was later replaced by the Schneiderian ones. Structured interview systems like PSE (Present State Examination) were developed and later diagnostic systems were developed that described schizophrenia as a chronic condition as defined by Kraepelin.

The above changes along with the widespread use of Lithium brought in the new imperium of affective disorder. It was proposed that all the phenomena of schizophrenia may also appear in affective (particularly bipolar) disorders. The emphasis changed to finding the more subtle forms of bipolar disorders. The category of bipolar disorder became progressively larger and the diagnostic threshold progressively lower. At first it was necessary to rule out schizophrenia to diagnose bipolar disorder, later, it was essential to rule out bipolar disorder to reach a diagnosis of schizophrenia.

To say that ADHD is the cause for all problems with attention is like saying fever is the commonest disorder or headache is the commonest 'disorder' for which people consult a doctor all over the world (as is the case of the omnibus label of depression). Like fever and headache which are symptoms that underlie many disorders and attentional problems are only sometimes a standalone disorder.

As discussed earlier, Leon Eisenberg, one of the first psychiatrists to study the effects of stimulants on attention deficit disorder in children, in his later years became an outspoken critic of what he saw as the indiscriminate use of psychoactive drugs.

Kandel (1998) put forth a new intellectual framework for psychiatry. He acknowledged that genes do contribute importantly to mental function and can contribute to mental illness. However, behaviour itself can also modify gene expression. Both Psychotherapy and pharmacotherapy may induce similar alterations in gene expression and structural changes in the brain.

Hari (2022) in his very well-articulated book *Stolen Focus* outlined six ways in which social-media sites currently operates and is harming our attention.

1. These sites and apps are designed to train our minds to crave frequent rewards. They make us hungry for hearts and likes.
2. They push us to switch tasks more frequently than one normally would.
3. They learn how to 'frack' you. They learn what you like to look at, what excites you, what angers you, what engages you. Social media knows exactly where to drill.
4. They make you angry a lot of the time and anger makes you think in a shallower and less attentive way.
5. They also make you feel that you are surrounded by other people's anger.
6. These sites set society on fire.

Sune (1986) noted that if one added up all the information blasted at the average human being – TV, radio, reading – it amounted to forty newspapers worth of information every day. By 2007, it had risen to the equivalent of 174 newspapers per day. The increase in the volume of information is what creates the sensation of the world speeding up. We are experiencing a more rapid exhaustion of attention resources (Quoted by Hari 2022).

Hari points to the collapse in reading books is in some ways a symptom of our atrophying attention and a cause of it. Anne said to him that she was worried that we are now loosing 'our ability to read long texts anymore' and we are also losing our 'cognitive patience…. (and) the stamina and the ability to deal with cognitively challenging texts'.

The guiding principle behind Twitter or most social media platforms is simple. (1) That you should not focus on one thing for long. The world can and should be understood in short simple statements of 280 characters. (2) The world should be interpreted and confidently understood very quickly. (3) What matters most is whether people immediately agree with and applaud your short, simple, speedy statements.

At Google, success was measured in the main by what is termed as 'engagement' which is defined as minutes and hours of eyeballs on the product. While designing products the emphasis is on engaging the maximum number of people as engagement equals more dollars through the ability to introduce more advertisements.

False claims spread on social media far faster than the truth because the algorithms that spread outraging material travel faster and further. A MIT study found that fake news travels six times faster on twitter than real news. As a result, we are being pushed all the time to pay attention to nonsense – things that just are not so.

This is destroying our sense-making, at a time when we need it the most. We live in a culture that gets us to walk faster, talk faster, work longer, and we are taught to think that is where productivity and success come from. Many of us have built our identities around working to the point of exhaustion. We call this success. Before the advent and widespread availability of smartphone it was not only hard but also unusual for bosses to contact their worker once they left office. In effect, the idea of work hours has disappeared and most of us are on call all the time.

Attention takes different forms, and they are layered. All these layers are now being stolen. Hari suggested that the first layer can be seen as the SPOTLIGHT (when you focus on 'immediate actions'). The second layer is the STARLIGHT. This is the focus you can apply to your 'longer term goals –

projects over time.' The third layer is your DAYLIGHT. This is the form of focus that makes it possible for you to know what your longer-term goals are in the first place. A fourth form is the STADIUM LIGHTS. It is our ability to see each other, and to work together to formulate and fight for collective goals.

The long covid-related lockdowns and working from home while also homeschooling children may have also put many under greater stress and increased need to adapt. This could have led to increased need for greater attention and concentration. Looking for a diagnosis and a simple cure may have driven some of the recent interest in attention deficit disorders.

Allen Frances (2013) warned against turning our passions into addictions. DSM 5 introduced the concept of "behavioural addictions." At present only pathological gambling will qualify for it. The rationale for this radical proposal is that compulsive behaviour is equivalent to compulsive substance use and is caused by the same brain pleasure centres. The term "addiction" is being stretched to include any passionate interest or attachment.

Behavioural addiction is likely to become a diagnosis used for all impulsive behaviours that have gotten someone into any sort of trouble. We will need to watch out for false epidemics of addictions to the internet (the candidate for imminent fad status), shopping, working, sex, golf, gardening etc.

ARE WE THROWING THE BABY WITH THE BATH WATER?

New referrals are dominated by request for a possible diagnosis of ADD or ADHD. This has been the trend for several years but has increased dramatically since the prolonged Covid 19 related lockdowns. Most of those seeking consultations claim to have diagnosed themselves by completing the checklist for these conditions which are readily available over the internet.

These checklists have been made available by drug companies selling stimulants. They are so worded that anyone who ends up completing them is more than likely to end up with a diagnosis. They have already noticed a potential gap between their performance compared to their desired performance. There is an inherent bias in such comparison as the desired performance is based on the false premise that 'everyone can do everything that they desire irrespective of their actual capability.'

The greater the gap between the observed and expected performance, the more the need to find a cause. The expectations are themselves misplaced and based on a hypothetical best-case scenario. Attention deficit disorder is handy as it is then a 'medical condition' that can be easily diagnosed by using a flawed checklist and can be equally easily treated by simply taking a pill. It absolves any obligation to change in behaviour. Like the rising rates of obesity in our world, ADHD is also now seen as a new epidemic. In both situations the epidemic is more likely to be a 'social' rather than a 'medical' one.

The truth as always may be somewhere in the middle. There may be some with childhood ADHD that were missed and there may be some who may have late onset disorder. ADHD has been associated with impairment in many aspects of life leading to educational underachievement, unemployment, unsuccessful marriage, and criminality. They are also associated with many comorbid psychiatric disorders. Whether ADHD is the primary condition or secondary to other psychiatric conditions is hard to determine.

Just because a diagnosis can be reached as they fulfill the diagnostic criteria laid out at a given time, does not by itself prove that are condition needs to be treated with a pill. Lifestyle and environmental factors may be playing a particularly key role in producing ADHD. The massive interest in the condition may also be linked to the changed narrative of our time. We have been drilled into thinking we can all do whatever we want to do. The key is the limit, and we are limited by those we impose on ourselves. Stories like this fail to account for the variations in various kinds of capabilities we are born with or have developed over time. Everyone cannot be an Albert Einstein or Steven Hawking.

We must prioritise our goals. We must accept our limitations while trying to get better at doing what we want to do. Humans are not robots and switching between tasks frequently has hidden costs. Our use and abuse of smart phones is often the most potent contributor towards our perceived attentional difficulties. We live in times of excesses. We all have a pool of mental energy to draw from.

Stimulants may help but they can also improve performance even in those without the disorder. Changes in managing the environment and lifestyle changes can also be amazingly effective. Adults who have been able to negotiate the challenges of development through childhood and adolescence into adulthood may be less impaired and may manage adequately with nonpharmacological attention enhancing measures.

ARE WE TRYING TO TINKER WITH VARIATIONS IN HUMAN BIOLOGY?

ATTENTION is the mental faculty of considering or taking notice of someone or something. ADHD as a disorder is characterised by attention deficit, hyperactivity, and impulsivity. Attention deficit disorder on the other hand is primarily concerned with one's difficulty paying attention as the primary symptom.

Attention is one of the basic mental processes and is an integral part of our cognition. There are four main types of attention that we use in our daily lives: selective attention, divided attention, sustained attention, and executive attention. It is hard to be certain about the precise point where someone who has one or more of these problems with attention turns to be one with attention deficit disorder.

Daniel Kahneman (2011) drew attention to the often-used phrase "pay attention." You dispose of a limited budget of attention that you can allocate to activities and if you try to go beyond your budget you will fail. It is the mark of effortful activities that they interfere with each other, which is why it is difficult or impossible to conduct several activities at once. You can do several things at once, but only if they are easy and undemanding. Intense focusing on a task can make people effectively blind, even to stimuli that normally attract attention.

One of the significant discoveries of cognitive psychologists in recent decades is that switching from one task to another is effortful, especially under time pressure. Internet and smart phones make us shift attention all the time. Our ability to control attention is not simply a measure of intelligence, it is also a measure of efficiency in the control of attention.

COGNITION plays an especially key role in the process of acquiring knowledge and understanding through thought, experience, and the senses. These mental processes relate to the input and storage of information and how that information is then used to guide your behaviour. It is in essence, the ability to perceive and react, process, and understand, store and retrieve information, make decisions, and produce appropriate responses. We need cognition to help us understand information about the world around us and interact safely with our environment, as the sensory information we receive is vast and complicated. Cognition is needed to distil all this information down to its essentials.

INTELLIGENCE can be defined as a construct that is made up of different cognitive abilities. These abilities allow people to acquire knowledge and solve problems. This general mental ability is what underlies specific mental skills related to areas such as spatial, numerical, mechanical, and verbal abilities. Intelligence is not only the ability to reason, but it is also the ability to find relevant material in memory and to deploy attention when needed.

Intelligence is distributed across the population as a bell-shaped curve. There are two tails of the bell. 94 to 98% of the population are in the middle of this bell. One to three percent are thought to lie on either tail of the bell (higher or lower than the average). General intelligence can be compared to athleticism. A person might be a very skilled runner, but this does not necessarily mean that they will also be an excellent figure skater. However, because this person is athletic and fit, they will perform much better on other physical tasks than an individual who is less coordinated and more sedentary.

The notion that intelligence could be measured and summarized by a single number on an IQ test was controversial even during Spearman's time. IQ and intelligence testing have remained topics of debate ever since. While influential, g factor is just one way of thinking about intelligence. Thurstone identified several aspects of intelligence which he termed as *primary mental abilities*: Associative memory, Number facility, Perceptual speed, Reasoning, Spatial visualization, Verbal comprehension. Gardner argued against the notion that a single general intelligence can accurately capture all human mental ability.

Gardner in his 1983 book *Frames of Mind: The Theory of Multiple Intelligences* proposed eight types of intelligences. These are: 1. Visual-Spatial Intelligence, 2. Linguistic-Verbal Intelligence, 3. Logical-Mathematical Intelligence, 4. Bodily-Kinaesthetic Intelligence, 5. Musical Intelligence, 6. Interpersonal Intelligence, 7. Intrapersonal Intelligence, 8. Naturalistic Intelligence. He suggested the possible addition of a ninth known as "existentialist intelligence." While a person might be particularly strong in a specific area, such as musical intelligence, he or she are more likely to possess a range of abilities. For example, an individual might be strong in verbal, musical, and naturalistic intelligence.

Gardner's concept of existential intelligence is of particular interest in this discourse. In its essence, existential intelligence is the ability to use intuition, thought and meta-cognition to ask (and answer) deep questions about human existence. Those of us who are inherently existential ask questions such as: Who are we? Why are we alive? Do we have a purpose? Why and how are we conscious? What is the meaning of life?

DYSLEXIA is a learning disorder that involves difficulty reading due to problems identifying speech sounds and learning how they relate to letters and words (decoding). Symptoms include late talking, learning novel words slowly and a delay in learning to read. It is a result of individual differences in areas of the brain that process language.

Attention like intelligence and ability to learn are aspects of our cognitive abilities. All of them lie on a continuum. Intelligence and learning ability can be influenced by several factors. There are no medications that can improve intelligence or ability to learn. However, most children with dyslexia can succeed in school with tutoring or a specialized education program. Similarly, attention problems can improve through specialized programs. Adults should be able to do it even better. We live in times that we want quick fixes, and we want to find a pill to cure our illnesses.

We live in times where we are bombarded with more information than we have ever been exposed to. Powerful forces are stealing our focus effectively taking over our life. We are living with an abundance of light that has extended our day greatly and have gadgets demanding significant time and have extended our expectations beyond our biological limitations.

John Hutton et al (2020) investigated the neurobiological effects of screen watching on children. They noted: "In a single generation, through what has been described as a vast 'uncontrolled experiment,' the landscape of childhood has been digitalized, affecting how children play, learn, and form relationships. Use begins in infancy and increases with age, and it was recently estimated at more than 2 hours per day in children younger than 9 years, aside from use during childcare and school." They point to the risks which include "language delay, poor sleep, impaired executive function and general cognition, and decreased parent-child engagement, including reading together." Increased screen time was associated with poorer white-brain matter functioning.

Mary Swingle (2019), a neuropsychologist, in her book, "*i-Minds: How and Why Constant Connectivity Is Rewiring Our Brains and What to Do About It*" has pointed to witnessing autistic-like characteristics in children without autism. Expressing concern about the impact of relentless screen exposure on brain development, she points to, "Less ability to focus on the normal, the baseline, including states of observation, contemplation, and transitions from which ideas spark-what many under the age of twenty now consider a void, proclaiming boredom. On a biological as well as cultural level, such brain changes affect learning, socialization, recreation, partnering, parenting, and creativity-in essence all factors that make a society and culture. The neuropsychological processes that regulate mood and behaviour are deregulating."

We need differently abled people to make our world. Are we then inventing diagnoses and expecting a pill that will extend our ability to overcome limitations? Are we seeking the impossibility of equality in basic cognitive skills for all? And if that was possible, will that enhance our ability to create another dystopia with further increase in the incidence of anxiety and depression?

THE STORY OF PERSONALITY AND ITS DISORDERS

'It's not the disease that comes to the doctor, but the person with the disease.' We are unlikely to make much progress in psychiatry unless we work towards a better understanding of what it means to be a person. Factors contributing towards the making of a person is fundamental to our understanding of personality.

Personality disorders came lower down the order in the hierarchy of psychiatric diagnoses (behind the organic psychoses, functional psychoses, affective disorders and psychosomatic disorders) because of the uncertainties regarding their biological underpinning. That may have also resulted in lesser focus on them.

Nature and nurture stand in reciprocity, not opposition (Eisenberg 2000). Studies have suggested that about 50% of individual differences in personality traits are genetically influenced. Genetic and environmental sources unfold their impact through many different pathways – from the biological micro to the sociological macro (McAdams, 2015). The relative influence of genes and environments are difficult to disentangle because they trans- and interact in many complex ways.

Epigenetics is a rapidly emerging area of research into how the environment affects children's experiences and the expression of genes. During development, the DNA making up our genes accumulates chemical marks that determine how much or how little of the genes will express itself in each person. The analysis of the net effects of genetic and environmental sources provides interesting insights into their roles for personality development. The proportion of genetic and environmental components in personality traits appear to change across the lifespan. Heritability appears to steadily decline as people get older, whereas environmental influences mount. (Kandler &

Zapko-Willmes, 2017). The present discussion concentrates on the existential factors involved in the development of personality and its disorders.

An existential perspective is essential to our understanding of what it means to be a person as exemplified by his/her personality. The basic tenets of existentialism were covered in Part II of the book.

COMING TO EXIST

The individual comes to exist through a long and complicated process of conception followed by a period of gestation leading to birth. The first breath signifies a transition from the foetus to an infant. Our bipedal stance led to a smaller birth canal and in a developmental context the human child has therefore a shorter gestation period to ensure an uncomplicated birth. This also means that the human body is most immature at the time of birth and entirely dependent on mothers and significant others for their basic survival. However, they do come endowed with innate social skills to create immediate chemistry with the adults around them. They turn their heads to fix a wide-eyed gaze on an adult's face, calm their crying when they hear their mother's voice, tightly grasp an adult's finger, or rest a tiny hand on the breast that feeds them.

They are hard wired to connect face-to-face, and adults are programmed to respond promptly to their crying, gazing and cooing (Susan Pinker 2014). The human infant hears the mother's voice repeatedly and is able to discriminate that voice from other female voices (DeCasper & Spence, 1986).

These attributes form the basis for an attachment between the baby and the mother, father and significant others as discussed earlier.

WHAT DEFINES A PERSON:

The literal use of the word 'Person' gives us a false sense of familiarity and definability. The basic human situation is that each person stands in the world as a finite individual, even though life is lived in a particular surrounding. The concrete reality in life is our body, our physical and mental abilities, the social order, and the other individuals around us. We are dependent but always with a possibility of activity within certain constricting bounds.

A brief look at the basic concepts of the individual and their identity and the parallels in the conceptual framework that shapes a person's evolutionary, religious, historical, cultural, and personal context can provide important insights.

THE INDIVIDUAL

The word individual is about being 'a single entity; the one that cannot be divided'. However, in effect that is a misnomer. Evidence suggests an individual is divisible on several counts. In one way of thinking there are at least two selves within us: 'the experiencing self' and 'the remembering self'. The two are intertwined.

Kahneman (2011) quoted Jeremy Bentham who opened his introduction to "*The principles of models and legislation*" with the famous sentence "Nature has placed humankind under the governance of two sovereign masters: pain and pleasure. It is for them alone to point out what we ought to do as well as to determine what we shall do." A strong majority favour reducing the memory of pain. The experiencing self is the one that answers the question: "Does it hurt now?" The remembering self is the one that answers the question: "How was it, on the whole?" Memories are all we get to keep from our experience of living, and the only perspective that we can adopt as we think about our lives is that of the remembering self.

The remembering self is sometimes wrong, but it is the one that keeps the scores and governs what we learnt from living, and it is the one that makes decisions. What we learn from the past is to maximise the qualities of our past experiences not necessarily of our future experience. This is the tyranny of the remembering self.

An individual is also divisible through their various key functions: cognitive, affective, and behavioural. At a different level, they are divisible based on the roles they assume in life at a given time or context: that of a child, sibling, friend, parent, a professional function, or their role as a citizen of the society they live in. The construction of a unified concept of identity is complex given the matrix of roles and responsibilities that a person assumes.

Many neuroscientists tend to believe that there is not a single self. My ***corporal*** self makes me aware that the body in which I am living is really my own body, my ***locomotive*** self tells me where I am at any given time, ***perspective*** self tells me that I am the centre of the world experienced by me, my "I" as experiential subject tells me that my sensory impressions and feelings are really my own and not those of others, my ***authorship and supervisory self*** makes it clear to me that I am the person who has to accept responsibility for my thoughts and actions, my ***autographical self*** makes sure that I do not step out of my own role and that I experience myself throughout as one and the same person, my ***self-reflexive self*** enables me to think about myself and play the psychological game of "I" and "me" and my ***moral*** self-works as a connection to tell me what is good and what is bad (Precht 2011).

IDENTITY

Identity denotes "This is the real me!". This involves the whole interplay between the psychological and social, the developmental and the historical for which identity formation is of prototypical significance (Erikson, 1968).

IDENTITY: EVOLUTIONAY PERSPECTIVE

Our feelings and thinking provide a coherent sense of self. Charles Darwin (1872) proposed: 'much like other traits in animals, emotions also evolved and were adopted over time.' As discussed earlier, according to modern evolutionary theory, different emotions evolved at separate times.

When young infants need food or comfort, they cry, and this typically results in a helpful adult response. The infant learns that as soon as he or she cries adults responds, so crying often becomes ritualized. Within the first few months of life infants also engage with others socially and share emotions.

Most infants begin acquiring language in the months around their first birthday. They point to request things (imperatives) and to share experiences and emotions with others (declaratives). During the second year of life, infants start using conventionalized gestures that they learn by imitating the adults. Novel arbitrary gestures and linguistic acquisition happen in the same way depending on the way adults introduce them in naming games and further learning. Earliest linguistic conventions tend to supplant pointing, which often supplements language, but iconic gestures operate in comparable manner to language. "Language is a social art. In acquiring it we have to depend entirely on intersubjectively available cues as to what to say and when" (Quine, 1960).

Affect perhaps remains the last frontier in our quest to understand the dynamics of human behaviour. Recent studies have showed that affect and cognition are not separate and independent faculties of the mind (Forgas, 2000). There is a fundamental interdependence between feeling and thinking in human social life. Our affective experiences are integrally linked with the way information about the world is stored and represented. In turn, experiences of even mild moods have a profound influence over the memories we retrieve, the information that we notice and learn, and the way we respond to social situations. Affect can influence both the process of thinking (how we deal with social information) and the content of thinking, judgements, and behaviour.

Existential Feelings: Ratcliffe (2008) drew attention to the concept of existential Feelings which provide the background orientations through which everything that we perceive, feel, think, and act upon is structured. They constitute "how we find ourselves in the world in general."

Stephan (2012) distinguished between two elements of existential feelings – elementary (or basic) and nonelementary (or non-basic). Elementary existential feelings are in the background of our affective lives and provide us with a sense of reality: of ourselves, our actions, other persons and objects, and the surrounding world. In contrast, nonelementary existential feelings alter without involving any severe distortion from normal mental functioning. They comprise feelings that concern one's own vital state (such as feeling healthy and strong versus feeling exhausted and weak), or that reflect one's own position within social environment (such as feeling welcomed and familiar versus feeling disrespected and rejected), or that manifest one's standing towards the world in general (such as feeling at home or as a participant in the tide of events versus feeling disconnected, like a stranger or not at home in the world).

Besides essential and nonessential feelings, there are atmospheric feelings which relates to specific events and situations. These feelings' pre-structure our interactions with others and the world. They also comprise self-related feelings, feelings that concern our social environment and feelings that relate to the world in general.

IDENTITY: HISTORICAL, CULTURAL, & POLITICAL PERSPECTIVE:

Our identity is no doubt shaped by our history which in turn affects culture. The political system is part of the cultural process and affects in many ways.

Physically the individual has not changed much since the advent of our species. But our perspective has continued to evolve through the millennia. For much of the last thirteen to fourteen thousand years of human history, most people lived in settled agrarian communities in which social roles were both limited and fixed. A certain hierarchy based on age and gender was accepted. Everyone had the same occupation (farming or raising children and minding a household). One's entire life was lived in the same village with a limited number of friends and neighbours. One's religious beliefs were shared by all in a particular community. Social mobility - moving away from a village, choosing a different occupation, or marrying someone not chosen by one's parents/family was impossible. Such societies had neither pluralism, nor diversity, nor choice.

Cultures change gradually. The Bible preached "everyone is born equal." The US Declaration of Independence (1776) included "the right to the pursuit of happiness" as one of the three unalienable human rights along with the right to life and the right to liberty. The Universal Declaration of Human Rights (1948), a humanistic manifesto passed unopposed by the United Nations General Assembly, has influenced most national constitutions written or modified thereafter. Lofty ideals but inequality remains widespread.

Enlightenment flowed out of the Scientific Revolution and the Age of Reason in the seventeenth century and spilled into the heyday of classical liberalism of the first half of the nineteenth (Steven Pinker, 2018). This view is disputed, and they may be talking about enlightenment of some not all. Non-European world may have been more enlightened much before that. It is just that lot of history has held a very Eurocentric views of development. The work of

Graeber and Wengrow (2021) concerning the basis of enlightenment has been highlighted in an earlier chapter.

There has been a seismic change in the perspective of life of humans particularly since industrialization. Developments over the last two centuries have been so swift and radical that they have changed the most fundamental characteristics of the social order. Traditionally, the social order was hard and rigid. Order implied stability and continuity. The pace of change has become so quick that the social order acquired a dynamic and malleable nature. It now exists in a state of permanent flux. Hence, any attempt to define the characteristic of the modern society is akin to defining the colour of a chameleon (Harari 2014).

Human history was driven by a struggle for recognition (Hegel). By the eighteenth century, the idea at the core of modern identity had evolved to take on a secular form. Fukuyama (2018) sees the modern concept of identity as uniting three different phenomena: (a) Thymos: a universal aspect of human personality that craves recognition of dignity, (b) The distinction between inner and outer self, (c) An evolving concept of dignity, in which recognition is due not just to a narrow class of people, but to everyone. Contemporary liberal democracies have not fully solved the problem of thymos: Isothymia (the demand to be respected on an equal basis with other people) and Megalothymia (the desire to be recognized as superior).

Modern democracies promise and largely deliver a minimum degree of equal respect, embodied in individual rights, the rule of law, and the franchise. It does not guarantee that people will be equally respected in practice, particularly members of groups with a history of marginalization. The recent resurgence of fascism and more orthodox views raising their head in distinct parts of the world is cause for concern. This was explored in Part II under the political story.

IDENTITY: FROM CHARACTER TO PERSONALITY

The word personality did not exist in English until the eighteenth century. The idea of "having a good personality" became widespread only in the twentieth century (Cain 2012).

Susman (1984) termed it as it a shift from a 'Culture of Character' to a 'Culture of Personality'. She wrote, "Every American was to become a performing self." The focus until then was on character formation. Attaining good virtues and living in harmony with one's family and society was of utmost importance. Americans embraced the "Culture of Personality." They now started to focus more on how others perceived them. They became captivated by people who were bold and entertaining (Cain 2012). The western world has continued to follow that trend and now the traditional Asian societies have gradually joined it too.

A cultural 'revolution' took place that reached a tipping point around the turn of the twentieth century, changing forever who we are and whom we admire, how we act at job interviews and what we look for in an employee, how we court our mates and raise our children. The recent story is that of the rise of the Extrovert Ideal, even though as Jung (1921) put it "there is no such thing as pure extrovert or a pure introvert."

Cultural historian Susan Warren believes that it was this move from a 'Culture of Character' to a 'Culture of Personality' that opened a Pandora's Box of personal anxieties from which we would never quite recover. In the culture of character, the ideal self was serious, disciplined, and honourable. What counted was not so much the impression one made in public as how one behaved in private.

IDENTITY: PERSONAL CONTEXT

The meaning of existence can be most clearly seen in the mirror of nonexistence. Melanie Klein (1921) considered the fear of death as the original source of anxiety. According to her even the very young child has an intimate relationship with death – a relationship that antedates by a considerable period his or her conceptual knowledge of death. The fear of death is present early in life and is instrumental in shaping character structure and continues throughout life to generate anxiety resulting in manifest distress and in the erection of psychological defences.

According to Eric Berne, the individual "decides" on a "life script", an unconscious blueprint for one's life course which encompasses personality variables and repetitive interpersonal interactions. Berne's life script has broad similarity to Adler's "guiding fiction "or Horney's "Idealized image system." Though it is more interpersonally based, it is also loosely equivalent to the Freudian concept of "character structure" (Yalom 1980). Life scripts are neither written at one specific time in life nor is it set in stone. Most people continue to revise their life script over time. Our life experiences and circumstances are the primary motivating factors to effect these changes. Sometimes we do it consciously at other times we change subtly and imperceptibly.

Identity is acquired initially through the process of identification. The mechanism of Identification (with significant others) is of limited use. Identity formation begins where the usefulness of identification ends (Erikson, 1968). Every individual goes through a process of separation and individuation that leads to the emergence of 'self.' The self is a complex matter. Historical and cultural factors provide the background, but life unfolds in the immediate precincts of the family unit.

No one has a perfect childhood. We cannot even be sure what that would be like. There is no such thing as a truly "grown up person." Parents do not take on the role of parenting with all the requisite wisdom. They themselves slowly evolve in their role. They are also greatly influenced by the prevailing social and cultural milieu. "Spare the rod and spoil the child" was once a laudable mantra and so was the notion that "children need be seen and not heard." Subsequent evidence proved without any semblance of doubt that these were farcical beliefs. The "goodness of the fit" model remains a truly relevant way of understanding the balance of probabilities for a given child. Parents being the adults and expected to be the ones with greater knowledge, experience and abilities need to work towards making that goodness of fit possible.

The type of attachment that the child develops with key persons in his surrounding is of critical importance. The contributions of John Bowlby (1969) have been covered previously under the topic of making of affective bonds earlier.

Childhood maltreatment (including physical, sexual, and emotional abuse, and neglect) appear to share nonspecific consequences. They can be conceived as errors of commission (abuse) and errors of commission (neglect). Neglect can be a subjective perception depending on the 'needs of a particular child' and the temperament of the 'caring adult'. The three Ls of parenting involve: Love, Limitation, and Letting them grow remain relevant. Parents often struggle finding a balance between appropriate 'Limitations' and need to 'Let them grow' and the inherent contradictions between the two. Thus, almost everyone is scarred to some extent.

Jean Liedloff (1985) noted: "The earliest established components of an infant's psychobiological makeup are those most formative of his lifelong outlook.' "What he feels before he can think is a powerful determinant of what kind of things he thinks when thought became possible."

Nelson (1993) takes the position that autobiographical memory is a social convention. He believes that early memories are transient and disorganised for two reasons: the child lacks the encoding experience to store them systematically, and in any case attaches no particular importance to them. At best they may remain in the "holding pattern" for up to six months.

Fivush and Hammond (1989) believe that the reinstatement of the event by the occurrence of a somewhat similar experience within the holding period would increase the potential longevity of such even memories. If there were no reinstatement within the holding period, the event memory will be lost. Tomkins' (1978) put forth the notion that a single event is in itself of little cognitive significance to a child, but further events can sometimes evoke the key process of 'magnification.' Several repetitions of similar events encourage the development of generic memories.

Fortunately, humans are also resilient in the face of adversity. Most of the maltreatment or trauma can be managed through other protective factors as well as our inherent resilience. "Trauma is not an event, not external to the individual, but rather is the subjective experience of the person. When integrative capacity of the individual is overwhelmed; this constitutes trauma, whether it involves actual abuse, the absence of experience (neglect) or an event that many others might experience as merely a stressful situation (such as being yelled at)" (Mosquera & Steele, 2017).

Humans are not stable but timeless entities. We are always a work in progress, a story in the process of being written.

IDENTITY: EMERGING SENSE OF SELF

Adolescence is the last stage of childhood. "The adolescence process, however, is conclusively complete only when the individual has subordinated his childhood identifications to a new kind of identification, achieved in absorbing sociability and in competitive apprenticeship with and among age mates" (Erikson, 1968).

The self is a mental representation of oneself. Alternatively, the self may be seen to represent 'our knowledge of ourselves.' As a conceptual structure the self is not unitary or monolithic. Our behaviour is broadly stable over time and consistent over space, and this stability and consistency reflect traits which lie at the core of personality.

The self consists of the stories we tell about ourselves – stories which relate to how we got where we are, and why, and what we have done, and what happened next. We rehearse these stories to ourselves to remind ourselves of who we are, we tell them to other people to encourage them to form a particular impression of ourselves, and we change the stories as our self-understanding, or our strategic self-representation, changes. The self is also a bundle of propositions about our abstract traits, and our specific experiences, thoughts, and actions in which semantic self-knowledge is represented independently of episodic self-knowledge (Kihlstrom & Klein, 1997).

As there are several selves, so there are also several ways of sizing up the self. No matter how neatly these states are distinguished, they blend within the brain. Precht (2011) saw the growth of the personality as being inextricably linked to the sense of self because people say 'I' when referring to themselves. It is assumed that approximately one-half of this personality development is closely linked to one's innate abilities. About 30 to 40 percent depends on impressions and experiences before the age of five. And only 20 to 30 percent of this development is significantly influenced by later influences in the home, or at school, and so forth. The functional self is usually conceptualized as a triangle: the three angles consisting of Thought (cognition), Feeling (emotion), and Behaviour (which could involve behaviour directed towards others and towards one-self).

Feelings and thoughts work together, sometimes in unison and at other times in opposition. Feelings can at times take over and rational thinking takes a back seat. At other times it is the thought process that tries to suppress or repress feelings. The two horses and the charioteer of Plato sometimes have a smooth ride or a bumpy ride. Our reasonable or emotional mind may be trying to take over or we can be in a 'wise mind' mode in our struggle to establish a coherent and authentic sense of self.

IDENTITY: FURTHER DEVELOPMENTS

A person is not a static being. He continues to live, experience, and grow. The ongoing lived experiences continue to shape and reshape them. The young narrator is in the process of mastering discursive and narrative techniques as he is undergoing the experiences to be integrated into his autobiography. They are unclear about a full range of things. A loving and nurturing environment is required to impart the skills to produce a satisfying and well-integrated story. Otherwise, the story itself may become disturbed and fragmented, containing indigestible lumps of experience which the discursive subject cannot assimilate adequately in his narrative.

Jaspers (1963) remarked, "Everything we experience and do leaves its trace and slowly change our disposition. People with the same disposition at birth may eventually find themselves in entirely different groves, simply through their life-history and experiences and the effects of their upbringing as well as of their own efforts at self-education. Once such development has taken place there is no point of return. In this lies the personal responsibility involved in every experience."

We do things to each other by speech and the interpersonal discourses constitutes reality of the subject When we consider what an individual personality appears in discourse, it is the precipitated residue of a lifetime of encounters with others. The subject is not fixed but is active, so that "it is in the relation between the subject's ego and the 'I' of discourse that you understand the meaning of this discourse" (Lacan 1977).

Words operate in shared practices and therefore link the responses of one person to those of others in normative ways. Many of our basic reactions are formed in close, indeed intense relationships where personal needs have been recognized or ignored and either met or unmet by those who care for us (Gillett, 1999).

PERSONALITY: NORMATIVE Vs PATHOLOGICAL

Personality difficulties are common, but personality disorders are much less common. The numbers depend on the criteria used to define it. The criterion keeps shifting over time. The latest version of the diagnostic systems have come up with a major shift in paradigm.

One of the widely acknowledged definition of personality is that proposed by Allport (1937). He saw: "Personality as the dynamic organization within the individual of those psychophysiological systems that determines his unique adjustment in his environment." He saw personality as constantly developing and changing, even though there is an organization or system that binds together and relates the various components of personality. He used the term 'psychophysiological to make sure that personality is seen as "neither exclusively mental nor exclusively neural. The word "determine" makes clear that personality is made up of determining tendencies that play an active role in the individual's behaviour (Hall & Lindzey, 1978). Being 'dynamic' also provides hope for the person to do better in the future and for clinicians to work towards a better outcome.

The construct of personality can be viewed in an existential perspective. Birth in a particular family setting which is part of a social and cultural setting defines the evolution of a sense of self which in turn defines the person and his personality. Debate has continued not only on the categorical versus dimensional construct of all psychopathologies, but even more in the context of personality and its disorders. The differentiation between personality traits and disorder is not easy and straight forward. The recent focus has changed to the severity as a major point to differentiate between what may be normal and abnormal personality.

Consensus has converged on a model with five dimensional factors that provides an adequate representation of normative personality (Goldberg, 1993). These five factors involve:

1. Neuroticism (a tendency to be depressed, anxious and stress reactive)
2. Agreeableness (an orientation towards empathy and getting along with other people)
3. Extraversion (a disposition to be outgoing, friendly, and emotionally positive)
4. Conscientiousness (a tendency to be orderly and achievement oriented)
5. Openness. (a tendency to be curious, imaginative and to try new change).

In general, personality disorders are characterized by high neuroticism, low agreeableness, and low conscientiousness. Categorical personality disorders as described in DSM 5 are fraught with problems, including excessive cooccurrence, heterogeneity within categories, arbitrary diagnostic thresholds, diagnostic instability over time, poor coverage of personality pathology, and criteria sets that are inconsistent amalgams of signs, symptoms, behaviours, traits, and even functional outcomes (Skodol, 2018).

Personality disorders are generally conceived as maladaptive conditions considered to be a type of mental disorder characterized by a rigid and unhealthy pattern of thinking, functioning, and behaving. A person with a personality disorder has trouble perceiving and relating to situations and people. This causes significant problems and limitations in relationships, social activities, school, and work. The connection between insecure attachment and a cascade of childhood maltreatment which may lead to an impaired sense of oneself and relationship with others is well-known. Problems in emotional regulation appear to play a critical role in the concept of personality but emotions and thinking always act in tandem (with emotions more often influencing thinking) and together they determine one's behaviour.

Personality disorders have been classified into various subtypes. DSM-III to DSM-IV and ICD-9 to ICD-10 described eight to ten distinct types. However, there is increasing recognition that a dimensional framework may be more relevant to describing personality pathology. Agreement appears to emerge that the severity of personality disorder is the strongest determinant of the degree of incapacity and prognosis of any mental disorder.

PERSONALITY DISORDERS: THE LOST FRONTIER

There is no ideal person or personality. 'The essence of man is in his incompleteness.' Karl Jaspers (1959) described 3 kinds of mental illnesses: (1) as a somatic process (Organic psychoses) (2) as a serious event which breaks the healthy life for the first time and procures a psychic change: a somatic base is suspected for this but is not known (Schizophrenia, Manic-depressive Illness, and Melancholia) (3) as a variation of human life far removed from the average and somehow undesired by the affected person or by his environment and therefore in need of treatment (The unwanted variations of human nature: The Personality conditions).

The Industrial Revolution was associated with a large scale move from agriculture to factory work, population growth, and urbanization. The old social order was disrupted. Mental patients were confined with other undesirables – paupers, criminals, orphans and intellectually infirm. The mad were considered less than full human. Philippe Pinel in the late eighteenth century saved the mentally ill and created the profession of psychiatry in the western world. He unchained the mentally ill, helped do away the medieval superstitions about mental illness and developed a new model of "asylum" care. That marked the end of the dark ages beliefs in mental disorder as caused by demonic possession.

In the late Nineteenth and early twentieth centuries, Kraepelin was seeing patients with psychoses in the hospital setting. He needed to look at patients rather than listen to them. For him diagnosis was prognosis, the course of patient's symptoms would tell what diagnosis they had. Freud on the other hand was treating patients in the community with neuroses. He was listening to his patients and working towards a theory. For him exploring the unconscious was the pathway to understanding psychopathology. How could they reach the same conclusion? Kraepelin's method would not work for Freud's patients, and neither would Freud's method for Kraepelin's patients. Different methods had been devised, correctly for different settings, conditions, and purposes. "They were both right; they were both wrong; for they were only partially right and universally wrong." What Jaspers discerned is that it is the nature of science that all knowledge is partial: no scientific theory can have validity outside of its chosen scope (Ghaemi 2010).

Personality disorders presented with too diverse symptoms to be of interest to Freud and the Freudians. Psychoanalysis did not work for those with personality disorders. In fact, it made them worse. Attachment issues and a multiplicity of traumatic experiences including sexual trauma and not the presumed problems with psychosexual development were involved. It was too "Non-Psychotic" for Kraepelin and the Kraepelinian. They did not fit into either of the major psychoses. They continued to float between these two streams of psychiatry and thus constituted a borderline (a protype of severe personality disorder) between the so-called psychoses and neuroses. When people with personality disorder were in hospital, they generated situations like *One Flew Over the Cuckoo's Nest* (1975) and when they reached the psychotherapist, it resulted in comic situations like *What about Bob*? (1991)

Life was tough for most people throughout history. Both physical and mental suffering was ubiquitous. The vagaries of nature, scarcity of food and resources, poor amenities, basic sanitation, and abundance of physical diseases with poor remedies made life precarious. Life expectancy was low, maternal, and infant mortality high, and people were more often caught up in the struggle to survive. Except for the privileged few, psychiatric disorders attracted attention only when they were so severe that there was no choice but to seek help.

To start with, psychiatrists worked only from mental asylums/hospitals. The gradual closure of mental hospitals, establishment of psychiatry departments in general hospitals and private psychiatry clinics helped liberate psychiatry itself from the high walls of the mental asylums. It paved the way for nonorganic, non-psychotic, and non-affective mental conditions to receive attention.

The growth of psychiatry as a speciality has been a slow grind marked by many milestones. The first milestone was the 'humane treatment of the mentally ill' in late 1880s, the second was the advent of Electroconvulsive therapy in the 1930s, the third (ironically) was the discovery of Penicillin (clearing the mental asylums of patients with neurosyphilis) in the 1940s, the fourth was the rather surreptitious discovery of the first antipsychotic and antidepressants in the 1950s, the fifth was the widespread adaptation of lithium as a mood stabiliser in the 1970s. The slow march towards the sixth and equally important milestone started with the Feighner criteria (Feighner et al 1972) and Research and Diagnostic Criteria (Spitzer and Robins 1978) and winding through the DSM-III in 1980s to DSM-5 and ICD-10 and ICD11. It is an ongoing process.

Disorders of personality remained a pariah to mainstream psychiatry until the advent of DSM-III. Massive changes in the two diagnostic systems and in particular the emergence of a dimensional system of categorising personality disorder constitutes a major advancement.

PERSONALITY DISORDER IN DSM:

The concept of multiaxial diagnosis was discussed in the European psychiatric literature since the 1940s (Williams 1985). The basic concept was that the individual is evaluated in terms of different domains of information that are assumed to be of high clinical value. It was not until 1980 that a bold initiative was undertaken in the organization of DSM-III by introducing a multiaxial system of classification. Axis II was dedicated to chronicle personality disorder and traits and was supposed to be part of the complete evaluation of a case. The decision to separate Axis I and II was to ensure that consideration was given to the possible presence of disorders that are frequently overlooked when attention is directed to the usually more florid axis I disorders.

DSM-III recognized that "personality disorders may co-exist with, predispose to, or result from axis I psychiatric disorders and also importantly influence their presentation, course, management, and response to treatment" (Frances1981). Accordingly, evaluators were encouraged to recognize both the clinical syndrome and personality disorder rather than being forced to arbitrarily make a choice between them (Frances 1981). Similarly, it was also meant to help ensure that a clinical syndrome was not overlooked when the diagnosis of personality disorder is made and focused on in treatment (Nakdimen 1981).

DSM IIIR and DSM IV continued the categorical concept of personality disorder with only minor modifications to the criteria. This approach to the description of personality were thought to have serious and practical considerations. Cloninger (1987) pointed out these limitations as: 1. An individual often has features of more than one personality disorder; 2. Clinical distinctions between maladaptive personality traits and personality disorders are somewhat arbitrary; 3. Adaptive impairment depends on both situational and temperamental variables; 4. The behaviours that are typically chosen as criterion variables in a particular culture are obviously not socially desirable or admirable, and consequently direct questioning often leads to guarded and defensive responses. He proposed three dimensions of personality defined in terms of basic stimulus-response characteristics of: 1. Novelty seeking, 2. Harm avoidance, and 3. Reward dependence.

There were obvious unresolved issues regarding diagnosis and differential diagnosis as well as causation. There will always be 'splitters' and 'lumpers' but, there is evidence to suggest that psychopathology is widespread with frequent overlap across categories and multiple diagnoses is the rule rather than the exception. The multiaxial system that was the dominant theme of DSM-III and DSM-IV (hailed as a major step forward) but was unceremoniously dumped by the DSM 5.

Debate on the categorical versus dimensional nature of personality disorder continues. DSM 5 as part of an ongoing review process included personality disorder in both section II (represents an update of same criteria as DSM IV) and section III (the proposed research mode that reflects the concept developed by the DSM 5 work group). Herein the core of the personality pathology is seen as a disturbance in self and interpersonal psychopathology. Self-functioning involves identity and self-direction. Interpersonal functioning involves empathy and intimacy. The level of personality functioning scale uses each of these elements to differentiate five levels of impairment.

PERSONALITY DISORDER IN ICD

Of the ten Personality Disorder in the ICD-10, two were used with a disproportionately high frequency: "Emotionally unstable personality disorder, borderline type" and "Dissocial (antisocial) personality disorder." Many categories overlapped, and individuals with severe disorders often met the requirements for multiple PDs, which Reed et al. (2019) described as "artificial comorbidity."

Modern personality disorder theories and research attempt to distinguish transdiagnostic impairments common to all of them. It has therefore been reconceptualized in terms of a general dimension of severity, focusing on five negative personality traits which a person can have to various degrees.

The ICD 11 model involves a measure of severity (mild. Moderate, and severe PD) as well as a subsyndromal condition called personality difficulty. There are five trait domains labelled Negative Affectivity, Detachment, Disinhibition, Dissociality, and Anankastic that further delineates personality function once the severity level has been determined (Tyrer 2016). The domains should only be coded if the features are prominent in an individual diagnosed with personality disorder. Kim et al (2016) showed good construct validity and test-retest reliability for the severity classification.

Tyrer et al (2016) reclassified personality status in their long-term Nottingham Study and reported that those with moderate to severe ICD 11 personality disorder had significantly worse outcome at both 2 years and 12 years than those with mild personality disorder or personality difficulty particularly with regard to social functioning. Bach et al (2017) used the DSM 5 alternative model personality disorder traits to describe the proposed ICD11 domains and reported that they were largely commensurate.

Personality difficulty have also been included and defined in ICD-II. They are conceived as occurring intermittently and often confined to limited situations. They are characterised by long standing difficulties (at least 2 years) in the individual's way of experiencing and thinking about the self, others and the world. These difficulties are manifested in cognitive and emotional experience and expression only intermittently. These are insufficiently severe to cause major disruption in social, occupational, and interpersonal relationships and may be limited to specific relationships or situations.

Doubts have been raised that the ICD-II classification has followed the still unproved idea that normal personality offers a valid bridge to the structure of abnormal personality (Gunderson and Zananini 2011). However, they have been shown to create distress, increase health service use, and impair social functioning and may be important in determining early personality pathology in adolescents (Tyrer 2019).

FACTOR ANALYTIC STUDIES: ONE, TWO, OR THREE FACTORS

Two latent dimensions have long been identified to describe psychopathology in children (Achenbach 1991). The internalizing dimension represents the propensity to experience inhibitory disorders such as depression, anxiety, panic, and phobias. The externalizing dimension is associated with disinhibitory disorders such as conduct disorder, substance abuse and antisocial personality disorder. The internalizing disorder have been found (Kessler et al 2010) to encompass two subfactors: distress and fear. The distress factor is associated with MDD, dysthymia, and GAD, while the fear factor is indicated by panic disorder, social phobia, and simple phobias.

Weston et al (2012) proposed a hierarchical organization of personality syndromes. Among patients with more severe personality pathology, they found three superordinate groupings or broad personality spectra, reflecting internalizing, externalizing, and borderline-dysregulated pathology. Patients in the internalizing spectrum are self-blaming and chronically prone to depression and anxiety.

Patients in the externalizing spectrum blame others and are chronically prone to anger and aggression. Patients in the borderline-dysregulated spectrum are qualitatively distinct from stable internalizers or externalizers. Their perceptions of self and others are unstable and fluctuating, and they exhibit an impaired ability to regulate emotion (often oscillating between emotions characteristic of internalizing and externalizing pathology, for example, depression, anxiety, and rage). According to Schmideberg (1959) people with borderline personality may best be described as "stably unstable."

Factor analytic studies have generally failed to support a putative personality disorder structure producing little evidence that BPD is a categorically defined diagnosis (Sharp 2016). It is also a highly comorbid disorder. One interpretation is that BPD criteria may capture the impairment in personality functioning defined in Criterion A in DSM 5 or the severity criterion in ICD11. Another possibility that has been proposed is that BPD is made up of three or more domains (Tyrer and Mulder 2018). There was considerable debate regarding this new dimensional model, with many believing that categorical diagnosing should not be abandoned.

In the ICD-11 committee there was disagreement about the status of borderline personality disorder. "Some research suggests that borderline PD is not an independently valid category, but rather a heterogeneous marker for PD severity. Other researchers view borderline PD as a valid and distinct clinical entity and claim that 50 years of research support the validity of the category. Many clinicians were aligned with the latter position. In the absence of more definitive data, there seemed to be little hope of accommodating these opposing views. However, the WHO took seriously the concerns being expressed that access to services for patients with borderline PD, which has increasingly been achieved in some countries based on arguments of treatment efficacy, might be seriously undermined." Thus, the WHO believed the inclusion of a Borderline pattern category to be a "pragmatic compromise" (Reed 2018).

Williams et al (2018) found that the two bifactor model – one confirmatory model with ten specific factors for each PD (acceptable fit) and one explanatory model with four specific factors resembling broad personality domains (excellent fit) – fit best and were compared via connections with external criteria. The general factor predicted interpersonal dysfunction beyond other kinds of psychopathology. The general factor also correlated with many pathological traits. Their study supported the validity of a model that included a general PD impairment dimension and separate individual difference dimensions.

Pettersson et al (2020) studied "g" factor using fifteen Weschler Adult Intelligence Scale subsets and "p" by analysing fourteen psychiatric diagnoses in many Swedish adults and adolescents and sixteen parent-rated psychopathology scale in children. Results indicated that the magnitude of "p" and "g" were remarkably similar. Controlling for "g", "p" significantly predicted later education. Controlling for "p", "g" significantly predicted later education and university entrance exam scores. Controlling "g", "p" significantly predicted all adverse outcomes. These findings support the notion that psychopathology indicators can be combined into a single score, similar to how intelligence subsets are combined into a general intelligence score.

THE BASIC SYMPTOMS OF PERSONALITY DISORDER

Borderline personality disorder (BPD) can be used as a prototype of severe personality disorder. This is in keeping with the suggestion that BPD is not an independently valid category, but rather a heterogeneous marker for personality disorder severity (Sharp et al 2015, Williams et al 2018). The dimensional approach to personality disorder raises the possibility that the borderline label may eventually become obsolete. However, the fact remains that BPD is the most widely researched category of personality disorder and treatment models exist with some proof about their efficacy. These can still be especially useful for the re-configured diagnostic categories envisaged in ICD 11 and alternative model of DSM 5.

A personality disorder with a 'Borderline pattern" qualifier that can be specified as 'mild', 'moderate' and 'severe' according to the prominence and impact of traits and symptoms on the individual's social and occupational functioning allows for further utilization of research so far and look at its generalizability to other types of personality disorders.

People with Borderline personality disorder are well known for their difficulties in managing emotions, especially anxiety and anger, their impulsive self-destructive behaviour, their lack of empathy, and their excessive use of maladaptive ego defence mechanisms. These are all suggestive of low emotional intelligence. Bar on (2001) found that those who scored low on EQ-I, score high on a borderline personality feature scale. People high in alexithymia tend to have insecure attachment styles (Taylor 2000). Kalpakci et al (2018) have proposed separating BPD into externalizing and internalizing subtypes of executive function. It is difficult to reconcile these findings with the concept of a distinct personality entity or domain as externalizing and internalizing characteristics belong to two opposite domains (Tyrer 2019).

BPD symptomatology (Severe PD) in an existential perspective

The basic structure of the self has often been depicted as a triangle with the three angles representing Affect (Emotions), Cognition (Thinking), and Behaviour (Action). Babies begin to feel earlier than they acquire an ability to think and develop language to express their feelings and thoughts. There is always a bidirectional and three-way interaction going on between emotions, thinking and behaviour (affect, cognition, and action). The subjective-self and the narrative-self reciprocally influence each other and determine overt behaviour. A normal trajectory of development results in a more stable self as seen in figure 1A.

The basic issue in the emerging BPD is the lack of a secure attachment starting from infancy and early childhood. Childhood maltreatment is more likely to be an accompanying problem. Both combine to create a battered and bruised sense of identity. If we compare the emotional system of a BPD patient to a car, then she or he may be driving the car with hypersensitive accelerator and poor brakes. In such a scenario, one would postulate the hypersensitive accelerator as the disordered emotional regulation and the poor brakes as the thought process. The impaired self-control and numerous interpersonal accidents are the behavioural outcome that result from the other two.

A person with borderline personality can also be seen as having a self like an inverted triangle (as seen in figure 1B) where-in the self is precariously balanced with the twin burden of unstable emotions and lack of a coherent remembering self (thinking). The behaviour of the person is unstable, and a lot of energy is spent in balancing emotions and thinking in a topsy turvy life. The degree of instability may depend on the degree of resilience available to contain their emotions or thoughts.

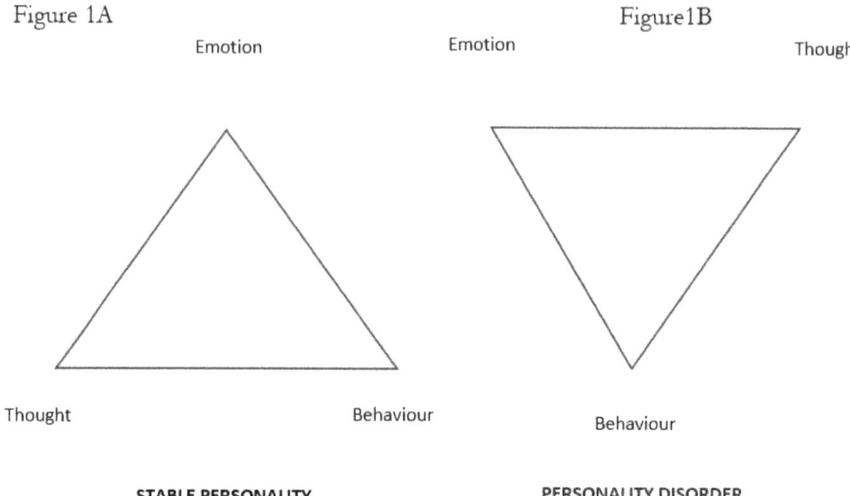

Behaviour can then be directed towards self and towards others. Lack of basic trust makes it hard to trust others around them. They rush towards a larger number of people to fill the gap. They start using people (including health providers) as objects to meet their unmet dependency needs. This rush makes it more likely to cause discomfort among others and thus perceived as rejection or abandonment based on the basic tenets of their insecure attachment.

A Borderline personality diagnosis is based on: (1) a pervasive pattern of instability of interpersonal relationships, self-image, and affects, and (2) marked impulsivity beginning by early adulthood and present in a variety of contexts, as indicated by at least five of the following:

1. Frantic efforts to avoid real or imagined abandonment; this does not include suicidal or self-mutilating behaviour covered in criterion 5.

2. A pattern of unstable and intense interpersonal relationships characterized by alternating between extremes of idealization and devaluation.

3. Markedly and persistently unstable self-image or sense of self.

4. Impulsivity in at least two areas that are potentially self-damaging (e.g., spending, sex, substance abuse, reckless driving, binge eating); this does not include suicidal or self-mutilating behaviour covered in criterion 5.

5. Recurrent suicidal behaviour, gestures, or threats, or self-mutilating behaviour.

6. Affective instability due to a marked reactivity of mood (e.g., intense episodic dysphoria, irritability, or anxiety usually lasting a few hours and only rarely more than a few days).

7. Chronic feelings of emptiness.

8. Inappropriate, intense anger or difficulty controlling anger (e.g., frequent displays of temper, constant anger, or recurrent physical fights).

9. Transient, stress-related paranoid ideation or severe dissociative symptoms.

The current conceptualization puts difficulties in interpersonal relationship at the top of the rung. This reinforces the notion that the condition is being designed primarily in terms of how it impacts on others rather than the person with BPD. Seen in this way, it appears to be an 'externalizing' rather than an 'internalizing' disorder. Evidence suggests that the person with BPD suffers intensely due to their affective instability and impaired sense of self. How they impact others can only be changed by helping them deal with the pathological processes within themselves. As impaired attachment and childhood maltreatment are likely to have contributed to the development of BPD, by emphasising the primacy to impaired relationship, we may covertly once again make them feel like being the perpetrator rather than the victim of failed social processes.

Each person is the centre of his or her universe. There are concentric circles that emerge from there. People depending on their closeness occupy different circles at a given time and may move from one to another circle for a variety of reasons. To start with the parents and siblings are in the most immediate circle. They may all be subject to similar factors may determine the pattern of interpersonal relationship issues that define the person's relationship with others.

In an existential format, the criteria could be conceptualized as a pervasive pattern of instability of affective control associated with impaired sense of self and instability of interpersonal relationships:

A. Instability in affective control would include Criteria 6 and 8
B. Impaired sense of self would include Criteria 3, 4, 5, 7 and 9.
C. Instability of interpersonal relationships would include Criteria 1 and 2

Diagnosis would include presence of both symptoms in clusters A and C and two or more from cluster B. Difficulty in affective control should be accorded the most significance. It is this aspect of the person that is more likely to lead to problems with self-image and in turn difficulties in interpersonal relationships.

It is commonplace for a diagnosis of personality disorder to be used to justify a decision not to admit someone to a psychiatric ward, or even to be accepted for treatment – a practice that understandably puzzles and irritates the staff of accident and emergency departments, general practitioners, and probation officers, who find themselves left to cope as best they can with extremely difficult, frustrating people without any psychiatric assistance (Kendell 2002).

Lewis and Appleby (1988) showed that suicide attempts and other behaviours by patients previously diagnosed as having personality disorders were commonly regarded as manipulative and under voluntary control. They were regarded as irritating, attention-seeking, difficult to manage and unlikely to comply with advice or treatment.

THE MANY BORDERS OF BORDERLINE PERSONALITY DISORDER

The term borderline first emerged in the 1950s. It was first used to describe patients lying on the border of psychosis and neurosis. Knight (1953) is credited with paving the way for the emergence of the modern concept of BPD. He pointed to some patients who developed psychotic symptoms during psychoanalysis. He considered it to be a clinical state related to schizophrenia and not a personality disorder. Kernberg (1967) was one of the most influential figures in describing borderline as a condition with enduring characteristics one sees in personality disorder.

Grinker and colleagues (1968) did a cluster analysis and produced four subtypes: (1) the psychotic border; (2) the core borderline syndrome; (3) the adaptive, affectless, defended, as-if person; and (4) the border with neuroses.

Gunderson and Singer (1975) proposed five aspects of the diagnosis: (1) affect (anger, depression, anxiety, and anhedonia); (2) behaviour (less impulse control and often with sexual problems); (3) brief psychotic episodes; (4) superficial relationships; and (5) deviant thought processes on projective testing. Perry and Klerman (1978) noted several problems with consistency while performing a comparison of all the models.

DSM-III (1980) came up with criteria set for BPD based on expert consensus. It provided a much-needed legitimacy and wider acceptance to borderline personality disorder.

Several factors influenced the wide-ranging interest in a diagnosis and treatment of borderline personality disorder:

1. The 1950s and 1960s had seen the emergence of several antipsychotic medications. There was a renewed interest in underpinning a biological root for common mental disorders. People with psychotic disorders were in long term care in mental hospitals. Psychiatrists were working from these facilities. Anything with a trace of psychosis was being labelled as schizophrenia and treated with antipsychotic medications.

2. In the 1960s and 1970s there was a growing conflict between those firmly entrenched in the psychoanalytic thinking and others with more biological leaning. The concept of borderline emerged from psychoanalytic school to underscore a new set of problems with greater psychological underpinning.

3. The 1970s saw a significant interest in the use of lithium. It gave rise to a new imperium of affective disorders. Anyone with a trace of a mood problem was seen to have some variant of affective/mood disorder. People with personality disorder responded poorly to medications and researchers were keen to exclude them from clinical trials.

4. The 1980s were marked by the arrival of DSM-III with a set of operationalized criteria for all disorders paving the way for research on borderline personality. Even though these criteria were derived through the consensus reached by 'experts' in their respective disorders, they acquired a great deal of legitimacy.

5. The 1990s saw the closure of all large mental hospitals. Psychiatry came to be practised from general hospitals and clinics and in government and private settings. Crisis assessment and treatment

(CAT) teams were set up to cover a perceived chaos that could follow as part of the massive shift in care provision. There was an expressed fear about what could happen when all those people with chronic psychosis were relocated in the community at large. Emergency departments of general hospitals were also exposed to people with severe mental symptoms and ill-equipped to deal with so many people suffering severe mental and behavioural problems. Crisis teams and acute response teams became the interface between the smaller psychiatric units and the community. The gate keepers jealously guarded entry into the system and people with BPD were seen as undeserving of the scarce resources.

6. As people who did not appear to be obviously psychotic or severely depressed, were turned away from emergency departments and by CAT teams a greater desperation ensued. Repeat presenters had to show even more extreme behaviours to gain attention and care. A set of patients with self-injurious behaviour were increasingly labelled as suffering from BPD.

7. Much of the notoriety of Borderline disorder was a result of Psychiatry itself being in a state of transition. Specialist services were created to deal with borderline personality disorder. These were driven by both political and economic consideration.

All forms of treatments have been tried for BPD, including low dose antipsychotics, antidepressants, mood stabilisers and various forms of therapy. From time to time the superiority of one over the other has been claimed. Treatment provided by specialist services do not appear to have a clear advantage. BPD remains terribly and unfairly stigmatized. Any reasonable treatment provided by reasonable clinicians in a reasonable manner has proven beneficial to persons with BPD (Zanarini).

At the core of all therapies is validation. This is achieved through an accepted treatment framework in which there is a consensus on the goals of treatment, a collaborative approach and consensus on how to achieve the goals and a therapeutic relationship. Therapy needs to be focused on achieving a change, not only in overt behaviour, but the whole person.

In the words of Yalom (1980): "Borderline is the word that strikes terror in the heart of the middle-aged comfort-seeking psychiatrist." What the specialist services were able to provide is training for many clinicians who would otherwise shy away from seeing anyone with a hint of BPD. The treatments most endorsed are therapies based on the principles of mindfulness.

Almost three decades since the closure of large mental hospitals society and the medical fraternity are no longer as tense about the predicted and feared mayhem. We are more at ease with people obviously mentally unwell living in our midst. The dreaded calls for help by patients with attempted self-harm has abated. We may have found a new equilibrium in the presentation of mental distress and our response to it.

Many specialist services for personality disorder continue to believe that severe personality disorder in general and borderline personality disorder in particular is a true illness. They cite genetic/familial data and some biological studies as the true biological underpinning for these disorders. They even believe that one day there could be a pill for these disorders. It is a surprisingly reductionist view of psychopathology. We are still seeking professional legitimacy by treating 'real' medical conditions.

As we have discussed throughout the book, biology is important in whatever works and does not work. Physiology is not all there is to human life. Physiology interacts with our experiential self as well as our physical, social, cultural, political world and our ability to make sense of all our experiences.

Our existence can never be reduced to any unidimensional mode of understanding.

All diseases may be biological, but everything biological is not disease. All human psychological experience is mediated by the brain which will always react biologically to every psychological experience. Showing MRI changes in borderline personality disorder does nothing to demonstrate a disease condition.

Psychiatry is a speciality always dealing with ambiguity. If we are unable to work with the complexity of human existence, then we should not be psychiatrists.

Nancy Andreasen (2001) pointed out: "I think most of us became psychiatrists because we are interested in what makes human beings tick. We choose psychiatry because we want to understand the human mind and spirit as well as the human brain. We choose to join a very clinical speciality because we are interested in people, and we want to work with them as individual people. We like to think about them within the social matrix they live to skilfully elicit a 'life narrative' that summarises their past and current experiences, and to use that information to understand how their symptoms arise and can be treated. Every person we encounter is a new adventure, a new voyage of discovery, a new life story, a new person. Although some patterns generalise across individuals, each patient is unique. This is what makes psychiatry challenging, intellectually rich, complex, and even enjoyable-despite the fact that we often care for people who suffer intensely and for whom we wish we could offer even more help."

THE CONTINUM OF PSYCHOPATHOLOGY

(ALL PSYCHOPATHOLOGY CAN BE SEEN AS AN EXTENSION OF PERSONALITY PATHOLOGY)

The importance of the person and hence the personality in all kinds of illness and their treatment has always been recognized. Hippocrates, universally regarded as the Father of Medicine (Circa 460 BCE to 370 BCE) said: 'It is more important to know, what sort of person has a disease than to know what sort of disease a person has.' William Osler (1849-1919) widely considered to be the modern Hippocrates, also taught students that they treat the person and not the disease. They needed to pay attention to the wishes, beliefs, and fears of the person who had the disease.

Abnormal personality types have been recognized and talked about for a long time. However, psychiatry as a speciality was caught up in trying to deal with the major mental illnesses in large mental asylums. Freud pioneered an increase in the scope of psychiatry by bringing the psychoneuroses in its gambit. Initial attention on various personality disorders focused on seeing them both as discreet entities as well as attenuated forms of major mental illnesses: paranoid, schizoid, and schizotypal disorder on the spectrum of schizophrenia; cyclothymia as attenuated forms of manic-depressive-illness, obsessive-compulsive personality on the spectrum of OCD, hysterical personality on the spectrum of psychoneuroses.

Personality disorders are thought to be underdiagnosed relative to their prevalence among people with various mental disorders. One thing that most clinicians and researchers in the field of personality disorder can agree on is that the current classification systems have serious limitations (Mulder and Tyrer 2019). Furthermore, there was no conclusive proof that there were 8-10 discrete categories of personality disorder.

The distinction between personality disorder and mental illness is complex. Wakefield (1982) argued that mental disorders were biological dysfunctions that were also harmful. The evidence that personality disorders are harmful is quite strong and not restricted to clinic population (Kendell 2002). Drake and Vaillant (1985) showed that compared to 283 men without personality disorders, 86 personality disordered men had poor mental health (79% to 14%), poor occupational performance and job satisfaction, and poor social competence (58% to 10%), and although alcohol dependence or misuse was partly responsible for their poor occupational performance, it made little contribution to their poor mental health and social competence.

People with personality disorders are at increased risk of several mental disorders, including depression and anxiety disorders, suicide and parasuicide, and misuse or dependence on alcohol and other drugs. Tyrer and Moulder (2022) conclude that all psychiatric disorders have high rates of cooccurrence with personality disorder – usually about 50%. This implies that personality disorders or behaviours encompassed by individual personality disorder categories are important conceptually, prognostically, and regarding treatment.

According to Kendell (2002), although it is difficult to provide irrefutable arguments that personality disorders are mental disorders, it is equally difficult to argue with conviction that they are not. The behaviour and attitudes that define personality disorders are graded traits present to a lesser degree in many other people, and quite different in different types of personality disorders. He concluded that the distinction between illness and personality disorder is starting to break down.

Most schizophrenic illnesses have the same time course as a personality disorder (onset in adolescence and persisting throughout adult life). The genetic bases of affective personality disorders and mood disorders, and of schizotypal personality disorders and schizophrenia have much in common.

Avoidant personality disorder has so much in common with the mental illness known as generalised anxiety disorder and social phobia. Recognition of these problems were responsible for many to question the value of distinguishing between Axis I and Axis II in DSM-III and DSM-IV.

The clinical utility of the severity classification of personality disorder has been demonstrated in recent studies. Research suggests that in common disorders like depression and anxiety, personality disorder of any severity hindered a positive outcome. Sanatinia et al (2016) in a study in which 381 (86%) had some personality dysfunction with 184 (41%) satisfying the ICD criteria for personality disorder. Those with no personality dysfunction showed no treatment differences and worse social function with CBT compared with standard care, whereas all other personality groups showed greater improvement with CBT maintained over 2 years. Less benefit was shown in those with more severe personality disorder. Costs were less with CBT except for non-significant greater differences in those with moderate or severe personality disorder. These findings remained true even at 5-year follow-up (Tyrer 2017).

It has been pointed out that the simplest plausible socio-political definition is that a condition be regarded as a disease, if it is agreed to be undesirable (an explicit value judgement), and, if it seems on balance that physicians (or health professionals in general) and their technologies are more likely to be able to deal with it effectively than any of the other alternatives (Kendell 2002). There is ample evidence for treatment to make a significant difference in the outcome for BPD. Therefore, WHO took seriously the concerns being expressed that access to services for patients with borderline PD, which has increasingly been achieved in some countries based on arguments of treatment efficacy, might be seriously undermined." Thus, the WHO believed the inclusion of a Borderline pattern category to be a "pragmatic compromise" (Reed 2018).

THE HYPOTHESIS OF A "P FACTOR" OF PSYCHOPATHOLOGY

Freud's biographer, Ernest Jones (1946) is credited to have first come up with the concept of a "p factor" in his valedictory address to the British Psychoanalytical Society. The p factor may underlie an individuals' propensity to develop all forms of psychopathology. Lahey et al (2012) provided the initial evidence for this model and it has been subsequently replicated by Caspi et al (2014).

The elaboration of the p-factor has been extrapolated from psychometric research in intelligence, which first proposed a general factor that is common to all items of mental tests. Cognitive abilities are dissociable into separate abilities, such as verbal skills, visuospatial skills, working memory and processing speed. Nevertheless, the general factor in intelligence (called the 'g' factor) summarizes those individuals who do well on one type of cognitive tests tend to do well on all other types of cognitive tests (Spearman 1904, Deary 2001). The g factor of cognitive abilities accounts for the positive correlation among all test scores.

Caspi and Moffitt (2018) in a landmark paper summarised the emerging literature that point towards the concept of a "One in all and all in one: The p factor." The correlated factor model identified propensities to specific forms of psychopathology (internalizing, externalizing and psychotic experiences), the general factor suggests that there is one common liability to all psychopathologies.

The p may represent: (1) a diffuse unpleasant affective state often termed '*neuroticism or negative emotionality*', or (2) '*poor impulse control over emotions*', or (3) '*deficits in intellectual function*'. Individuals with high levels of p experience greater cognitive problems in their everyday life according to people who know them well.

This is possible because: (1) low cognitive ability is a marker of neuroanatomical deficits that increase vulnerability to multiple different common psychiatric disorders. (2) low cognitive ability increases both exposure and vulnerability to life stressors. (3) low cognitive ability reduces mental health literacy, which precludes early help-seeking, prevents access to evidence-based care, and reduces treatment adherence. (D) A fourth hypothesis is that p captures the disordered form and content of thought that permeates the extreme of practically every disorder.

Disordered thought process occurs in the context of affective disorder, anxiety disorders, eating disorders, post-traumatic stress disorder, somatoform disorders, dissociative disorders, substance use disorders, and antisocial disorders.

Disordered thought processes are illogical, unfiltered, tangential, and reality distorted and distorting cognitions. Examples include not only delusions and hallucinations but also thought problems such as difficulty making decisions, ruminations, body image disturbances, intrusive thoughts, intrusive fears, reexperiencing trauma, dissociative states, belief that something terrible will happen if a behaviour is not performed. It appears possible that the symptoms of disordered thought process will prove to be the most diagnostic elements of p.

Caspi and Moffitt (2018) hypothesised that many young children exhibit diffuse emotional and behavioural problems, fewer go on to manifest a brief episode of an individual disorder, still fewer progress to develop a persistent internalizing or externalizing syndrome, and only a very few individuals progress to the extreme elevation of p, ultimately emerging with a psychotic condition, most likely during late adolescence or early adulthood. A developmental progression model would anticipate that when individuals are followed long enough, those with the most severe liability to psychopathology will tend to move in and out of diagnostic categories. This hypothesis is consistent with evidence that sequential comorbidity is the rule rather than the exception (Cerda et al 2008) and that individuals experiencing sequential comorbid disorders also exhibit more severe psychopathology.

A stress-diathesis model is used to explain the phenomenon. It involves stress embedding, generation, sensitization, and sensitivity. *(1) Stress embedding* occurs as neural changes in threat system lay down a vulnerability to later disorder. (2) *Stress generation* occurs as individuals who are maltreated behave in ways that contribute to the occurrence of other negative events in their lives, including further and new forms of victimization (revictimization). (3) *Stress sensitization* occurs as individuals who are exposed to early maltreatment are more vulnerable to disorders that are triggered by later, proximal stressors, many of which are brought about through stress generation. (4) *Stress sensitivity* (a process distinct from stress sensitization) suggest that some individuals are more sensitive to stress due to a putative, most likely genetically mediated trait.

AN EXISTENCIAL APPROACH SUPPORTS A CONTINUM OF PSYCHOPATHOLOGY

Psychopathology is limited, according to Jaspers, in that there can be no final analysis of human beings, since the more we reduce them to what is typical and normative the more we realise there is something hidden in every individual that defies recognition. We have to be content with partial knowledge of an infinity that we cannot exhaust.

The individual's personality could possibly be the p factor of psychopathology. Existential feelings are background orientations through which everything that we perceive, feel, think, or act upon is structured (Ratcliffe 2008). They constitute how we find ourselves in the world in general. According to Gross (2002) emotion regulation refers to the processes which influence which emotions we have, when we have them, and how we experience and express them. Hence, one of life's great challenges is successfully regulating emotions. Stephan (2012) added the additional task of successfully regulating existential feelings as they pre structure many, if not all our encounters with the world.

Fear of death or 'ceasing to exist' is particularly important for those who are conscious of their existence. Otto Rank in his essay, "Life Fear and Death Fear" talked about a basic dynamic that illuminates the relationship between the two defences. Rank felt that there is in the individual a primal fear that manifests itself sometimes as a fear of life sometimes as a fear of death. By "fear of life" Rank meant anxiety in the face of a loss of connection with a greater whole. The fear of having to face life as an isolated being. The prototypical fear was "birth" the original trauma, and the original separation. By "fear of death" Rank referred to the fear of extinction, of loss of individuality, of being dissolved again into the whole.

Between these two fear possibilities, these poles of fear, the individual is thrown back and forth all his life. Life anxiety emanates from the defences of specialness. It is the price that we pay for standing out, unshielded from nature. Death anxiety is the toll of fusion, when one gives up autonomy, one loses oneself and suffers a kind of death. Death anxiety is the starting point of all stress and how well we cope with that anxiety underlies all aspects of life and illness. Avoiding anxiety is like choosing to be frozen in adolescence.

It is possible that psychopathology may come in two forms: (1) psychopathology limited and (2) psychopathology unlimited. This may be determined by the balance between degrees of vulnerability and protective factors operating in an individual. When the balance favours the protective factors, they may present with more specific psychopathology e.g., MDD, specific phobias, specific anxiety disorder. With increasing disbalance they may present with two or more domains of psychopathology. Someone with severe personality disorder is likely to show the whole gamut of psychopathology, either at once or at separate times, or in various combinations.

Several converging lines of evidence point to a continuity between aspects of personality (difficulty and disorder) to all forms of psychopathology. Human existence is governed by the concerns regarding life and death; a state of being and non-being. The exceedingly high chance of comorbidity is a major challenge to the specificity and reliability of diagnostic categories. The age of onset of most major mental disorders is in the teens and early adulthood.

A Danish register study (covering nearly two decades and nearly 6 million individuals) showed that patients do meet the criteria for many different diagnoses in turn, every mental disorder diagnosed was associated with an increased risk that the patient will be diagnosed at another time with other disorders, both inside and outside the index disorder's family (Plana-Ripoll 2019).

In the Dunedin longitudinal study, the onset of a mental disorder occurred by adolescence for 59% of the participants (Caspi et al 2020). This is also the age of greatest vulnerability for a maturing personality. It follows that a chink in personality development may be an incredibly significant factor in producing further psychopathology. The study also replicated the Danish register findings that patients in psychiatric clinics tend to experience diverse disorders in turn, and every disorder is associated with elevated risk for every other disorder.

A secure attachment allows one to develop a sense of security and explore our world comfortably. We develop a good sense of self and develop resilience and competence. We are on a path to greater self-reliance and self-actualization. Lack of a secure attachment and childhood maltreatment may predispose us to significant vulnerability. Diverse kinds of vulnerability and protective factors may underlie the kind of psychopathology one develops. We can start by trying to understand the person before we try to understand the symptoms they display and hence a categorical diagnosis. Otherwise, we can first work on the immediate cause for concern and then look at the meaning of the symptoms. A third and possibly the best approach is to see both person and the illness at the same time. One cannot understand why a person presents with a particular set of symptoms, without a good understanding of what it means to be that person at this time.

The boundaries demarcating the different disorders are ever so much fuzzier in real life than they appear on paper (Frances 2013). Diseases may be real objective entities, but they happen to individual human beings with feelings, power to think and repertoire of behaviour. Mental disorders are too heterogeneous in presentation and in causality to be considered simple diseases; instead, each of our currently defined disorders will eventually turn out to be many different diseases (Frances 2013). Sometimes these are not disease states but a disorder of personality which predisposes one to feel, think, and act in a certain way. It is possible that one or more personality traits that predispose to increased problems of living and the emergence and elaboration of certain forms of psychopathology.

In an influential article *On Being Sane in Insane Places* Rosenhan (1973) illustrated some of the difficulties in psychiatric diagnoses. Eight sane people gained secret admission to twelve different hospitals located in five different states of US complaining of hearing voices. Soon after admission the 'pseudo patients' ceased simulating any symptoms of abnormality and behaved normally. All of them (with only one exception) were admitted with a diagnosis of schizophrenia and each was discharged with a diagnosis of schizophrenia 'in remission.' The length of admission varied from 7 to 52 days, with an average of 19 days. The conclusion drawn was that physicians operate with a strong tendency towards type 2 error (being more inclined to call a healthy person sick) than type 1 error (call a sick person healthy).

Rosenhan commented: "Whenever the ratio of what is known to what needs to be known approaches zero, we tend to invent "knowledge" and assume that we understand more than what we actually do. We seem unable to acknowledge that we simply do not know." "Rather than acknowledge that we are just embarking on understanding, we continue to label patients 'schizophrenic', 'manic-depressive', and 'insane', as if in those words we have captured the essence of understanding."

The difficulties in diagnostic distinction between distinct categories of mental disorders and the distinction between mental disorders and personality disorder remain unresolved problems. The view in the ICD II group was that if categories were to be used, they had to be part of a dimension, not independent elements, and this can be argued for all psychiatric disorders (Tyrer 2019). These dimensions may independently and in various combinations predispose us to diverse kinds of psychopathology and play a role in our response to various kinds of treatment. The person that we are is the most significant fact of our lives. It exists even when we are asleep or casting no shadows anywhere. Life, growth, senescence, health, and illness all occur within the self that characterise us as a person.

Suris et al (2016) concluded that "in the foreseeable future, we will continue to diagnose psychiatric disorders the old-fashioned way: by taking history and assessing the currently accepted criteria to make diagnoses as they are provided in the established classification system." Without accurate diagnosis, appropriate treatment cannot be selected, the prognosis cannot be known, communication about disease between clinicians and scientists in medical field will suffer, and research will not advance – ironically, the very biologic research that the field needs to further advance the diagnostic criteria of psychiatry.

From an existential viewpoint: "Psychopathology is a vector – the resultant of anxiety and the individual's anxiety-combating defences, both neurotic and characterological" (Yalom 1980). Humanism is individual and existential. Humans are complex beings. We not only exist, but we are also possibly most conscious of both our existence as well as have a concept of non-existence. Our consciousness includes not only a sense of self, but also that of other people, other living beings, vegetations, objects and the environment. We develop a narrative of self and all our surroundings. We continuously observe through our senses, make mental impressions of what we observe, create images, analyse, and interpret them through the passage of life. Our experiences shape us from birth to death and we also try to imagine what would happen to us beyond death and to those who will survive us.

We are incessant narrators of stories about almost anything in our lives (Damasio 2018). We happily colour our narratives with all the biases of our past experiences and our likes and dislikes. So much of what we commit to memory concerns not the past but the anticipated future, the future that we have only imagined for us and for our ideas. We live part of our lives in the anticipated future.

Personality disorders refer to a stable pattern in how someone's sense-making goes astray over time. Sense-making refers to how the world is opened to me, to how I experience the world, and this is what is disordered in the case of personality disorder.

I THE BASICS OF EXISTENCE

We have no basic concept in terms of which we can define man nor any theory that would wholly cover his actual, objective existence (Jaspers 1959). We have no psychic master-plan. Freedom of action, conscious reflection and qualities of intellect and spirit can be considered as the fundamentals of humanity.

Feelings describe our subjective perception of emotional states and their accompanying somatic responses. The existence of feelings can at present only be assessed by verbal report – and therefore is currently uniquely accessible to study only in humans (Anderson and Adoloph 2014). Feelings are possibly the most important aspect of our existence that makes us uniquely human. According to modern evolutionary theory, different emotions evolved at separate times. Humans possess a small set of so-called "basic" emotions, including happiness, anger, disgust, and sadness. Besides them, we also possess primal, filial, and social emotions and they have been discussed in previous sections.

Damasio (2018) in his book "The strange Order of things" has elaborated on 'life, feelings, and the making of cultures.' Humans are biological, psychological, as well as social entities and the three aspects of their existence are always interacting with each other and influencing each other in return. "There is no being, in the proper sense of the term, without a spontaneous mental experience of a life, a feeling of existence." He believes that feelings have not been given the credit they deserve as motives, monitors, and negotiators of human cultural endeavours.

"Feelings are the mental expressions of homeostasis, while homeostasis, acting under the cover of feeling, is the functional thread that links early life forms to the extraordinary partnership of bodies and nervous systems. Feelings tell the mind whether any situation or process is in good or bad direction. This happens intuitively without the need for any spoken words."

II EXISTENCE AS A PHYSIOLOGICAL CONSTRUCT

Humans are multicellular organism with multiple organs and systems which are intricately linked and interdependent. These systems have evolved over a long time from unicellular organisms to multicellularity of increasing complexity. The emergence of the nervous system enabled homeostasis to be better modulated. Any good understanding of our existence must start with a functional physiological system. Our body, brain, and mind are part of the physiology.

Feelings are also part of our physiology. They provide valuable information about the state of life. The experience of feeling is imbued with valence which is its defining element. "Valence" translates the condition of life as good, bad, or in between. When we experience a condition that is conducive to the continuation of life, we describe it in positive terms and call it pleasant. Repeated encounters with the same class of triggering situations and consequent feelings allows us to internalize the feeling.

The Intellectualization of feelings is an exercise in the economy of the time and energy necessary for the process. Feelings are for life regulation. They tell us about risks, dangers, and ongoing crises that need to be averted. They play a role in our decisions and permeate our existence.

III EXISTENCE AS A PSYCHOLOGICAL CONSTRUCT (Mind)

Besides being a biological being, we also have a psychological existence. We have a brain and a mind. Brain is the organ of the mind and mind is one of the many functions of the brain. When we say mind, it does not make it any less biological. All human psychological experiences are mediated by the brain, and each person has one brain; therefore, the brain will always be biologically changing as we have psychological experiences (Ghaemi 2007).

Our mind can be imagined as a musical performance, played by several hidden orchestras. There are two groups of instruments. First, the main sensory devices with which the world around and inside an organism interacts with the nervous system. Second, the device that continuously respond emotively to the mental presence of any object or event. The devices are known as drives, motivations, and emotions. Over the 'playing time,' their actions result in certain kind of music, the music of our thoughts and feelings and of the meanings that emerge from the inner narratives that they help construct (Damasio 2018).

Feelings and reason, Damasio explains, are involved in an inescapable looping, reflective embrace. The embrace can favour one of the partners, but it involves both. The collections of questions, explanations, consolidation, discoveries, and inventions required a motive. Alleviation of pain and suffering particularly in contrast to pleasure and flourishing provided the necessary incentive. Humans developed extended cognitive and language abilities, the ability to think beyond what could be immediately perceived, the ability to interpret and diagnose a situation as well as understanding cause and effects.

IV EXISTENCE AS A SOCIO-CULTURAL CONSTRUCT (Being part of a society and culture)

Besides our biology and psychology, we also live in a social matrix. Our social connections are determined by our biology and psychology. Most drives, motivations, and emotions are inherently social. Their field of action extend well beyond the individual. Desire and lust, caring and nurturing, attachment, and love, all operate in a social context. The same applies to most instances of joy and sadness, fear and panic, anger or of compassion, admiration and awe, envy, and jealousy and contempt. Conscious feeling and creative intelligence helped in the rise of human cultures. They in turn helped tame aggression. Humans are social animals and there is an ongoing struggle between the self and the collective self. We learn the art of mutual coexistence.

Most provoked feelings result from engaging emotions that relate not just to the isolated individuals but to the individual in the context of others. Beneficial sociality is rewarding and improves homeostasis, while aggressive sociality does the opposite (Damasio 2018). Nature and nurture stand in reciprocity, not opposition (Eisenberg 2000). Children inherit, along with their parents' genes, their parents, their peers, and the communities they inhabit (Eisenberg 1995).

The ontogenetic niche (West and King 1987) is a legacy that structures development, a crucial link between parents and offspring, an envelope of life changes. Whether a child acquires any language at all, let alone a specific language, is determined by the child's linguistic community. The degree of linguistic competence attained is a function of nature, nurture, and niche (Eisenberg 1995).

Humans are unique in the extent of their reliance on socially transmitted information in coping with physical and social environment. An important class of emotions consist of those which mediate the acquisition, use, and dissemination of cultural information. On a larger scale, conformity to cultural values, beliefs, and practices makes behaviour predictable and allows for the advent of complex coordination and cooperation. Shame and pride motivate an assessment of prevailing norms and awareness of the presence of observers and conformity to pervasive expectations under observation (Anderson and Adoloph 2014).

Our experiential base is dependent on our family, society, and culture. These experiences shape us and make us to a substantial extent the person we become. They also help us in our ability to make sense of everything. Our coping skills or the lack of it is significantly influenced by them.

Two hundred years ago, Pinel wrote about the psychiatric risks associated with unexpected reverses or adverse circumstances, and his initial question to newly admitted psychiatric patients was: "Have you suffered vexation, grief or reverse of fortune?" Since the beginnings of psychiatric practice, there has been a recognition that negative life experiences and stressful happenings may serve to precipitate mental disorders (Garmezy & Rutter, 1985). There is a very impressive literature on the link between adverse life experiences and mental disorders. Eugene Paykel (1980) worked out a Life Event Scale that has been widely used over the years.

However, adverse factors are not a sentence to doom. Every child of parents who are alcoholics do not turn out to be alcoholic. Rutter (1985) in an elegant study on 9 to 10 years old in the Isle of Wight and the Inner London borough, showed that children often show remarkable resilience in the face of adversity.

The theme of the 2021 Mental Health Services Conference in October and the 2022 Annual Meeting in May was "Socio-political Determinants: Practice, Policy, and Implementation" to highlight the social determinants of mental health. Vivian Pender, the President of American Psychiatric Association emphasised that the risk factors for many common mental disorders were heavily associated with social inequalities, whereby the greater the inequality, the higher the inequality in risk." In other words, people do not necessarily start with the same opportunities or resources (inequity), and social factors further divide us. This suggests that our psychiatric patients suffer from biopsychosocial determinants that could have been prevented in the first place.

These social determinants of mental health more generally encompass multiple co-occurring factors, such as:

- **Social factors**, including racism, adverse childhood experiences, discrimination, and social exclusion based on race, ethnicity, gender, age, or mental illness; health care inequity due to lack of access to care; and exposure to violence and the criminal justice system.

- **Economic factors** related to resources, lack of education, employment insecurity, and neighbourhood poverty that have cumulative effects on an individual.

- **Built-environment factors**, including housing; pollution of the air, water, and ground; and climate change.

- **Structural factors**, including cultural norms; systemic policies; and laws and regulations that institutionalize disparities for populations, such as Black, Indigenous, Hispanic, rural, and other minority communities.

V INTERACTIVE MODEL OF EXISTENCE

Of central interest to psychiatry is the fact that evolution has shaped the development of the brain, the organ of mental functions or what we call the mind (Guze 1989). He asserted that 'there is no such thing as a psychiatry that is too biological.' All brain functions, including perception, learning, thought, memory, emotions, communication, language etc. reflect the results of such evolution. However, people learn differently, perceive differently, and think differently as the result of different genotypes interacting with different and constantly varying environments (both internal and external to the organism).

There is no mental function without brain, mind, and a social context. There is no existence without a physical/physiological self, but the 'I' that exists would be quite different, if the context in which it exists were different. A brainless or mindless psychiatry or either of the two without a social construct of the brain provides an incomplete picture of our existence. None of the three makes psychiatry any less biological. Kety (1960) had pointed out: 'It requires as much oxygen to think an irrational thought as to think a rational one.'

Daniel Kahneman (2012) in his book *Thinking Fast and Slow* distilled a lifetime of work on the engine of human thinking. He showed our brains to be highly evolved to perform many tasks with great efficiency. However, they are often ill-suited to accurately carry out some tasks. He introduced the two ways in which our mind operates: "(1) System 1 operates automatically and quickly, with little or no effort and no sense of voluntary control. (2) System 2 allocates attention to the effortful mental activities that demand it, including complex computations. The operations of System 2 are often associated with the subjective experience of agency, choice and concentration." These two systems somehow co-exist in the human brain and together help us navigate life. They are not literal or physical systems but are only conceptual. System 1 is an intuitive and cannot be turned off. It helps us perform most of the cognitive tasks that everyday life requires, such as identify threats, navigate our way home on familiar roads, know that 2+2=4, recognize friends, and so on. System 2 can help us analyse complex problems, do math exercises, do crossword puzzles, and so on. Even though System 2 is useful, it takes effort and energy to engage it. So, it tends to take shortcuts at the behest of System 1. Lot of times we use system 2 thinking only to justify our system 1 thinking.

Whatever is easier for System 2 is more likely to be believed. Ease arises from idea repetition, clear display, a primed idea, and even one's own good mood. It turns out that even the repetition of a falsehood can lead people to accept it, despite knowing it is untrue, since the concept becomes familiar and is cognitively easy to process. Our System 1 is "a machine for jumping to conclusions" by basing its conclusion on "What You See Is All There Is" (WYSIATI). WYSIATI is the tendency for System 1 to draw conclusions based on the readily available, sometimes misleading information and then, once made, to believe in those conclusions fervently. The measured impact of halo effects, confirmation bias, framing effects, and base-rate neglect are aspects of jumping to conclusions in practice. One example is confirmation bias, where we are more open to and looking for evidence that supports our beliefs, rather than what does not. Rationally, we should look for evidence that contradicts beliefs since that will subject our belief system to greater scrutiny. But outside of the rigors of pure science, such an approach is uncommon. (In the sciences, one methodology is to construct a so-called null hypothesis, the rejection of which proves the original claim. The alpha is usually set at 0.05, which still means that there is one in twenty chances of it being false).

Kahneman saw humans as a product of their evolutionary environment and in many ways ill-equipped to deal with a rational, science-based, logical world. Worse, they are at constant risk of repeating the same cognitive errors and biases, easily manipulated, and riven by irrational beliefs and fears. In a reality that is dominated by science and statistics, most of humankind lacks the basic knowledge and experience to thrive. A tiny minority with those capabilities can manipulate others and command great wealth. As a result, global wealth inequality has continued to rise over modern times.

Eisenberg (1986) observed that there is not now, nor can there be, a technical service capable of transducing brain structure or chemistry into social meaning. Neither a brainless or mindless psychiatry or either of the two without a social construct of the brain can provide a complete picture of our existence.

Minds depend on the presence of nervous systems charged with helping life run efficiently in their respective bodies, and on a host of interactions of nervous system and bodies. The minds are enriched by feelings and subjectivity, image-based memory, and the ability to enchain images in narratives that probably began as nonverbal film-like sequences but eventually, after the emergence of verbal language, combined verbal, and nonverbal elements. The ability to generate images opened the way for organisms to represent the world around them. Advanced nervous systems as ours fabricate images of the outside world and images of the world inside us. For this we use our senses. The location of four of the five specialised senses is in the head. And they are both physically and physiologically close to each other. The specialization of each of these sense organs is truly remarkable (Damasio 2018).

We return to the four-dimensional model of human existence which includes: 1) the physiological self, 2) the experiential self, 3) the sociocultural self, and 4) the existential self. It is the consciousness of our existential self that necessitates having to make sense of all that is within and around us. Usually, psychiatric disorders involve in some way or the other all the four aspects of our existence. However, not all criteria need to be fulfilled in all disorders. In different disorders the emphasis may be on distinct aspects and the suffering and problems with the existential stance may even be absent. Neither normality nor psychopathology has strict boundaries.

De Haan (2020) identified the four general characteristics of pathological sense making:

THE APPROPRIATENESS OF SENSE-MAKING: Sense-making is always about something specific and in a particular situation. What makes an experience, reaction, or sense-making pathological is the context. For example, grief is a way of relating to one's situation, but depression is not a meaningful connection to the world.

Our sense-making is, to a significant extent, just 'common sense'. Sensemaking has: (1) universal aspects (we all have a body but we are also social creatures, with similar needs and vulnerabilities), (2) sociocultural aspects (we are brought up in a certain community with specific norms and practices), and (3) idiosyncratic aspects (depending on our specific life histories and experiences).

THE FLEXIBILITY OF SENSE-MAKING: Psychiatric disorders often involve a 'freezing' of a certain sense-making. Self-fulfilling prophecies can create a vicious circle rigidifying a particular pattern of thinking and interaction. People who think nobody will find them interesting will (unconsciously) make themselves invisible.

People may withdraw as: (1) a direct result of their disorder (such as social anxiety or depression and schizophrenia), (2) an experience of estrangement (of being out of tune with the rest of the world), (3) practical reasons to avoid social situations (OCD with fear of germs, eating disorder with dread of eating socially), and (4) being ashamed of their condition.

THE FLEXIBILITY OF STANCE-TAKING: Our existential stance provides the freedom to maintain a flexible and relative stance. We can take a different perspective on oneself and one's situation. That flexibility may be 'hijacked' by a psychiatric disorder. Depression not only affects the primary interactions with the (social) world, but also one's existential stance so that one cannot imagine even being happy again. Delusions often involve improbable, inept, or even bizarre notions held with conviction.

THE EXPERIENCE OF SUFFERING: People whose stance-making has become stuck in a rigid pattern and thus out of tune with their actual situation often suffer as a result. At times it may be that people closest to them are the ones suffering most from their affliction.

Sense-making discloses a world significant to the person. It offers to them various possibilities for action. Many actions may be performed unthinkingly, while others are motivated by specific goals we may pursue. Van den Berg (1972) said '. . .when the psychiatric patient tells what his world looks like, he states, without detours and without mistakes, what he is like. This is because 'our world is our home, a realization of subjectivity.' They reflect our relation to time, to others, and to our surroundings in general.

Life experiences are the foundations on which our stories are formed. Once composed in our mind, a story sticks in our memory. For the person, 'understanding' means retrieving these stories and applying them to new experiences. For the listener it means mapping the speaker's stories onto the listener's stories. Different people understand the same story differently precisely because the stories they already know are different. People are constantly questioning themselves and each other to find out why someone has done what he has done and what the consequences are likely to be. A therapist is better equipped to understand the stories and help make better sense of them and help the patient arrive at a better story about himself one freer of morbidity and self-condemnation.

TREATMENT CONSIDERATIONS

Ayurvedic medicine (the ancient Hindu system) was based on a balance between the various forces in the body. Other ancient systems also emphasised balance. According to humoralism, four bodily fluids—blood, yellow bile, black bile, and phlegm—determined a person's temperament and an imbalance led to certain sicknesses dependent upon which humours were in excess or deficit. The germ theory led us to a dream-world of simplicity that we have failed to replicate in most conditions as there are no germs to be found. We keep looking for simplicity and try to shy away from embracing the complexity of our existence.

It would be simplistic to expect that there is one solid diagnostic entity (such as Major Depressive Disorder) which can be explained by one causal factor (chemical imbalance of one or more neurotransmitters) that can be remedied by the administration of a chemical agent (one of the many antidepressants) or a physical method of treatments (ECT or TMS). Such fairy tales do not exist in real life. We are unlikely to once again find another situation that arose from the discovery of Treponema pallidum as the cause for the General Paralysis of the Insane and then find penicillin that will lead to a cure and empty large chunks of mental hospitals beds that these patients once occupied.

In recent times psychiatry has gone through a kind of existential crisis of its own. Psychiatric services have been renamed as Mental Health Services. This is an ambitious leap of faith. We are still struggling to define and understand mental illness and that is a far cry away from understanding mental health. Part of the reason for the change could be the democratization of services. Psychologists and social worker may be more comfortable with the title 'Mental health services' where they feel like being equal partners as opposed to working within 'psychiatric services' which may convey a sense of working under the leadership of psychiatrist.

An unfortunate consequence of this move is the use of the terms like 'client' and 'service provider.' Using the language of the market economy may have the undesired consequence of a rarefied therapeutic relationship. Let us be honest about our limitations. Psychiatry is a limited speciality, and psychiatrists are trained in mental disorders. The gulf between mental disorders and mental health is quite wide. There are many shades of grey between the black of mental disorders and the white of mental health. Medicine is not labelled as physical health. It is hard to imagine how branches like Surgery and Obstetrics and Gynaecology can be named alternatively.

Creation of iconic institutions like the National Institute of Mental Health (NIMH) may have contributed towards this trend in psychiatry. Visiting the NIMH website illustrates the point well. It states that "The National Institute of Mental Health (NIMH) is the lead federal agency for research on mental disorders." The wide gulf between the banner and underlying function is obvious.

Users of the so called public funded "Mental Health Services" treat only mental disorders and that too only those which are considered severe. In practical terms a well-accepted pre-requisite for acceptance into the services is that the patient is either psychotic or suicidal with few exceptions. They are to a significant extent those at risk to themselves or others. The usual refrain is that they are only 'funded to serve such client group.' The pertinent question then is what purpose the veneer of 'mental health' serves? Does that make us feel-good, or it serves a political purpose?

Even our treatment outcome stops at sufficient reduction of symptoms rather than return to health. Concerns have been raised about the skill base of psychiatric trainees who are historically trained in such facilities where there is limited opportunity to see patients with less severe illness and disorders that are more highly prevalent in the community. In recognition of such limitations, a public-private partnership in training in psychiatry is being implemented. They are steps in the right direction.

There can be no confusion that psychiatrists are the leaders of psychiatry which is the branch of medicine that deals with mental disorders. However, if a psychiatrist wants to be just a psychopharmacologist, then they are possibly in the wrong speciality. Psychiatrists are best placed to be in the leading role working in collaboration with psychologists, social workers, welfare agencies, neuroscientists, pharmacologists, and people with lived experiences.

On the other hand, we must concede that knowing about mental disorder does not qualify us to be experts in mental health. Physical health cannot be defined as just the absence of a physical illness but depends on a variety of other factors which includes appropriate nutrition, good sanitation, good hygiene, proper education to name just a few. Similarly, mental health is not about the absence of a mental disorder but depends on many social, cultural, political, and other factors. Most of these are outside the purview of psychiatry.

As Charlton (1990) very succinctly put it: "Scientific specialities are no God given, eternal, immutable; they just happen to be the way we divide things up at present with particular purposes in mind so that we can understand and predict them". "Each science is a system of linked metaphors. To combine science will need a new system of metaphors: there is no point in mixing metaphors." All disciplines differentiated themselves from Metaphysics or Philosophy and once sufficiently differentiated, look for a philosophy of their own.

TWO OUNCES OF PREVENTION BEFORE EMBARKING ON A POUND OF CURE

Using an approach towards Mental Health can have two components: primary prevention and secondary prevention. Psychiatry will be better served if we do not try to assume a leadership role in primary prevention, because in doing so, we are making several assumptions that are likely to be controversial.

THE FIRST OUNCE OF PREVENTION: PRIMARY PREVENTION

Primary prevention is a huge undertaking. It needs a wholehearted commitment by the society at large and be embraced by the governments across the world. This would mean investment and not just creating slogans. At the basic level, primary prevention needs to start at two points.

The first point of primary prevention needs to target parents before they start embarking on to parenthood. It is so ironical that people need at least some training even to serve coffee or alcohol, but no training is required to undertake parenting, a task that is possibly the most complex, challenging, time-consuming, and life-changing that one would undertake. Out of all the role-transitions in life the transition to parenthood is the most complex and challenging. Antenatal classes occur only after a woman is pregnant and mostly concentrates on the birthing process. It is assumed that parenting just comes naturally to people as humanity has grown only through procreation. Many do have an intuitive understanding about it but that does not ensure a smooth ride. Lifestyle and processes have become increasingly more complex over time. The number of mothers who end up with a diagnosis of post-natal depression and anxiety is quite high. There is increasing recognition about fathers also suffering similarly.

A decision to become a parent is a tough one that is often taken more out of a societal expectation or a matter of course rather than a carefully considered decision. It is a choice that changes one's life altogether and forever. No one can ever be sure what the child would be like and how good the fit would be between the child's temperament and that of the parents. We need to create programs that allows people to understand what it means to be parents. Such programs could also explore why a couple wants to be a parent and the degree of commitment they have towards each other and about parenting.

The second point for primary prevention needs to focus on an ongoing education about health in general including mental health. Well informed parents can take the lead in an age-appropriate manner, setting reasonable limits and proper education and understanding. Such an effort should commence in primary school. We teach children prime numbers, algebra, and trigonometry and many more that the majority will never use over a lifetime but not enough about healthy life-styles, emotions, thoughts, wellness, and resilience. We need to take this with greater seriousness and sincerity. We need the skills of developmental and educational psychologists, social workers to provide leadership in collaboration with teachers and parents to devise age-appropriate teaching material and guidelines. These should become part of every educational institution and they need to be carefully monitored over time. Some work has been going on but there is a need for this to be taken more seriously and implemented uniformly.

Life is a continuous learning process and having the attitude: 'a student of life, and a student for a lifetime' can serve as a good model. Until we die there is still one learning to do and that is how to breathe our last, for no one can do it a second time.

THE SECOND OUNCE OF PREVENTION: SECONDARY PREVENTION

Based on the story highlighted so far it is necessary to accept the complexity inherent in our life and illness. There are many factors that play an important part in maintaining good health. These need to be seen as worth addressing as lifelong projects.

Our body is the basic unit of our existence. A healthy lifestyle is essential for our physiological integrity. This includes a good diet, regular exercise routine, maintaining a good sleep-wakefulness cycle, and avoiding an excess of everything. Keeping a regular schedule is not as easy as it seems. We have abundance of human-made light ready to disturb our sleep-wakefulness cycle and along with that the other biological rhythms. Gadgets available to us like television, computer, internet, and smartphones are major distracting forces. We are also encouraged to be driven towards greater achievement and to try and stretch ourselves towards creating a bigger splash on the world stage.

When people are stressed for whatever reason, two processes are happening simultaneously. There is a need to improve our ability to overcome the stressful situation, but at the same time stress makes us less efficient in doing so. A viscous cycle ensues, and all biological rhythms are likely to be out of tune. Stress is a major factor in burnout and that is drawing increased attention. These should be seen as an important part of clinical consultations and not be accorded just a passing interest. Developing good attitudes towards self and people around us (family, neighbours, and members of the society) allows for developing close confiding relationships and a sense of connectedness.

Our physiology works on a template that was formed about 40 to 50 thousand years ago. But the lifestyle we lead now is far removed from the times our body evolved and our current lifestyle emerged. To start with physical activity was driven by the need to hunt, gather, find water and shelter. Even after changing to growing food and looking after the other necessities of life, we were still using the only power available, and that was our body. Thanks to the gradually more organized life and societies that we live in where all our needs are met by technology and human cooperation and collaboration, we now need much less physical effort than ever. Lazarus (2020) suggested that many of the so-called 'Diseases of Ageing' could better be understood as 'Exercise Deficiency Diseases.' It is estimated that only about a quarter of the population is exercising.

We eat a lot more than what our physiology requires. We have more per capita food available than we ever had. We have much better production, distribution, storage, and preserving strategies than we ever had. We consume more than we need. We eat because it is time to eat rather than because we are hungry or need more nutrition. The result in a marked increase in proportion of the population that is overweight or obese.

Religion may play an important part in the life of many. It is worth trying to find out how significant is that for an individual. It is good to be able to support the functional aspect of their belief system and pay some attention to what may be causing distress. We must not forget that besides religious matters they also represent great philosophical traditions of their time and may hold significant benefit for some. If patients need religious counselling, then they can get it through their religious resources and systems. We must remember that people come to a psychiatrist because we are medical specialists and are renumerated for our specific skills in treating mental disorders.

TREATMENT OF MENTAL DISORDERS

The word patient comes from the Latin word *patiens*, which means 'one who suffers.' It signifies the vulnerable position of the one with problems find themselves. The person is the basic unit of all treatment endeavours. Their personality provides the background where psychopathology develops, expresses itself and affects them and secondarily affects those who make their physical, psychological, and social network. In an existential context, the person is at the centre of their universe.

E.H. Carr (1961) suggested: "study the historian before you begin to study the facts. When you read a work of history, always listen to the buzzing. Facts are like fish swimming about in a vast and sometimes inaccessible ocean; and what the historian catches will depend, partly on chance, but mainly on what part of the ocean he chooses to fish in and what tackle he chooses to use – these two factors being determined by the kind of fish he wants to catch." This applies to psychiatry history taking as well. It is hard to make sense of what ails the person until we can understand the person who is relating the story, and we have a framework broad enough to understand the whole person.

The treatment favoured at any time reflects the ideas that are currently in favour and shapes what those administering treatment believe would provide relief. These beliefs may not invariably be shared by those receiving treatment. The disconnect may be partly because of the nature of illness itself (the hopelessness and helplessness of depression or the lack of trust in those with paranoid symptoms) or the lack of trust in the model of service provision.

Every form of treatment comes with its own rationale and is supported by clinical studies as well as the backing of current opinion leaders. Frontal lobectomy, malaria therapy, insulin coma therapy, and many others had their own hey days and were later discarded for good. The classic psychoanalytic psychotherapy also has very few takers now as are many of the other modalities of treatment which were once heralded as a great stride forward.

All measures outlined under secondary prevention remains quite relevant, not only in the management of an index episode being treated, but in the prevention of future relapse and maintaining well-being.

VARIOUS MODALITIES OF TREATMENT:

As outlined above, an existential formulation has a place for every treatment modality available that can help ameliorate symptoms and gradually lead towards full remission and better integration of the person that could prevent a relapse. They can be used in conjunction leading finally to a better understanding of existential issues in sickness and life.

We have too many patients whose mental disorders remain inadequately treated. Some of the causes for their unmet needs may be due to our quest for simple answers that do not exist. The aphorism: "As simple as possible, but not simpler" sums it appropriately. We must treat symptoms through all the means available. An existential approach that helps the person to reconstruct a new sense of self offers the best chance to gain full recovery.

It is facile to divide the world of psychiatric patients into: (a) the first-class citizens, who can achieve their cure or salvation by will power, or by behaviour modification, insight, psychoanalysis, and (b) those who are weak in their mental fibre and need a crutch in the form of psychopharmacologic agent. Gerald Klerman (1972) used the term, "pharmacological Calvinism" to say that any drug that makes people feel good is something bad. Advocates of medication worry about the underuse of antidepressants. What Klerman calls the "Calvinist" view of psychotropic medication leads a substantial proportion of the public to resist taking drugs because they associate their use with weakness: characterological, moral, or some other kind.

Paul McVaugh (2006) wrote about psychoanalytic excess that led to the suicide of a Harvard medical student and termed it as "Psychotherapy Awry." Ghaemi (2010) pointed out that the excess of psychoanalysis has ended but has been replaced by an equally dogmatic psychopharmacological extremism. He called it "psychopharmacology Awry." He pointed out: "when a single dogma is applied to all of psychiatry, treatment-resistant syndromes will abound. It matters little whether the dogma is Freud or Effexor." Patients come seeking help for what bothers them. They put their hope and expectations on the professionals to help them and we must strive to understand their condition and help them as well as we can. We must have an open mind and be vigilant against all kinds of dogmas.

John Markowitz and colleagues (2022) lamented that the definition of treatment resistant depression (TRD) was overly narrow. No uniform definition for TRD exists, but they are mostly defined as repeated failure to respond to antidepressants with or without physical methods of treatment (such as ECT or TMS). This is despite demonstrated efficacy of different forms of therapy. Psychotherapy may not only help with depression but also "emotionally alter a patient's self-regard, distinguishing self from illness: recognizing they are not 'defective', as they often believe, but ill."

The initial psychiatric consultation must not be hurried. It is important for the professional to try and run as much on time as possible. Patients not having to wait for long conveys the professionals positive regard for them and their time. Many coming for their first appointment with a psychiatrist, or other mental professionals may be apprehensive about the consultation. They may also have symptoms that make it difficult to concentrate well enough or otherwise struggle to provide all the details that may be required by the professional. Much of the therapeutic alliance is formed during the initial interview. By the end of that initial consultation, one should in most instances be able to come to an initial shared view whether medication need to be prescribed immediately or can wait until further evaluation.

There are two important considerations that help decide on medication at this stage. One is the presence and severity of the physiological symptoms and the extent to which the patient sees them as a significant problem. Prescribing needs to be a mutual and participant decision. Explaining the choices available and the pros and cons of these choices will help in forming a positive regard for the patient.

The placebo effect operates even in the most "scientifically proven treatment." We must not get too swayed when the patient comes for the first review and reports a massive improvement. What it more often means is that a basic degree of trust has been formed, and it is possible for them to work with you towards a resolution of their condition. Life is complicated and all mental disorders are complex. All medications like all forms of therapy take time to work.

LIVING BETTER CHEMICALLY: PSYCHOPHARMACOLOGY

Humans live in their body and everyone's body is an amalgamation of their anatomy and various physiological systems. Pathology (including psychopathology) implies disordered physiology. Our body, brain, and mind are all based on our physiology. So, it makes sense that there would be a role for medications that could help to restore disordered physiology. All forms of psychopharmacological agents can be used where needed but these need to be targeted towards specific symptoms rather than to cure any presumed basic condition.

By acknowledging that existence is embodied, the importance of our physiology is well recognised. Judicious use of medication is vitally important. We must pay heed to Philip Pinel who as far back as 1806, warned: 'In diseases of the mind......it is an art of no little importance to administer medicine properly, but it is an art of much greater importance and more difficult acquisition to know when to suspend or altogether omit them.' Targeting the most troublesome symptoms frees us to an extent in the choice of psychotropic medications in each situation.

The pharmacological method often uses the flawed logic of working backwards. The effect of the drug is taken to mean that what was changed must be the cause of the condition. No drug has a single site of action, and many drugs can induce the same effect as can purely psychosocial interventions. Antidepressants are the most used drugs for long term treatment of anxiety and yet depression and anxiety are seen as independent diagnoses.

SSRI group of medications are useful in most anxiety-based disorders including generalized anxiety disorder, panic disorder, phobic disorders, obsessive-compulsive disorder, and post-traumatic stress disorder. Medication, cognitive-behaviour therapy, and even simple behavioural activation have been shown to be effective in depression and show similar changes on fMRI.

We must acknowledge that in psychiatry we have the so-called antianxiety medications (for they are only useful for the short term treatment of anxiety), the so-called antidepressant (as besides depression they have been used for all types of anxiety-based disorders), the so-called antipsychotic medications (besides psychosis they are widely used as mood stabilizers, augmenting agents in depression and small dosage in difficult to treat anxiety-based disorders), and so-called mood stabilizers (besides bipolar disorder they are used as augmenting agents to antipsychotics and antidepressant in a variety of situations, including for impulsivity in mood disorder). Such non-specificity also puts a question mark on the naïve view of our biological treatment being disease specific. They also could point to the limitations of the diagnostic categories themselves.

Medications undoubtedly have a useful role to play in the treatment of mental disorders as these disorders encompass a physiological dimension. Sleep, appetite, weight loss, energy, motivation, agitation etc can all improve with targeted treatment. They may be even unavoidable in the acute stages of the illness. No psychological therapy of any sort can be effective if the person is so sleep deprived that he is unable to attend to and concentrate to what is going on in therapy. When faced with an acute disturbance of mental function medication has a lot to offer. The situation may even be dangerous for the person and others around them. These are many clinical situations where it is not possible to just wait for therapy to be effective. Resolution of significant vegetative symptoms require immediate treatment and with-holding them would be negligent.

By the time a patient has come to see a psychiatrist they have usually crossed several hurdles. The first one is their own recognition of a problem and a decision to seek treatment. This is followed by seeing a general practitioner who would have a significant role to play in deciding that there is a mental condition that requires attention. They may themselves prescribe some medication or made an assessment that the person be referred to a psychologist or counsellor rather than a psychiatrist. Thus, it is much more likely, at least in the advanced economies that a patient coming to see a psychiatrist has crossed several barriers to care and seen as someone who needs the medical expertise of a psychiatrist. Pharmacotherapy is of limited benefit without combining it with therapy that the psychiatrist feels most comfortable with.

Because antidepressants help with the vegetative and some of the nonvegetative symptoms does not necessarily imply that depression is what the antidepressant ameliorates. The reality is that depression is a complex disorder, and it includes features that cannot be fully understood on the basis physiology alone.

Whitwell (2005) in “Recovery Beyond psychiatry” used the designation of ‘naïve psychiatry’ which was based on the ‘illness-treatment-recovery model.’ The hope or myth took root that medical treatments if carried out with significant vigour would not only get people into remission but also get them into recovery. He observed that myths were powerful ideas that exert powerful influence because we think they are true. They come to be seen as ‘myths’ only when we start examining them closely. It is then that we can see their feet of clay.

No psychiatric condition has so far been ‘cured’ by medication. Every new medication adds to the range of treatment available but does make a difference for some people only and not all. The success rates of most antidepressant for example is one in three.

An ambitious study was "The Sequenced Treatment Alternatives to Relieve Depression (Star*D trial 2007). Outpatients with nonpsychotic major depressive disorder were enrolled and treated prospectively in a series of randomized controlled trials. These were conducted in representative primary and psychiatric practices. Remission rates for treatment steps 1 to 4 based on the 16-item Quick Inventory of Depressive Symptomatology Self report were 37%, 31%, 14%, and 13%, respectively. There were no differences in remission rates or times to remission among medication switch or among medication augmentation strategies at any treatment level. Participants who required increasing numbers of treatment steps showed greater depressive illness burden and increasingly greater relapse rates in the naturalistic follow-up period (40%-71%). Prognosis was better at all levels for participants who entered follow-up in remission as opposed to those who entered with response without remission. These results highlight the prevalence of treatment resistant depression and suggest potential benefit for using more vigorous treatments in the earlier steps. Some of the reservations about the results of the study has been highlighted in the section of affective disorders.

The quest for newer psychotropic medications continues. Psychedelics are currently being under intense trial. Esketamine has already been approved by the FDA for the treatment of depression. Psilocybin and LSD are touted as potential wonder drugs. Are we going to see a new generation of drug addicted mental patients in near future?

However, we must accept that mental disorders like all other chronic medical conditions are complex disorders. There are no fairy tales to tell ending with, 'they happily lived thereafter.' Despite all the limitations pointed out so far, psychiatry was and will remain a medical speciality. Few basic tenets of pharmacological treatment should always be kept in mind. Start with one medication as far as feasible. Start low and go slow. Before adding another medication, always reassess whether the ones already in use is serving any purpose or can be tapered off or discontinued. Treatment must be cost-effective which means that side effects of the medication must not be more than the distress associated with the illness. At the same time, the index patient is suffering now, and treatment needs to be chosen from the various alternatives available to us now.

We also got to acknowledge that our nosology needs further work, and we may not yet know how the different treatments work. We are not the only speciality that is faced with such problems. As Agus (2011), an oncologist pointed out "Despite chemotherapy being widely used treatment for cancer, nobody has ever shown that most chemotherapy actually touches a cancer cell. It has never been proven.' We must be careful about drawing fixed conclusions based on what is observed in a very controlled petri dish. Chemotherapy clearly benefits cancer patients, yet frequently we cannot explain why. We must openly admit that we cannot always explain how things work.

Dysfunctional uterine bleeding is a condition that is associated with vaginal bleeding to occur outside of the regular menstrual cycle. The main cause of dysfunctional uterine bleeding is an imbalance in the sex hormones. Heavy and prolonged bleeding accompanied by a thickened uterine lining can often be treated by dilatation and curettage (D & C). No one can be sure why the scraping of the target tissue should remedy a condition that is of hormonal origin. However, the fact remains that the procedure works and is also one of the widest used procedures in gynaecology.

We need not get overexcited when a new medication hits the market. We must not panic when any study or meta-analysis shows that medication is ineffective. Clinical practice should be like an old woman in her kitchen. Unlike the novice they know exactly where her pots and pans are. She also knows her pantry well. She goes about her work with a sense of calm assurance and is likely to make a lot less noise.

Changing a patient to the newest available medication should be a carefully considered decision. Every new medication that hits the market goes through a honeymoon period. Often after that it could take one of the three trajectories: 1) Better than existing medications for a select group of patients, more often due to better tolerability rather than efficacy. 2) As effective as others (most medications now go through a non-inferiority trial rather than efficacy trial). 3) Toxic and may be withdrawn from the market.

LIVING BETTER PHYSICALLY

Taking stock of our physical self is an essential part of living better. This involves firstly our level of physical well-being. It also includes physical methods of treatment for mental disorders. These treatments are part of our armamentarium in providing adequate care.

LIVING BETTER BY NORMALISING PHYSIOLOGY

Deep breathing exercises, Progressive muscle relaxation exercises, Yoga, Pranayama, Taiichi, Pilate and even gym, cycling, running, swimming can all be powerful tools. Anything that gives us a sense of "Flow" can help the mind to focus on to something better than the trap of a negative mind set. Negative cognitions, like pain, tends to fill all the time available for it.

To be living needs the persistent activity of our heart, lungs, brain, and all other parts of the body. More critically, brain activity cannot survive even beyond just a few minutes of the cessation of our cardio-respiratory functions. Our mind is very vulnerable to symptoms of cardio-respiratory dysfunction. It raises concerns about our very existence.

Pranayama is the practice of breath regulation. It is a main component of yoga, an exercise for physical and mental wellness. In Sanskrit, "prana" means life energy and "yama" means control. The practice of pranayama involves breathing exercises and patterns. One is required to inhale, exhale, and hold your breath in a specific sequence.

The word 'Yoga' is derived from the Sanskrit root 'Yuj', meaning 'to join' or 'to unite'. It is an ancient Indian system to train the body and mind to self-observe and become aware of their own nature. In yoga, pranayama is used with other practices like physical postures (asanas) and meditation. Together, these practices lead to the many benefits of yoga.

Breathing exercises and progressive muscle relaxation exercises are based on similar principles. They help with the vicious cycle of physical dysregulation and increasing anxiety and panic. Proper use of all forms of exercises can also provide similar benefits as yoga. The process is important and can best be achieved when these activities are performed within the limits of one's physiology. The limits can be enhanced over time. Awareness of our body changes works like a biofeedback mechanism.

Csíkszentmihályi (1975) brought to focus the old concept of a flow state. It is the mental state in which a person performing some activity is fully immersed in a feeling of energized focus, full involvement, and enjoyment in the process of the activity. Being able to reach such stages may have significant benefits and we should encourage each person we treat to find for themselves what gives them a sense of flow.

Mood and sleep processes are deeply connected with circadian function and there is growing interest in targeting circadian pathways and sleep regulation for treatment of mood disorders. Bright light therapy, sleep deprivation, melatonin agonist and behavioural interventions to address the dysregulation have been found to be useful.

LIVING BETTER ELECTRICALLY:

Electroconvulsive therapy (ECT) has been around for a long time. No treatment survives for nearly nine decades without being useful. The idea was based on the misplaced notion that those with epilepsy did not suffer from schizophrenia. Initially used to calm down markedly agitated patients with psychosis, it came to be used quite indiscriminately for all psychiatric disorders.

Over time the ECT machines became more sophisticated, administration under anaesthesia made it a more humane and its use is now mostly restricted to severe depression not responding to medication or where the person may be at severe risk. It is still being occasionally used for other condition when they have not responded to standard treatment.

ECT does retain a role in the treatment of severe mental illnesses where less invasive treatments have been ineffective. Anyone who has seen dramatic improvement in patients with severe depression can vouch for its effectiveness. Like any treatment there is no guarantee of its effectiveness.

LIVING BETTER MAGNETICALLY:

Transcranial Magnetic Stimulation (TMS) is another physical method of treatment that has come to play a significant role in the treatment of mental disorders. It was initially developed as a more humane form of stimulation technique to replace ECT for the treatment of depression with fewer side effects.

They are being trialled for the treatment of anxiety disorders, obsessive-compulsive disorder, PTSD, and more. Protocols of administration vary from centre to centre, consultant to consultant, and patient to patient. Lot of research is still required regarding its indications, procedure, placement etc. As long it still helps some, it must be part of our treatment armamentarium.

LIVING BETTER COGNITIVELY

The Stoics may have been the true protagonists of cognitive behaviour therapy. Spinoza in the 17th century put forth the idea that anxiety was a problem of logic. Informal CBT has however been used by all good parents, teachers, elders of any community, and mentors. Einstein (1950) observed that "science is nothing but refined everyday thinking".

Cognitive behaviour therapy has been successfully used for a wide range of conditions. These include depression and a full range of anxiety disorders. They have also been used for schizophrenia and other conditions with somewhat limited benefit. Emotions may be even more important determinant of behaviour. Cognition is to a considerable extent also governed by emotions. They are interconnected processes. If cognition is the head emotions may be the neck and it is the neck that determines where the head would turn.

CBT may be of limited benefit in severe personality disorder. "Primal emotions" such as fear are associated with ancient parts of the brain. Fear of death is one of the basic causes of all anxiety and in an existential formulation the basic cause of all forms of psychopathology. They are much more resistant to change. "Basic" emotions including happiness, anger, disgust, and sadness may be more amenable to therapy. In CBT the focus is on cognitions and behaviour. The person and his/her personality are an important part of whatever mental illness they present with.

CBT can be challenging when depression or various forms of anxiety-based disorders are associated with personality disorder. The minds of people with personality disorders/difficulties are possibly too caught up in their "emotional-mind" and unable to shift to a "reasonable-mind" set where CBT works. However, it may be of some benefit as an adjunct to other forms of therapy and may be of even greater use after mindfulness-based therapies has helped them to be more in the "wise-mind" set. As a result of such insights, mindfulness based cognitive behaviour therapy and similar innovations re gaining increasing attention.

LIVING BETTER INTERPERSONALLY

Interpersonal therapy is based on three theoretical underpinnings: 1) Attachment theory (humans have an intrinsic instinctual drive to form interpersonal relationships). 2) Communication theory (communication is one manifestation of attachment). 3) Social theory (a deficiency in social relationship is cause for distress and current interpersonal distress leads to psychopathology).

Within all relationship individuals negotiate three aspects of their relationship such as affiliation, dominance, and inclusion. Interpersonal therapy focusses on problem areas of grief and loss, interpersonal disputes, role transitions, and interpersonal sensitivity.

The four essential tasks are to: (1) create a therapeutic environment with high inclusion and affiliation, (2) recognize patterns of interpersonal communication, (3) identify maladaptive communication, and (4) assist the patient in building better social support network.

A wide range of methods are used including those that focus on transactional analysis. The effectiveness of interpersonal therapy is well established in several problem areas.

LIVING BETTER MINDFULLY

Epictetus believed: "People are not disturbed by things but by the view they take on them." The 'view taken' may in fact denote 'sense-making.' Seneca wrote: "There are more things to alarm us than to harm us, and we suffer more in apprehension than in reality." Anxiety is apprehension of what could go wrong and in depression hopelessness is about a loss of a worthwhile future. Therapy involves learning to live better in an unknown future.

Mindfulness is a central theme in Buddhism. Buddhist philosophy is based on the Four Noble Truths. The first truth is called "Suffering" (everyone in life is suffering in some way). The second truth is "Origin of suffering" (all suffering comes from desire). The third truth is "Cessation of suffering" (it is possible to stop suffering and achieve enlightenment). The fourth truth, "Path to the cessation of suffering" (the adoption of Middle path, which are the steps to achieve enlightenment). Mindfulness based therapies have been framed on these broad principles of Buddhist philosophy.

Dialectical Behaviour Therapy (Linehan 1993) has been widely used in the treatment of BPD. The success of the therapy in one of the most dramatic and difficult to treat condition has led to the growth of several other therapies that have been group together a variety of therapies broadly referred to Mindfulness Based Therapies.

Several psychotherapeutic approaches are effective in the treatment of BPD and cost-effective in the short-term (Murphy et al 2019). These include Dialectic Behavioural Treatment (DBT – for which the largest evidence-base data exists), Mentalisation-Based Treatment (MBT), Transference Focused Psychotherapy (TFP), Schema Focused Therapy (SFT), and Systems Training for Emotional Predictability and Problem Solving (STEPPS). All target the four psychopathological domains of BPD (Emotional Regulation; Impulse Control; Behavioural and Interpersonal Skills) (Rao et al 2020).

Bateman (2012) summed up the characteristics of the therapies that make them effective. These therapies 1) provide a structured manual that supports the therapist and provides recommendations for common clinical problems; 2) are structured so that they encourage increased activity, proactivity, and self-agency for the patients; 3) focus on emotion processing, particularly on creating robust connections between acts and feelings; 4) increase cognitive coherence in relation to subjective experience in the early phase of treatment by including a model of pathology that is carefully explained to the patient; and 5) encourage an active stance by the therapist, which invariably includes an explicit intent to validate and demonstrate empathy and generate a strong attachment relationship to create a foundation of alliance.

The landmark McLean Study of Adult Development (MSAD) entered its 24th year, after publication of 10, 14- and 16-year follow-up data. This study, with 290 patients and seventy-nine controls, conducts assessments every 2 years. All patients had severe BPD at recruitment and continued to receive psychotherapy and medications throughout the follow-up period. After 16 years, 99% of patients had achieved remission lasting at least 2 years; 78% had a remission lasting 8 years (Zananini et al 2010, 2012).

The effectiveness of mindfulness-based therapy transcends diagnostic categories. Such transdiagnostic therapies are gaining appeal for good pragmatic reasons. Some psychotherapies (e.g., DBT) developed for one disorder have become transdiagnostic because they were subsequently found to be effective for several other disorders. Other psychotherapies have been deliberately designed to treat multiple related disorders. Their increasing use and demonstrated effectiveness also point to the possibility of a continuum of psychopathology in real life.

Several tools used in mindfulness-based therapies can easily be adapted in existential therapy. They do address issues that are the core of existentialism. These include the concept of the wise mind:

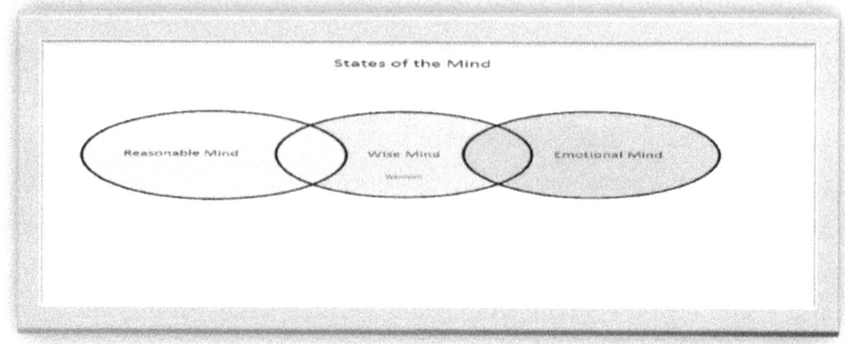

The reasonable mind is like the concept of thoughts/cognition, the emotional mind signifies affects/emotions, and the wise mind is the joint operation of cognition, emotion, wisdom which includes insight and sense making. Parallels can easily be drawn to Plato's white horse, black horse, and the charioteer. Working on specific skills that can help people to be in a wise state of the mind can be rewarding.

The concept: "We are all imperfect people, and we live in an imperfect world" can be used quite broadly and effectively. "We must give up the hope of a better past."

LIVING BETTER EXISTENTIALLY

We need to first look at a detailed existential formulation which can then be used to be a guide to existential therapy.

AN EXISTENTIAL CASE FORMULATION

A diagnosis is shorthand for an illness or disorder but also a starting point towards finding appropriate management. A diagnosis or, more frequently, diagnoses are like labels, often concealing more than they reveal. A label does not tell us what one is doing and why, but a formulation does. A case formulation is an explanation of how the patient's problems have developed, what maintains them and what can be done to address them. A good formulation will guide us towards the development of an appropriate treatment plan.

Jaspers distinguished between two types of understanding: one involved tracing the causal origins of various psychic events and states and the other involved their meaning to the patient. The former is linked to natural processes which may or may not be biologically explicable. The latter concerns the meaning of the event to the person. He further differentiated 'rational' from 'empathic' understanding: the former can only reveal contents of the mind linked by the rules of logic, whereas the latter brings us into contact with a person's individual psychology or autobiographical narrative.

Jaspers identified the role of psychiatrists as, in part, participation in the process of extending the knowledge of the patient so that it embraces areas of unnoticed mental life playing a role in his behaviour but not consciously appreciated.

Assuming that psychiatric disorders are caused by events outside the realm of meaning (such as changes in neurotransmitters or other biological variables) and the only objective way to understand them, then the stage is set for us to neglect the meaning of the disease to the patient. Meaning, in that context, can only be regarded as an epiphenomenon having no role in correcting changes leading to his dysfunction. The individual physiology is without doubt an important driving force, influenced by our physical reality as well as past experiences while continuously interacting with his social and cultural milieu. Such interactions also lead to changes in our physiology.

Yalom (1980) described four main existential concerns we need to come to terms with: (1) the knowledge of our death and the fear this evokes, (2) our condition of freedom and the responsibilities implied, (3) our isolation and the difficulties in relating to oneself and others, and (4) our quest for meaning. These depend on our stance-taking capacities, but the enactive model sees stance-taking to be even broader than just these concerns.

The concerns raised by Yalom above may be a more limited formulation, better suited to a practice involving patients who can be treated through psychological therapy alone. In psychotherapy practice with less seriously disturbed patients, Yalom found the diagnostic process largely irrelevant, and believed that the contortions psychotherapists must go through to meet the demands of the insurance companies for precise diagnoses are detrimental to both therapist and patient.

In real time clinical psychiatry, we obviously need a broader formulation useful for the initial assessment of a case in all areas of clinical practice so to help us draw a comprehensive treatment plan. The Existential Dimension is best represented as the way people relate to and make sense of themselves and their situation. It is a special form of the experiential dimension and so important for psychiatry that it constitutes a dimension of its own (de Haan 2020). We do not just experience things, but also relate to our experiences. We can take a stance on the situation at hand and ourselves; on what we do, think and feel.

Enactivism envisions an existentially informed therapy. It tries to understand the basis of our existence as a cognitive process considering all our physiological, experiential and socio-cultural factors. This helps us make sense of all those. It is a major step towards an integrative view of psychopathology and its treatment. The four dimensions included are:

1. The Physiological Dimension including genetic, anatomical, biochemical and neurological aspects of psychiatric disorders.

2. The Experiential Dimension referring to a patient's lived experience.

3. The Sociocultural Dimension refers to the fact that humans do not live in a vacuum: that 'no man is an island'; that they are always in interaction with their environment. We are part of specific sociocultural communities including our social network of family, friends, and acquaintances. Their norms, habit and self-interpretations are all shaped by the practices of the social group to which we belong. The individual's psychiatric problems cannot be understood in isolation from their social context, both currently and in the past. No action, thought, perception or feeling is in and of itself pathological; it always depends on context. Their appropriateness can only be assessed within the specific situation of the person.

4. We can also relate to our experiences, take a stance on the situation at hand and on ourselves; on what we do, think, and feel.

The "genetic, anatomical, biochemical, and neurological aspects of psychiatric disorders" described in the enactive model appears to point towards a psychiatric diagnosis as described in Diagnostic and Statistical Manual or International Classification of Diseases. The limitations of these systems have been discussed before. Lost under the veneer of psychiatric diagnoses are the unique characteristics of the person presenting with the disorder. They need to be used for official purposes such as Medicare, Insurance, Medico-legal, statistics, and further research, but may be of limited benefit in real-time clinical practice.

From a practical and clinically useful standpoint one can conceptualise:

1. *Existence as Embodied* in our physiology (and anatomy) residing in a physical and emotional environment.

2. *Existence as Experiential*

3. *Existence as Embedded* in our social, cultural and political milieu.

4. *Existence as a process of Making Sense* of what it is to be me in relation to my identity, role functioning and in respect to everyone else. Sense-making is more than a cognitive process. Emotions play an especially important part in our cognitive processes. Part of the emotion is that which can be conveyed in words (feelings), but some remain at just visceral level. There is a fundamental interdependence between feeling and thinking in human social life. Our affective experiences are integrally linked with the way information about the world is stored. Affect can influence both the process of thinking and the content of thinking.

In keeping with such an existential framework, a case formulation would include:

1. The physiological dimension including:
   a. Diagnosis, which is necessary mainly for administrative purposes.
   b. Evaluation of significant vegetative symptoms, emotional and other behavioural that the person presents with and their severity, which may help choose medication.
   c. Any significant associated medical disorders that may cause an overlap of symptoms and require medical intervention.

2. The significant experiential traumas affecting the person.
3. The social and cultural factors of clinical significance.
4. The person's comprehension of their condition including the dominant cognitive and emotional distortions playing a part in their sense making.

An adequate understanding of sense-making will be helped by the assessment and recording of the five dimensions of personality:

1. Neuroticism (a tendency to be depressed, anxious and stress reactive),

2. Agreeableness (an orientation towards empathy and getting along with other people),
3. Extraversion (a disposition to be outgoing, friendly, and emotionally positive),
4. Conscientiousness (a tendency to be orderly and achievement oriented),
5. Openness. (a tendency to be curious, imaginative and to try new change).

EXISTENTIAL THERPAY

Therapies reflect, and are shaped by, the pathology they seek to treat. In therapy the person looks at the "meaning" of life thereby implying a search for coherence. In conventional usage it is the same as "purpose" of life (which refers to intention, aim, or function). In real terms, we can forego the question: "Why do we live?" but we must confront the question: "How shall we live?" (Yalom 1980).

"Man, not only exists but knows that he exists. In full awareness he studies his world and changes it to suit his purposes. He is not merely cognisable as excitant, but himself freely decides what shall exist. Man is mind, and the situation of man as man is a mental situation" (Jaspers 1933). Thus, every individual, inasmuch as he exists, is something more than a mere member of the masses. He must not be merged with the masses in such a way as to forfeit his right to independent existence as a human being. Existentialism for Jaspers was a biological existentialism and not a social constructionist, postmodernist, antimedical perspective.

The self consists of the stories we tell ourselves – stories which relate to how we got where we are, and why, and what we have done, and what happened next. Once we are past a particular moment, hour, or day all we have is the mental image and impression of the time gone by. We store them as a story of the time which becomes part of the larger story of our life. We rehearse these stories to ourselves to remind us of who we are, we tell them to other people to encourage them to form a particular impression of ourselves. The most important ingredient of any meaningful relationship is for it to be close and confiding.

We can and do change the stories over time as our self-understanding, or our strategic self-presentation changes. Sometimes, stories are assimilated to our self-understanding, on other occasions, our self-understanding must accommodate itself to the new story. When this happens, the whole story of our life changes. "The telling of a narrative can be disrupted in various ways, and we must be sensitive in clinical life to the fact that a person's narrative can get broken" (Zaner 1998).

Immanuel Kant (1781) in *The Critique of Pure Reason* asserted: "All representation I devise of the world are representations in my head. My sense enables me to gain experiences, which my understanding turns into representations, and my reason helps me to sort out and assess them. But I know nothing of what lies completely outside of the world of my sensory experience." Existentialism involves understanding the whole person through the process of phenomenological understanding. (The study of "phenomena": appearances of things, or things as they appear in our experience, or the ways we experience things, thus the meanings things have in our experience. Phenomenology studies conscious experience as experienced from the subjective or first-person point of view). It does not believe in the kind of experimentation treating the person as an object or thing to be pushed and pulled around in a laboratory.

Mind thinks in images but, to communicate with any other person, it must transform image into thought and then into language. This march from thought to language can be treacherous. The richness of images, their plasticity, flexibility, and emotional quality may be lost when converted into language. We are selective about what we choose to disclose. Most existential therapists tend to focus less on the past and more on the future. Existential therapy traces the behaviour of the individual to their projects and the values that they have adapted to guide them through these projects. The therapist aims to develop an existential understanding of the origins of the problems and helps the person to overcome them.

Gillett (1999) believes psychiatry must take an inclusive stance to understand the three-way interaction between biology, cognition and interpersonal activity. The mind is a narrative told by a person from the engagement between their brain and the world. The person as the teller of this tale is primarily and inescapably a 'being-in-relation-with-others.' These are the main themes shaping a discursive account of psychiatric disorders as disorders of relational narrative beings. We depend on our brains as the information processing organ realizing and mediating our interactions with the physical interpersonal, and cultural world around us.

Psychiatric disorders concern one's capacities for adequate perceiving, thinking, feeling, and acting; experiences at the heart of who you are. And as we are stance-taking, reflective beings, our stance on ourselves and our situation co-determines the way we feel, perceive, think and act. One can argue that psychiatric disorders emerge from this stance-taking ability of persons (Fuchs 2011).

We receive information from the outside world through our senses and use this input to construct an inner model of the world. We need to consider the dynamic character of life and its developmental trajectory. Notions like 'mental', 'mind' and 'cognition' are best understood in terms of sensemaking: the embodied and embedded activity of organisms and persons who evaluatively orient themselves in their environments or worlds.

Tew et al (2011) reviewed published literature and identified five inter-locking processes characterising recovery: (1) empowerment and reclaiming control over one's life, (2) rebuilding positive personal and social identities, (3) connectedness (both personal and wider aspects of social inclusion), (4) hope and optimism about the future, and (5) finding meaning and purpose in life. All these aspects of life are intimately related to existential issues.

Psychiatric disorders refer to problems with this sense-making. On a very general level we can say that how the person makes sense of his/her world is biased in a certain direction. For psychiatric patients their world changes in character to the extent that their sense-making is out of tune.

The individual "decides" on a "Life Script" – an unconscious blueprint of one's life course which encompasses personality variables and repetitive interpersonal interactions. A script is a set of expectations about what will happen next in a well understood situation. There are many situations in life where people play their respective roles like a drama. Scripts are useful in several ways. They make mental processing easier, by allowing us to think less. They clarify the actions of others if we know the script they are following. However, people also have many very personal scripts which others do not share. In certain situations, our life scripts distort perhaps because of our past or present life experiences or the social-cultural milieu of which we are part. They may also have been revised by changes to our physiology from, say, a major medical condition.

Working on the dysfunctional aspects of life scripts (trait dependent) or recently modified scripts (state dependent) is a significant part of therapy. Existential therapists attempt to understand the private world of the patient and not how the person deviates from the presumed norms. "The analyst should approach the patient phenomenologically; that is, he or she should enter their inner world. Various existential analysts agree on one fundamental procedural point; that is, he or she must enter the patient's experimental world and listen to the phenomena of that world without the presuppositions that distort understanding" (Yalom 1980).

The success of any therapy is, to a significant extent, also dependent on what the patient brings to the sessions. Some are good at telling their stories and some less so. Some are better at recognising relevance while the degree of openness in revealing their inner thoughts and feelings may vary.

Jaspers was critical of the Freudian view that "man is the puppet of his unconscious, and (that) when the latter has had a clear light thrown upon it, he will become master of himself." He thought that: "the self-examination of a sincere thinker, which after the long-lasting Christian interlude attained its climax in Kierkegaard and Nietzsche, is in psychoanalysis degraded into the discovery of sexual longings and typical experiences of childhood; it is the masking of genuine but hazardous self-examination by the mere rediscovery of familiar types in a realm of reputed necessity wherein the lower levels of human life are regarded as having an absolute validity."

Consciousness consists of two aspects, the pre-reflective and the reflective. The pre-reflective awareness is only implicit (non-positionally) awareness of what is going on around one's sphere. The subject is present but is almost 'in the wings.' Reflective consciousness occurs when one responds to the situation consciously. Sartre believed that we are always implicitly self-aware in every conscious act and this self-awareness is occasionally made explicit by subsequent reflection.

Existentialists reject the Freudian concept of the unconscious underlying our consciousness since this, in turn, compromises our responsibility. This also avoids the wild-goose chase of reflection to infinity so as to grasp the consciousness of self. Every conscious act is self-aware whether implicitly or explicitly and hence is our own responsibility. The pre-reflective awareness was seen to mean 'comprehension.' Sartre believed we comprehend more than we know. If we take knowledge to denote reflective awareness, it will mean being aware of more than what we know.

Yalom (1980) pointed to a generation of young adults who have been nursed and spoon-fed according to a compulsively permissive regimen. Structure, ritual, boundaries of every type are being relentlessly dismantled. The picture of psychopathology has changed accordingly. The classical psychoneurotic syndromes have become a rarity. Today's patient has to cope more with freedom than with suppressed drives.

Sartre was particularly critical of Freud's conceptions of the inferiority complex, which centred on an overactive ego. Sartre saw perceived inferiority as a project.

Some people present to themselves and to others as intrinsically inferior, either to carve out a distinct identity or to evade taking responsibility for their lives. They either set goals that they cannot hope to achieve or go about pursuing achievable goals in hopeless ways. Either the end is the problem, or the means, or both.

The "inferiority project" stems from the distorting and reinforcing behaviour unlikely to produce satisfying results. Sartre held there were two kinds of reflection on one's own experience. Pure reflection is the way the world seems and so it does not ascribe any motivation to oneself. Impure reflection, on the other hand, views one's experience as a relation between the way the world seems and one's own motivation. Inferiority projects follow the general structure of 'bad faith.' This 'type of being in the world' tends to perpetuate itself. It structures one's experience of the world in such a way that other people's behaviour appears as expressing their fixed natures. One can pursue the project of bad faith which also helps in hiding it from themselves.

de Beauvoir's (1949) 'The Second Sex' is regarded as the first major application of existentialist psychotherapy. She saw the origins of woman's femininity in the 'feminine condition' designed to 'freeze her as an object.' 'One is not born, but rather becomes woman.' Boys and girls are behaviourally and psychologically different because of differences in how they develop their 'projects.' She was also critical of Freud's construction of the individual as a collection of disparate basic drives.

Sartre saw the inferiority complex as an individual's chosen project, but Beauvoir took it as a 'sedimented' social meaning. Thus, the underlying cause of an individual's problem can be found in a conflict between the values they explicitly endorse and the sedimented meaning that implicitly structures their desire. Beauvoir held that the individual's chosen projects become progressively more embedded, limiting their outlook, constraining the range of projects they might choose, and that any change of projects could only be gradual.

Fanon (1952/2008) in his book *Black Skin, White Masks* drew attention to the collective inferiority project among the Black people. In a colonial environment the Black man is a slave to his inferiority and the white man to his superiority. He enumerates the various ways that the black man is made to feel inferior. "A normal Black child, having grown up with a normal family, will become abnormal at the slightest contact with the white world." They are made to feel responsible for not only their body but also for their race and their ancestors.

The black problem is not just about Black people living among Whites, but about the Black man exploited, enslaved and despised by a colonialist and capitalist society that happens to be white. Many colonized Black people try to escape from their feeling of inferiority by metaphorically wearing a mask identifying them with the white colonizers. However, the mask periodically slips as it is ill-fitting. The problem in wearing the mask is not that the colonizer controls the features of the masks, but that the colonizer classifies as inferior whatever features the mask has.

Webber (2018) classified the version of the idea that 'existence precedes essence' articulated more fully in Beauvoir's *The Second Sex*, Fanon's *Black Skin, White Masks* and Sartre's *Saint Genet* as 'the canonical form of existentialism.' They reflect the values enshrined in our projects, which we can change but which becomes progressively sedimented as they are deployed in cognition and action. Socialization in childhood has a profound and lasting influence but can be reduced over time through recently endorsed values.

This theory of the structure of human existence has two dimensions. One is the psychoanalytic theory that some form of distress can be traced to the mistaken idea that people have fixed personalities. The second dimension of existentialist ethics is a moral requirement to value the structure of human existence. Authenticity is of therapeutic value. The human individual combines the freedom to revise the values shaping their outlook with the sedimentation of their projects over time.

Humans can be seen as not stable but timeless entities. Whatever identities we have is either imposed from outside or sustained by our own ongoing, self-defining existential project, our fundamental choice. We are always a work in progress, a story still being written. Existential therapy cannot be manualised, as it is concerned with notions of facticity, transcendence (project), alienation, authenticity and bad faith all of which are addressed in therapy. A manualised approach will be antithetical to the notions of authenticity and free will. Becoming an existential individual is to accept responsibility for our actions.

Relationship is at the heart of all doctor-patient relationship. In psychotherapy this relationship forms the very basis of treatment. "What is left as the ultimate thing in the doctor-patient relationship is existential communication, which goes beyond anything that can be planned or methodically staged. The whole treatment is thus absorbed and defined within a community of two selves who live at the possibilities of existence itself, as reasonable beings.....Doctor and patient are both human beings and as such are fellow travellers in destiny.... There is no final solution" (Jaspers 1913/1959).

In existential therapy, the therapist begins with a neutral listening to the patient. His role is to understand the patient in terms of his mental state and his conscious awareness of his existence. Most existential therapists tend to focus less on the past and more on the future. Psychological reality is different from historical reality.

The fundamental choices we make provides us with the unifying meaning and direction of life. Choice is pre-reflective. It is what we are and not just what we do. We come to reflective consciousness having already made this choice. Its concrete expressions are the many choices articulating this project. We are a story in the making and not a disconnected set of events. It is a project that unifies our experiences and the multiple options following upon this choice.

The problem of the past is a problem of memory and therefore a problem of consciousness (Rank 1936/1978). We can usually recall only a minor fraction of our experience and can only selectively recall and synthesise the past to achieve consistency with our present view of ourselves. "You have power over your mind – not outside events. Realize this, and you will find strength." (Marcus Aurelius 1749).

The emphasis is on the decisions that need to be taken and the goals that lie ahead. Guilt and misgivings about the past are hard to disappear. One must learn to forgive oneself and others for the guilt and hurt from the past. One must give up the hope for a better past.

A powerful tool for clinicians is to follow the advice of Nietzsche. He asked people to carry out a thought experiment. The question to ask oneself: How you have not lived well? What regrets do you have about your life? What can you do now in your life so that one year or five years from now, you will not look back and have similar dismay about the new regrets that you have accumulated? In other words, can you find a way to live without continuing to accumulate regrets? Often collecting injustices and regrets can become the 'self-fulfilling prophecy' and a barrier to recovery.

While somatic diseases threaten the precariousness of person's self-organization, psychiatric disorders result from threats to the existential self. In the former, the physical integrity is at risk, but in the latter their very integrity as a person is at stake. Our existential self is at least as important as our physical self, if not more so. All meanings of life are derived from that existential self, but no meaning can be derived in the absence of a body and its physiology. "Life is realisation through the process of creation and adaptation, through struggles and resignations, compromises, and fresh efforts at integration. The content of the person's lifestyle can be classified according to his attitude to reality, and the meaning this acquires for him in the course of time" (Jaspers 1913/1959).

Man is not condemned to be free, as initially proclaimed by Sartre. Humans tend to have a yearning to be free, but this can only happen should they aim to be free. This freedom is not absolute. We can select our goals in life and the path to follow to achieve these goals. If we change our goal posts, then we must have the freedom to make choices. Humans cannot exist in a vacuum. We are social animals and need a sense of belonging. However, we also have the freedom to choose to whom we can be close and to what extent. Life is a journey of a solitary person who carries his 'me' from birth to death. Many co-travellers join the individual in this journey for variable periods of time and in many roles. We were born alone and finally we will die alone. We all hope that we die a 'timely death', an 'appropriate death', and a 'dignified death.'

Fanon, a psychiatrist recognized: existentialism neither needs, nor could have, a single central theoretician of the forms of psychiatric distress. Psychological difficulties are grounded in the collective unconscious and no individual thinker could hope to understand all cultural realities.

Simone Beauvoir and Merleau-Ponty saw existentialism as a philosophy of ambiguity. These subjective and objective factors cannot be weighed and measured with precision. This was in keeping with the Aristotelian belief that it was a mistake to seek a greater degree of clarity than a subject matter allows. One cannot look for mathematical precision in moral matters.

We live in times, where individuality is seen as the most important aspect of life and are encouraged to see all aspects as "projects": physical, mental, emotional, career, social and all else. Yet, we take shelter in unverified and unverifiable beliefs like essentialism, biological determinism etc. to avoid taking responsibility for the life we live.

An individual can be said to be in a situation. In some instances, situations are unconscious, and become effective without awareness on the part of the person concerned. The situation does not lead automatically to something inevitable, but rather it indicates certain possibilities and the limits of what is possible. What happens as a result of it is partly determined by the person who is in the situation, and by what he thinks about it. The grasping of a situation is the first step in the direction of its mastery; since to scrutinise it and to understand it arouses the will to modify its being (Jaspers 1933).

The central point in existential therapy is to identify the 'I' or 'Me' as the centre of my universe. I may have a family I was born into; I may have a family that I have created, and I have a social network in which I live, but how much closeness or distance I will keep with each of them is a decision that only I can take. Man is what he does. The only reality is in action. Man is nothing other than his own project. He exists only to the extent that he realizes himself, therefore he is nothing more than the sum of his actions, nothing more than his life."

Some of the central themes of existentialism has been described in some detail in previous chapters. These include:

Facticity: The kind of person that I am cannot be defined in factual or third person terms. It is the first-person account of the person and is also defined by the stance I take towards my facticity.

Transcendence: The ability for a person to take a stance towards their own characteristics and their practical engagement in the world. Through transcendence a person acquires an agent's perspective with the ability to make choices and decisions.

Alienation: The estrangement of the self both from the world and from oneself. While it is through 'my projects' that the world takes meaning, the world itself is not brought into being through my projects.

Authenticity: The attitude with which I engage in my projects as my own. It reflects my choice of myself, a commitment I make to be a person of this sort.

***Freedom*:** It is the ethical theory placing freedom at the core of human existence. It fosters an authentic stance towards values based on engagement and commitment. It is not simply a matter of the ability to pursue one's projects but includes the freedom not to pursue these projects.

One needs to believe in a 'free will', even though that freedom to free will comes with caveats. Our need for affiliation to familial, social and cultural groups dictates limits to free will but we also have the ability and need to put our own caveats on such expectations. To lead an authentic life, we must believe in our need for autonomy and self-direction. At every corner of life, we reach a crossroad and the direction we choose to take makes a difference.

Engagement/Responsibility: Values acquire significance only if I am at some level engaged. The world acquires significance only through the way the individual constitutes it. Many avoid personal responsibility by displacing on to others. Accepting personal responsibility is one of the important factors in the recovery process.

The therapist operates with the assumption that a patient has created his or her own distress. People can make their own distorted scripts, which can become "self-fulfilling prophecies." In therapy, the role a patient plays in the creation of his own dilemma is explored as is also the kind of excuses used to avoid taking responsibility for them. One can and often does get afflicted by the curse of 'excuse-itis' (the tendency to find excuses). In therapy they can be helped to make appropriate changes.

Bad faith: signifies our usual inclination to deny responsibility for our situation. It is seen as a form of self-deception that is quite well spread. From an existentialist stand-point, the therapist teaches the patient how to conceptualize their 'inferiority project' or 'project of bad faith' they were unaware of. The patient needs to be encouraged to take responsibility for their feelings (both pleasant and unpleasant) as well.

The therapist faces the task of determining the role the patient plays in their own dilemma. They must then find ways to communicate this to the patient. Realization of this connection affords the opportunity for change. Once a patient realizes: "Only I can change the world I have created," a window of opportunity to recovery is created. They need to reconstrue what they cannot alter. They also need to understand this responsibility to be ongoing. One does not create one's situation in life once and for all; rather one is continuously recreating oneself.

My existence includes:

My body: It has a physiology. It forms a continuum with my physical environment. Perturbation in my physiology needs to be reset. This can be achieved with certain medications as well as living a balanced life, in tune with the environment.

My past experience: My past consists of memories. They are my memories, and I can reshape them. I must give up the hope for a better past. I live in the present and this is where I can take a stand that affords me a better life.

My social and cultural milieu: They do influence me in many ways, but I can also have a role in shaping it. Society and culture are also not static, and I can see how they have changed over time. There is a macro-culture and a microculture, and we usually live in a microculture which is more conducive to my healthy living. I can subscribe to help and develop a more fulfilling relationship within it.

My sense-making and stance taking enables me to live a better existence. It gives a perspective to everything. I have the freedom to make choices and draw and redraw my life script. To live my life authentically, I must take responsibility to what happens to me in the present and future.

Using the existential formulation in therapy, one could keep working on making sense of persons' lived experiences, conceptualization of their social and cultural factors and their stance on their condition. The formulation may need to be revised periodically. This is likely to not only help with amelioration of our current state but also help build resilience for further life situations where there may be potential for relapse.

INSIGHT, STANCE TAKING AND SENSE-MAKING

The term insight lacks a clear definition and remains a rather problematic notion meaning different things to different people. For some time, an important distinction was made between those having a psychotic condition with lack of insight as opposed to those with neurotic conditions. As the joke went: A neurotic was one who built castles in the air, a psychotic was one who wanted to live in the castle, and a psychiatrist was one who collected rental from both.

Sir Aubrey Lewis (1934) disputed this view and saw lack of insight occurring in both psychosis and neurosis. Originally it meant internal sight, i.e., seeing with the eyes of the mind, having inner vision and discernment. He pointed to numerous instances of grossly defective insight into physical disorders. In any mental disorder, whether mild or severe, continued or brief, alien or comprehensible, it is with his whole disordered mind that the person contemplates his state or his individual symptoms. 'His judgements and attitudes can therefore never be the same as ours because the data are different, and his machine for judging is different in some respects.'

According to David (1990) insight should not be regarded as an 'all or nothing' phenomenon but as having three distinct overlapping dimensions: 'the recognition that one has a mental illness, compliance with treatment, and the ability to relabel unusual mental events as pathological.' He called for the assessment of insight to be standardized.

Several ways of measuring insight have been used. Lincoln et al (2007) suggested a one-item measure might suffice for a screening of overall insight in schizophrenia or other severe mental disorders. *The Scale to Assess Unawareness of Mental Disorder* measures current and previous awareness of having a mental illness, the effect of medications, consequences, and the signs and symptoms of the illness (Amador and Kronengold 2004). It includes seventy-four items forming four subscales (current awareness, retrospective awareness, current attribution, retrospective attribution). *The Birchwood Insight Scale* (Birchwood et al 1994) measures three dimensions of insight (ability to relabel symptoms, awareness of mental illness, and recognition of a need for treatment).

The concept of insight has expanded recently and is used often to measure outcome of different modalities of therapy. In cognitive behaviour therapy insight relates to becoming aware of automatic negative thoughts. *The Beck Cognitive Insight Scale* (Beck et al 2004) measures patient's capacity for distancing themselves from and re-evaluating anomalous beliefs and misinterpretations. It has two subscales (nine items tapping self-reflectiveness and six on self-certainty).

In a psychodynamic formulation insight refers to the patient's understanding of associations between past and present experiences, typical relationship patterns, and the relation between interpersonal challenges, emotional experience, and psychological symptoms. A systematic review and metanalysis found a significant, moderate correlation between insight and the outcome of psychotherapy (Jennissen et al 2018). The magnitude of the correlation was comparable to the effect sizes of established treatment factors such as therapeutic alliance, positive regard and empathy.

Insight in existential terms relates to the concept of sense-making and stance taking. It captures a formulation based on existential understanding better than the concept of insight. Only humans can take a stance on themselves and the situation they are in. It shapes the way we relate to ourselves and our world while also shaping our behaviour. People relate to themselves and their situation thereby affecting their sense of the world.

A decision to recognize having a problem, consult someone about it, agree to treatment, and decide on the preferred type of treatment involves stance taking. In therapy, insight or sense-making helps change the person's stance taking. In Cognitive Behaviour Therapy it helps change their cognitions and behaviour. In mindfulness-based therapies it promotes a non-judgmental recognition of the situation one is in, not the one that is comfortable, and not the one they would prefer. The existential stance offers another framework for change. While doing so, it also recognizes the importance of our physiology.

One needs to make sense and take an appropriate stance to the physiological changes as well as other non-physiological aspects of life.

An existential approach provides very important insights into human lives, personality, the mental disorders they suffer and their treatment. The physical (climate, population, pollution, water resources, iron, iodine, lithium etc) is on a continuum with our physiology and the body, brain and mind are part of the same complex. The physical and physiological are both affected by life experiences and the society and culture inhabited. True insight includes not just intellectual and emotional insight but must be associated with existential insight to be truly transformational.

Insight involves sense-making, and it is usually related to a specific aspect of life and in a particular situation. It is often the context that makes an experience, reaction, or sense-making pathological. Psychiatric disorders involve in a sense the 'freezing' of a certain kind of sense-making. Suffering results when people are stuck in a rigid and dysfunctional style of stance taking which is out of tune with their actual situation. Existential therapy aims at providing the freedom to maintain a flexible and relative stance. We can take a different perspective on oneself and one's situation with better outcome.

We live in times when most aspects of life are seen as projects (an individual or collaborative enterprise that is carefully planned to achieve a particular aim). Examples include health projects, well-being projects, financial projects, developmental projects etc. Similarly, we can see life itself as a project as suggested by existentialism. This will allow us to live an authentic life where we embrace freedom to make choices that are our own. Most of the constraints of life can be overcome through our wholehearted commitment to our project. Authenticity can be gained only by giving up the fantasy of an all-knowing and all-powerful creator who can also do the double act of the ultimate rescuer.

LIFE IS FULL OF PARADOXES

Kierkegaard (1833-1855) and Nietzsche (1844-1900), pioneers of existentialism, were seen as eccentric characters during their lifetime. There is little evidence to suggest that they knew about each other's work. Many of Kierkegaard's earlier works were written pseudonymously. His work was translated decades later and are widely followed.

Nietzsche was a complex and sensitive man whose outlook was at least partly coloured by his experience of being repeatedly rejected in love. Nazis quoted him selectively to claim Nietzsche to be endorsing their viewpoint. There is however truly little evidence to support such a viewpoint. Nietzsche was shunned by his colleagues due to his rather controversial claims for the time he lived in. He gave up his academic position at least partly because of his poor physical health. He moved a lot through Europe over the years in search of warm weather. His work received a lot more attention posthumously.

Martin Heidegger translated Kierkegaard work. He rose to fame with Being and Time (1927). This work, which shaped philosophical existentialism, claimed Western culture had lost touch with what he portentously called the "Meaning of Being." Heidegger joined Adolf Hitler's Nazi Party in 1933. He is known to have given a series of fiery public speeches in favour of the Nazi regime. After the war, Heidegger was subject to a teaching ban under denazification. He tried to downplay his engagement with Nazism after the end of World War II and never apologised for his role in legitimising the Nazi seizure of power.

This was not the only blemish in his life. Heidegger also had a torrid affair with one of his students Hannah Arendt. She had later moved to Heidelberg to study under Karl Jaspers for her doctoral dissertation. She would later flee to US and become a distinguished and influential scholar. Interestingly, she continued to correspond with Heidegger, and it was Arendt who made a valiant effort to resurrect the image of Heidegger after the war.

Jean-Paul Sartre and Simone de Beauvoir the two leading figures in existentialism and advocates of "freedom" ended up challenging all social conventions. They were involved in several love triangles. As a young man Sartre was hugely influenced by Heidegger's assertion that we are thrown into the world at a point of history beyond our control, and that we have to fashion the best life we can from this contingency.

Sartre found Nazism appalling. He was convinced it could not last very long. After the outbreak of World War II Sartre served briefly in the French army before becoming a prisoner of war from 1940 to 1941. It was during the war that Marxism became his second intellectual love. Although he never joined the French Communist Party, he was one of France's best-known communists. He often spoke out in support of the USSR and its policies. In 1954, he visited the Soviet Union.

After the invasion of Hungary by Soviet forces in 1956, Sartre denounced the Soviet intervention and the submission of the French Communist Party to the dictates of Moscow. He condemned the Soviet invasion wholeheartedly and without any reservation. He however continued to advocate Marxism and sought to develop a new kind of socialism in *Search for a Method* (1960). A final break with the Soviet Union came in 1968 with the Soviet suppression of Czechoslovakia.

While Heidegger tried rigorously to regain his claim to fame, Sartre refused the 1964 Nobel Prize in Literature on the grounds that a writer "should refuse to allow himself to be transformed into an institution."

As far as sexual indiscretions go Heidegger, Sartre, and de Beauvoir were in august company. Warren Ward (2022) in his book Lovers of philosophy summarised how the intimate life of seven philosophers (Kant, Hegel, Nietzsche, Heidegger, Sartre, Foucault and Derrida) shaped modern thought.

The compelling story of Victor Frankl finds a good resonance in an existential context. Frankl and his family were arrested in the mid-1900s and sentenced to slavery in one of Nazi Germany's concentration camps. He was deprived of all of his belongings, beaten into submission, and forced to work to the point of exhaustion every day. He along with his campmates were stripped naked, their heads shaved, and their identities reduced to little more than a number tattooed on their forearms. They retained nothing more than their bodies, which became withered and bruised before long. His wife and children killed, home destroyed, and the bundles of paper that contained his entire life's work were burned.

Frankl survived until the camp was liberated. After being liberated he went on to develop a psychological theory known as Logotherapy, "a concept based on the premise that the primary motivational force of an individual is to find a meaning in life." *"What was really needed was a fundamental change in our attitude toward life. We had to learn ourselves and, furthermore, we had to teach the despairing men, that it did not really matter what we expected from life, but rather what life expected from us."*

EXISTENTIAL FORMULATION

Name Age Occupation Date

1. The physiological (biological) dimension including:

   a. Diagnosis

   b. Significant vegetative (physical or bodily) symptoms

   c. Any significant associated medical disorders

2. Significant experiential trauma(s) that may have had a bearing on you:

3. The social and cultural factors that may have had a significant impact on you:

4. How do you understand your condition?

This is a template on which the patient is encouraged to work on. It may take several revisions to complete an existential formulation. This becomes their workbook. Sense-making is an ongoing process that can be visited and revisited over time.

PART V

THE CRUX OF THE PROBLEM IN PSYCHIATRY

Why are we where we find ourselves in our understanding of mental illnesses? Why do we so often find ourselves being so near and yet so far? The real problem could be that we are constantly trying to find simple solutions to problems that cannot be simplified. The WHO definition: "Health is a state of complete physical, mental, and social well-being and not merely the absence of disease or infirmity" sets impossibly lofty standards.

The realm of the "Normal" has been shrinking as an expanding psychiatry stretches easily across its elastic boundary. Diagnostic inflation has been the worst consequence of structured diagnostic systems. They have been called a splitter's dream and a lumper's nightmare. "Normal" has no universal meaning and it can never be defined with precision. It is very much in the eye of the beholder and changeable over time, place, person and culture. But each change makes it harder to know how to assimilate all previous research based on what has changed now. An interaction of the biological and psycho-social factors is abundantly clear from various points of view.

More than a hundred years ago, Karl Jaspers observed: "Biological and psychological investigations of the mind were like the exploration of an unknown continent from the opposite directions, where the explorers never meet because of impenetrable country that intervenes." They should complement one another and make each other stronger. Although we keep attempting to find a constructive collaboration between the biological and psychological but, like boxing matches, after each round, opponents retreat to their side of the ring. The dogmatist within is always worse than the perceived enemy outside.

For Guze (1989): "The conclusion appears inescapable to me that what is called psychopathology is the manifestation of disordered processes in various brain systems that mediate psychological functions. Psychopathology thus involves biology. Biology's scientific strategies are directed at understanding how organisms have evolved and how they develop and function within a genotype environment interaction framework."

Ghaemi (2007) on the other hand, pointed to our tendency to confuse the term "biological" with "disease." All things biological are not disease, even though we can define disease in such a way that all diseases are biological. All human psychological experience is mediated by the brain, and each person has one brain; therefore, the brain will always be biologically changing as we have psychological experiences. So, showing MRI changes in any condition does nothing to demonstrate that those conditions are diseases. Here the biological changes could easily be the effect and not the cause. Similar views have been expressed by many others like Burton and Frances mentioned before.

Are we following "the story of the man who is searching at night for a lost key, not in the dark alley where he dropped it but under the lamppost where the light was better?" (Yalom 1980). It is a person who develops a disorder, and hence the attributes that constitute his personality is the core of all psychopathologies, the edifice on which all other forms of psychopathology develop. Personality can best be described in a context making the task of defining other mental disorders much more complex than our current diagnostic systems suggests. The way we use current diagnostic categories is to simplify things. We may do well to keep reminding ourselves of the aphorism: "As simple as possible but not simpler."

The limitations of our current approach are borne by our paradox and predicament. Frances (2013) lamented: "We have not yet found ways of translating basic science into clinical psychiatry. None of the promising biological findings has ever qualified as a diagnostic test. Mental disorders are too heterogeneous in presentation and causality to be considered simple diseases; instead, each of our currently defined disorders will eventually turn out to be many different diseases. It may also explain the high incidence of treatment-resistant conditions seen across the board not only in psychiatry but all of medicine. Our diagnostic approaches may have created their own limitations by looking more at discreet diagnostic entities while not giving enough attention to the person who has the condition. One must be aware of the risks of self-diagnosis, fad diagnoses and drug companies. Time and resilience are good healers too."

A biologically deterministic position can both be a blessing and a curse. The blessing may come in the form of not having to take any responsibility for one's condition while allowing treatment and the treaters to provide all the answers. If all mental illnesses were based on our genes and neurobiology, then it is not the person who is either responsible or has any control. It provides a negative narrative: try as hard as one may, the biology of the condition will always reign supreme. But we know that even gene expression can be altered by environmental influences and thus also by changes to the way we live.

A more open and pragmatic approach taking an existential perspective provides the best opportunity for a sense of partnership between the person and his physiology. The person is in charge, at least to an extent, of his social and cultural circumstances and making sense of the meaning of his existence.

HUMILITY NOT HUBRIS

We may be following on the story of the blind men who have never come across an elephant before. Each blind man feels a different part of the elephant's body, but only one part, such as the side or the tusk. They then describe the elephant based on their limited experience and their descriptions of the elephant are different from each other. The moral of the story is that humans tend to claim absolute truth based on their limited, subjective experience.

For every complex problem there is an answer that is clear, simple, and wrong. (H. L. Mencken in a 1920 collection of essays called "Prejudices: Second Series"). We must admit that we still do not understand the causes of mental illness. It is often claimed that specialisation is the process of knowing more and more about less and less. We can add: It is also knowing more and more about what we don't know. The rest of medicine deals with much simpler organs than the brain/mind duo, but the causes of most of the physical illnesses also remain far from clear. Human diversity has its purpose otherwise it would not have survived the evolutionary rat race. It was good to have some who would avoid dangers, others who would ruthlessly exploit them. We must also give up the utopic vison that one day we will be able to reduce all mental disorders into chemical disturbances in the brain and cure it with a pill.

Thomas Hobbes (1588 – 1679) said human life was solitary, poor, nasty, brutish, and short. In the last two hundred years billions of people are suddenly rich, well nourished, clean, safe, and healthy. In 1964 Isaac Asimov (much acclaimed for his works on science fiction) forecasted that psychiatry would be the largest medical speciality in 2014 due to the millions of people who found themselves adrift in the sea of "enforced leisure" (Bregman 2017). There is a sharp increase in self-esteem since the 1980's. The younger generation considers itself smarter, more responsible, and more attractive than ever. It is a generation in which every kid has been told, you can be anything you want, you are special." We've been brought up on a steady diet of narcissism. (Jean Twenge 2017). This narcissism however conceals the vast uncertainties of life. We have also become a lot more fearful over the last decades. Never have so many people (children as well as adults) seeing a psychiatrists, psychologist, or counsellors, having career burnouts, and are being prescribed psychotropic medications, and committing suicide.

History is often shaped by exaggerated hopes (Harari 2015). Ambrose Bierce noted in *The Devils Dictionary* that the mind has nothing but itself to know itself with and it may never feel satisfied that it understands the deepest aspects of its own existence, its own subjectiveness (Pinker 2018).

Are we treating mental disorders (which are of limited validity and reliability) rather than what ails the human existence? All illnesses (particularly mental) are in effect failures of proper adaptation to our ever changing personal (physical and psychological) and social milieu. The aim of treatment should not just stop at the abolition of symptoms but promoting a better fit between the person and the world they live in. If psychiatric disorders are seen as existential crises, treatment would be directed at addressing the existential concerns of the patients and not just target their brain and its neurotransmitters.

Despite all of us being imperfect people living in an imperfect world, we can continue to strive towards greater perfection. However, we will always remain a work in progress. The reason for our inability to ever be perfect lies in our emotional mind. If life is a triangle, it is an inverted triangle, with its inbuilt instability. The horizontal part of the triangle is the self as seen through our overt behaviour, that meets the world around us. This is supported by the two other arms, the cognition and emotion.

The developmental process over time and particularly from the ape to modern humans has been an incredible journey. Most of our cognitive, scientific, industrial, and technological advances have been evolutionary and have served us well. The journey of life is an emotional journey. "If one were born with all the wisdom, what would one do for the rest of his/her life" may be an apt saying. One can only be born as an infant and then grow through the several stages of life.

Each step in the developmental process is unique for the person going through the process. There is the person, significant others in their lives and the social milieu around them, each playing a dynamic dance of life. Wisdom consists of learning how to keep getting better at managing emotions. Each stage of life has its own challenges. One must go through those stages, make one's mistakes, and learn along the way. "We must also learn from the mistakes of others. You can never live long enough to make them all yourself."

Cognitive advances can change behaviour in major ways for the whole or large segments of the population at once. They have made tremendous difference to the way we live our lives. Emotions on the other hand is governed by phylogenetically older part of the brain. They originated at an earlier stage of the evolutionary process. They were at first nociceptive response. Gradually they became more differentiated. Humans show a large variety of emotions, but they can be summed as positive and negative emotions. The scope of our emotional life evolves through the various stages of life.

In discussing the meaning of health and illness, Jaspers thought value judgements are unavoidable. Values are part of the illness process, but it does not necessarily follow that those illnesses are nothing but values. Jaspers believed: "A precise definition of health seems pointless if the essence of man is his incompleteness." All cognitive instructions aimed at containing emotions is helpful. Many cultural institutions prescribe norms for living a better life but play a subsidiary role in the management of personal emotions.

Our brain can be lazy. It likes shortcuts and a diagnosis may just be a way of labelling to maintain an economy of scales. Defining illness, without defining health of course runs the risk of over pathologizing, overdiagnosis, social construction and abuse of medical power. Disease, though real objective entities in the natural world, happens to individual human beings. And sometimes there is no disease at all, but only problems of living.

WHERE TO FROM HERE?

We should never stop asking questions, because a combination of learning and enjoyment is the key to a fulfilled life. Learning without enjoyment wears you down, and enjoyment without learning is mind-numbing. Nietzsche said that a man's worth was determined by how much truth he could tolerate. You are by no means only what you already know. You are also that which you could know, if only you would.

Our existence is too complex, and no one can know themselves completely. We all contain wisdom that we cannot fully and consistently comprehend. We have a self-narrative and it is a coherent story with manageable contradictions and conflicts. When our stories go haywire for whatever reason, we need help. An existentially informed therapy can be used to help us. We must continue to try and fix what we can fix using the current state of available knowledge. Patients cannot wait until we know all we need to know to help them ideally.

Mental or psychiatric disorders are not the only disorder of the brain, or of the body, but they pertain to the person. We can understand personality disorders when we look at the persons in their interactions with their world. The complex person-world system over time helps us understand its dynamics. Understanding human life is both an art and a science. Osler viewed 'medicine as an art based on science.' It makes sense that without science medicine would be empty, without art medicine would be irrelevant.

Sense-making develops by interacting in certain ways with the world. Depending on how others react, a person will develop a certain style of interacting in various preferred types of reacting in specific situations. In this continuous cycle of action and reaction, patterns emerge. A person's sensemaking is shaped by the people they interact with and the sociocultural practices shaping these interactions, while the individual, in turn, also shapes them. These emergent patterns are not carved in stone, new paths of interacting develop through new experiences – although patterns developed early in life may be very persistent.

In some cases, such as traumatic events, or poor development of attachment in early life, the original contributing factor may not be alterable anymore. All interactions take place in a certain context, and their effect will depend on how they are taken up by the whole person/world system. Because of the interconnectedness of the factors involved in sense-making and the potential feedback loops between them, both positive and negative spirals can occur. Psychiatric disorders dissolve if one succeeds in changing one's way of interacting with the world, opening up one's sclerotic pattern of sensemaking.

There have been five major anatomical changes in our species: Becoming bipeds, acquiring the perfect oppositional movement between the fingers and thumb, a unique ear apparatus, the large forebrain, and an appropriately positioned vocal cords. They have been complimented by the acquisition and increasing elaboration of four major virtues: the 4 Cs: Critical thinking, creativity, communication, and collaboration. The combination of these have set humans on a Path of Perpetual Progress. Millions of neurons act as units which functions in unison to form a mind which is in turn influenced by its past experiences and interacts with their social and cultural to derive a set of meanings. Our cognitions, metacognitions and emotions are intertwined and create our unique existential reality.

A healthy mind in a healthy body falls short in its reach to a good life. We cannot expect to be born with an ideal body and in a perfect familial, social, and cultural milieu. We cannot expect never to experience stress and adversity. However, we can try our best to make sense of the basics of our existence and what lead to the dis-ease or predicament we are faced with.

We can become the agent of change for our personal, social, and physical reality. We are 'temporary residents' of this world but must try to be 'good tenants' to play our part in making a better future in which our children and grandchildren can live and flourish. Leaving them a better world than the one we inherited is our most significant immortality project.

As we have discussed throughout this book, to be meaningful and effective, our life story should make sense, be congruent and internally consistent. Beliefs explain behaviour independently of their truth or falsity. A person's false belief explains his behaviour just as effectively as his true ones (Gaita 1999). Stories can be adaptive and maladaptive but only people with maladaptive stories present for treatment. Therapy helps turn maladaptive stories into adaptive ones. Until and unless there is a fundamental change in the way the person makes sense of life and its problems, they are likely to repeat behaviours leading to the condition for which they required treatment.

We must try to differentiate between mental disorders and mental health. Psychiatrists can be participants in the mental health movement, which can at best be seen as being in its infancy. However, they should refrain from trying to lead it. Mental health involves what is described in the previous chapter as an ounce of primary prevention. It is a gigantic enterprise and will need the joint effort of everyone. Besides psychiatrists, politicians, bureaucrats, economists, developmental and educational psychologists, social workers, welfare organisations, self-help groups and community at large must be partners in the movement. It will need lot of money and dedication and the goals will take a long time to attain.

Psychiatrists are best equipped to deal with mental disorders but must take an existential stand to do it well. An existential formulation is elaborate, informative, and considers all the complexities of what constitutes a mental disorder. They can form the basis of a treatment plan that includes the role of medications to deal with the vegetative symptoms associated with the disorder but also addresses the world of experiences, social and cultural factors, and our disordered sense-making.

An existentially oriented psychiatric treatment offers the best hope not just for recovery from the current disorder but a more integrated person capable of living a better life.

REFERENCES

Achenbach, T. M. (1991). *Manual for the child behavior checklist.* University of Vermont Department of Psychiatry.

Adler, A. B., LeardMann, C. A., Roenfeldt, K. A., Jacobson, I. G., Forbes, D. (2020). Magnitude of problematic anger and its predictors in the Millennium Cohort. *BioMedicine Central Public Health, 20*(1), 1168-1178.

Adler, A. B., LeardMann, C. A., Villalobos, J., Jacobson, I. G., & Forbes, D. (2022). Association of problematic anger with long-term adjustment following the military-to civilian transition. *Journal of the American Medical Association Psychiatry, 5*(7).

Agnew-Blais, J. C., Polanczyk, G. V., Danese, A., Wertz, J., Moffitt, T. E., & Arseneault, L. (2016). Evaluation of the persistence, remission, and emergence of attention deficit/hyperactivity disorder in young adulthood. *Journal of the American Medical Association Psychiatry, 73*(7), 713–720.

Agus, D. B. (2012). *The end of illness.* Simon & Schuster.

Alliance Development Works. (2013). *World risk report 2013.*

Allport, G. W. (1937). *Personality: a psychological interpretation.* Holt.

Amador, X. F., & Kronengold, H. (2004). Understanding and assessing insight. In X. F. Amador & A. S. David (Eds.), *Insight and psychosis: Awareness of illness in schizophrenia and related disorders* (pp. 3–30). Oxford University Press.

American Psychiatric Association. (1952). *Diagnostic and statistical manual of mental disorders* (1st ed.).

American Psychiatric Association. (1968). *Diagnostic and statistical manual of mental disorders* (2nd ed.).

American Psychiatric Association. (1987). *Diagnostic and statistical manual of mental disorders* (3rd ed., rev.).

American Psychiatric Association. (1994). *Diagnostic and statistical manual of mental disorders* (4th ed.).

American Psychiatric Association. (2000). *Diagnostic and statistical manual of mental disorders* (4th ed., text rev.).

American Psychiatric Association. (2013). *Diagnostic and statistical manual of mental disorders* (5th ed.).

American Public Health Association. (1890). *The Bertillon classification of causes of death*. R. Smith Print Company.

Anderson, D. J., & Adolphs, R. (2014). A framework for studying emotions across species. *Cell, 157*(1), 187–200.

Andreasen, N. C. (1995). Posttraumatic stress disorder: Psychology, biology, and the

Manichaean warfare between false dichotomies. *The American Journal of Psychiatry, 152*(7), 963–965.

Andreasen, N. C. (2001). *Brave new brain: Conquering mental illness in the era of the genome.* Oxford University Press.

Andrews, J. B. (1891). Traumatic hysteria from railroad injury. *American Journal of Psychiatry, 48*(1), 37–42.

Angell, M. (2011). The illusions of psychiatry. *The New York Review of Books, 58*(12), 20–22.

Angelou, M. (1969). *I know why the caged bird sings*. Random House.

Aristotle. (2013). *Politics* (2nd ed.). University of Chicago Press.

Arnold, T. (1786). *Observations on the nature, kinds, causes and prevention of insanity, lunacy or madness* (Issue v. 2). G. Ireland.

Aron, E. (1996). *The highly sensitive person: How to thrive when the world overwhelms you.*

Carol Publishing Group.

Asimov, I. (1964). Visit to the World's Fair of 2014. *New York Times, 16*.

Auden, W. H. (1947). *The age of anxiety: A baroque eclogue*. Random House.

Aurelius, M. (1749). *The meditations of the Emperor Marcus Aurelius Antoninus* (T. Gataker, Trans.). Robert & Andrew Foulis.

Australian Bureau of Statistics. (2022). *Religious affiliation in Australia (2021).*

Bach, B., Sellbom, M., Kongerslev, M., Simonsen, E., Krueger, R. F., & Mulder, R. (2017). Deriving ICD-11 personality disorder domains from dsm-5 traits: Initial attempt to harmonize two diagnostic systems. *Acta Psychiatrica Scandinavica, 136*(1), 108–117.

Bacon, F. (1620). *Novum organum scientiarum*. Unknown.

Bar-On, R. (2001). Emotional intelligence and self-actualization. In J. Ciarrochi, J. P. Forgas,

& J. D. Mayer (Eds.), *Emotional intelligence in everyday life: A scientific inquiry* (pp. 82–97). Psychology Press.

Bateman, A. W. (2012). Treating borderline personality disorder in clinical practice. *The American Journal of Psychiatry, 169*(6), 560–563.

Beck, A. T., Baruch, E., Balter, J. M., Steer, R. A., & Warman, D. M. (2004). A new instrument for measuring insight: The Beck Cognitive Insight Scale. *Schizophrenia Research, 68*(2–3), 319–329.

Becker, E. (1971). *The birth and death of meaning: An interdisciplinary perspective on the problem of man*. Free Press.

Becker, E. (1973). *The denial of death*. Free Press.

Bentham, J. (1789). *Principles of morals and legislation*. Batoche Books.

Bernard, C., & University College, London. L. S. (1865). *An introduction to the study of experimental medicine*. Schuman.

Berne, E. (1964). *Games people play: The psychology of human relationships* (Issue v. 10). Grove Press.

Birchwood, M., Smith, J., Drury, V., Healy, J., Macmillan, F., & Slade, M. (1994). A self-report Insight Scale for psychosis: Reliability, validity and sensitivity to change. *Acta Psychiatrica Scandinavica, 89*(1), 62–67.

Bodkin, J. A., Pope, H. G., Detke, M. J., & Hudson, J. I. (2007). Is PTSD caused by traumatic stress? *Journal of Anxiety Disorders, 21*(2), 176–182.

Bolton, D. (2008). *What is mental disorder?: An essay in philosophy, science, and values.* Oxford University Press.

Bonanno, G. A. (2022) *The End of Trauma: How the new science of resilience is changing how we think about PTSD.* Basic Books.

Bower, G. H. (1981). Mood and memory. *American Psychologist, 36*(2), 129–148.

Bowlby, J. (1969). *Attachment and loss* (Issue v. 1). Penguin Books.

Bowman, M. L. (1999). Individual differences in posttraumatic distress: Problems with the DSM-IV model. *The Canadian Journal of Psychiatry, 44*(1), 21–33.

Bracken, P. J. (2001). Post-modernity and post-traumatic stress disorder. *Social Science & Medicine, 53*(6), 733–743.

Brawman-Mintzer, O., Lydiard, R. B., Emmanuel, N., Payeur, R., Johnson, M., Roberts, J., Jarrell, M. P., & Ballenger, J. C. (1993). Psychiatric comorbidity in patients with generalized anxiety disorder. *The American Journal of Psychiatry, 150*(8), 1216–1218.

Bregman, R. (2017). *Utopia for realists: And how we can get there.* Bloomsbury Publishing.

Bregman, R. (2019). *Humankind: A hopeful history.* Bloomsbury Publishing.

Brown, G. W. (1981). Life Events, psychiatric disorder and physical illness. *Journal of Psychosomatic Research, 25*(5), 461-473.

Bryant, R. A., Galatzer-Levy, I., & Hadzi-Pavlovic, D. (2022). The heterogeneity of posttraumatic stress disorder in DSM-5. *Journal of the American Medical Association Psychiatry, 80*(2), 189–191.

Burgess, A. W., & Holmstrom, L. L. (1974). Rape trauma syndrome. *The American Journal of Psychiatry, 131*(9), 981–986.

Burton, R. (1621). *The anatomy of melancholy.* John Lichfield and James Short.

Burton, R. A. (2008). *On being certain: Believing you are right even when you're not.* St. Martin's Press.

Burton, R. A. (2013). *A skeptic's guide to the mind: What neuroscience can and cannot tell us about ourselves.* St. Martin's Press.

Cain, S. (2012). *Quiet: The power of introverts in a world that can't stop talking.* Penguin Books Limited.

Carr, E. H. (1961). *What is history?* Vintage Books.

Caspi, A., & Moffitt, T. E. (2018). All for one and one for all: Mental disorders in one dimension. *The American Journal of Psychiatry, 175*(9), 831–844.

Caspi, A., Houts, R. M., Ambler, A., Danese, A., Elliott, M. L., Hariri, A., Harrington, H., Hogan, S., Poulton, R., Ramrakha, S., Rasmussen, L. J. H., Reuben, A., RichmondRakerd, L., Sugden, K., Wertz, J., Williams, B. S., & Moffitt, T. E. (2020). Longitudinal assessment of mental health disorders and comorbidities across 4 decades among participants in the Dunedin Birth Cohort Study. *Journal of the American Medical Association Network Open, 3*(4).

Caspi, A., Houts, R. M., Belsky, D. W., Goldman-Mellor, S. J., Harrington, H., Israel, S., Meier, M. H., Ramrakha, S., Shalev, I., Poulton, R., & Moffitt, T. E. (2014). The p factor: One general psychopathology factor in the structure of psychiatric disorders? *Clinical Psychological Science: A Journal of the Association for Psychological Science, 2*(2), 119–137.

Cerdá, M., Sagdeo, A., & Galea, S. (2008). Comorbid forms of psychopathology: Key patterns and future research directions. *Epidemiologic Reviews, 30*(1), 155–177.

Charlson, F., Ali, S., Benmarhnia, T., Pearl, M., Massazza, A., Augustinavicius, J., & Scott, J. G. (2021). Climate change and mental health: A scoping review. *International Journal of Environmental Research and Public Health, 18*(9), 4486.

Charlton, B. G. (1990). A critique of biological psychiatry. *Psychological Medicine, 20*(1), 3– 6.

Churchill, W. (1940). *Their finest hour.* Saskatoon Star-Phoenix.

Cipriani, A., Furukawa, T. A., Salanti, G., Chaimani, A., Atkinson, L. Z., Ogawa, Y., Leucht, S., Ruhe, H. G., Turner, E. H., Higgins, J. P. T., Egger, M., Takeshima, N., Hayasaka, Y., Imai,

H., Shinohara, K., Tajika, A., Ioannidis, J. P. A., & Geddes, J. R. (2018). Comparative efficacy and acceptability of 21 antidepressant drugs for the acute treatment of adults with major depressive disorder: A systematic review and network meta-analysis. *Focus, 16*(4), 420–429.

Clifton, J. (2022, June 18). Unhappiness is soaring around the world, laments Jon Clifton. *The Economist.*

Cloninger, C. R. (1987). A systematic method for clinical description and classification of personality variants: A proposal. *Archives of General Psychiatry, 44*(6), 573–588.

Coper, E. (2022). *Facts and other lies: Welcome to the disinformation age.* Allen & Unwin.

Cosgrove, L., & Krimsky, S. (2012). A comparison of DSM-IV and DSM-5 panel members' financial associations with industry: A pernicious problem persists. *Public Library of Science Medicine, 9*(3).

Critchley, S. (2017). *What we think about when we think about football.* Penguin Publishing Group.

Crowell, S. (2020). Existentialism. In *The Stanford Encyclopedia of Philosophy.* (Summer 2020 Edition).

Csikszentmihalyi, M. (1975). *Beyond boredom and anxiety.* Jossey-Bass Publishers.

Dahlgreen, W. (2015, August 12). *37% of British workers think their jobs are meaningless.* https://yougov.co.uk/topics/society/articles-reports/2015/08/12/british-jobsmeaningless

Damasio, A. (2003). Feelings of emotion and the self. *Annals of the New York Academy of Sciences, 1001*(1), 253–261.

Damasio, A. R. (2018). *The strange order of things: Life, feeling, and the making of cultures.*

Pantheon Books.

Darwin, C. (1872). *The expression of the emotions in man and animals.* John Murray.

Darwin, C. (1891). *The origin of species by means of natural selection.* John Murray.

Das, A., & Khanna, R. (1993). Organic manic syndrome: Causative factors, phenomenology and immediate outcome. *Journal of Affective Disorders, 27*(3), 147–153.

David, A. S. (1990). Insight and psychosis. *The British Journal of Psychiatry, 156,* 798–808.

Dawson, E., Moore, T., & McGainty, W. (1972). Relationship of lithium metabolism to mental hospital admission and homicide. *Journal of Central Nervous System Disease, 33*(8), 546–556.

de Beauvoir, S. (1949). *The second sex.* Gallimard. de Beauvoir, S. (1966). *She came to stay.* Penguin Books.

de Botton, A. (2014). *The news: A user's manual.* Penguin Books Limited.

de Botton, A. (2016). *The course of love.* Simon & Schuster.

de Haan, S. (2020). Bio-psycho-social interaction: An enactive perspective. *International Review of Psychiatry, 33*(5), 471–477.

de Haan, S. (2020). *Enactive psychiatry.* Cambridge University Press.

de Jong, K., Mulhern, M., Ford, N, van der Kam, S., Kleber, R. (2000). The trauma of war in Sierra Leone. *Lancet,* 355, 2067-2070.

de La Rochefoucauld, F. (1645). *Reflexions ou Sentences et maximes morales.* Chez Claude Barbin.

Deary, I. J. (2001). Human intelligence differences: A recent history. *Trends in Cognitive Sciences, 5*(3), 127–130.

DeCasper, A. J., & Spence, M. J. (1986). Prenatal maternal speech influences newborns' perception of speech sounds. *Infant Behavior & Development, 9*(2), 133–150.

DeJong, C., Aguilar, T., Tseng, C.-W., Lin, G. A., Boscardin, W. J., & Dudley, R. A. (2016). Pharmaceutical industry-sponsored meals and physician prescribing patterns for Medicare beneficiaries. *Journal of the American Medical Association Internal Medicine, 176*(8), 1114–1122.

Diamond, J. M (1997). *Guns, germs, and steel: The fates of human societies.* Vintage

Dobbs, D. (2009). The post-traumatic stress trap. *Scientific American, 300*(4), 64–69.

Dohrenwend, B. P., Turner, J. B., Turse, N. A., Adams, B. G., Koenen, K. C., & Marshall, R. (2006). The psychological risks of Vietnam for US veterans: A revisit with new data and methods. *Science, 313*(5789), 979–982.

Douglas, S. J. (1989). *Inventing American broadcasting, 1899-1922.* Johns Hopkins University Press.

Drake, R. E., & Vaillant, G. E. (1985). A validity study of Axis II of DSM-III. *The American Journal of Psychiatry, 142*(5), 553–558.

Dückers, M. L. A., Alisic, E., & Brewin, C. R. (2016). A vulnerability paradox in the cross-national prevalence of post-traumatic stress disorder. *The British Journal of Psychiatry: The Journal of Mental Science, 209*(4), 300–305.

Dunner, D. L. (2001). Management of anxiety disorders: The added challenge of comorbidity. *Depression and Anxiety, 13*(2), 57–71.

Durkheim, É. (1912). *The elementary forms of the religious life: A study in religious sociology.* Allen & Unwin.

Eastmond, M. (1998). Nationalist discourses and the construction of difference: Bosnian Muslim refugees in Sweden. *Journal of Refugee Studies, 11*(2), 161-172.

Einstein, A. (1950). *Out of my later years.* Thames and Hudson.

Eisenberg, L. (1986). Mindlessness and brainlessness in psychiatry. *The British Journal of Psychiatry, 148*, 497–508.

Eisenberg, L. (1995). The social construction of the human brain. *American Journal of Psychiatry, 152*(11), 1563–1575.

Eisenberg, L. (2000). Is psychiatry more mindful or brainier than it was a decade ago? *The British Journal of Psychiatry, 176*(1), 1–5.

Ekman, P. (1976). Movements with precise meanings. *Journal of Communication, 26*(3), 14–26.

Ekman, P. (1992). An argument for basic emotions. *Cognition and Emotion, 6*, 169–200.

Ekman, P., & Friesen, W. V. (1971). Constants across cultures in the face and emotion. *Journal of Personality and Social Psychology, 17*(2), 124 –129.

Ellingson, T. (2001). *The myth of the noble savage* (Vol. 1). University of California Press.

Enard, W., Przeworski, M., Fisher, S. E., Lai, C. S., Wiebe, V., Kitano, T., Monaco, A. P., & Pääbo, S. (2002). Molecular evolution of FOXP2, a gene involved in speech and language. *Nature, 418*(6900), 869–872.

Engel, G. L. (1977). The need for a new medical model: A challenge for biomedicine. *Science, 196*(4286), 129–136.

Erikson, E.H. (1968). *Identity: Youth and crisis.* Norton & Co.

Esquirol, J. (1838). *Mental maladies: A treatise on insanity.* Unknown.

Fanon, F. (1952). *Black skin white masks* (R. Philcox, Trans.). Grove Press.

Faraone, S. V., Biederman, J., & Mick, E. (2006). The age-dependent decline of attention deficit hyperactivity disorder: A meta-analysis of follow-up studies. *Psychological Medicine, 36*(2), 159–165.

Fava, M., Alpert, J. E., Carmin, C. N., Wisniewski, S. R., Trivedi, M. H., Biggs, M. M., Shores Wilson, K., Morgan, D., Schwartz, T., Balasubramani, G. K., & Rush, A. J. (2004). Clinical correlates and symptom patterns of anxious depression among patients with major depressive disorder in STAR*D. *Psychological Medicine, 34*(7), 1299–1308.

Feifel, H. (1977). *New meanings of death.* McGraw-Hill.

Feighner, J. P., Robins, E., Guze, S. B., Woodruff, R. A., Winokur, G., & Munoz, R. (1972). Diagnostic criteria for use in psychiatric research. *Archives of General Psychiatry, 26*(1), 57–63.

First, M. B. (2010). Paradigm shifts and the development of the diagnostic and statistical manual of mental disorders: Past experiences and future aspirations. *Canadian Journal of Psychiatry, 55*(11), 692–700.

Fisher, W. R. (1988). The narrative paradigm and the interpretation and assessment of historical texts. *The Journal of the American Forensic Association, 25*(2), 49–53.

Fivush, R., & Hamond, N. R. (1989). Time and again: Effects of repetition and retention interval on 2-year olds' event recall. *Journal of Experimental Child Psychology, 47*(2), 259–273.

Forgas, J. P. (2000). *Feeling and thinking: The role of affect in social cognition.* Cambridge University Press.

Frances, A. (2009). A warning sign on the road to DSM-V: Beware of its unintended consequences. *Psychiatric Times, 26*(8).

Frances, A. (2013). *Saving normal: An insider's revolt against out-of-control psychiatric diagnosis, DSM-5, big pharma, and the medicalization of ordinary life.* William Morrow & Co.

Frankl, V. E. (1946). *Man's search for meaning.* Hodder & Stoughton.

Franklin, B. (1868). *Autobiography of Benjamin Franklin: Edited from his manuscript.* Lippincott.

Fromm, E. (1963). *The art of loving.* Unwin.

Frueh, B. C., Grubaugh, A. L., Elhai, J. D., & Buckley, T. C. (2007). US Department of Veterans Affairs disability policies for posttraumatic stress disorder: Administrative trends and implications for treatment, rehabilitation, and research. *American Journal of Public Health, 97*(12), 2143–2145.

Fuchs, T. (2011). Are mental illnesses diseases of the brain? In S. Choudhury & J. Slaby (Eds.), *Critical neuroscience: A handbook of the social and cultural contexts of neuroscience* (pp. 331–344). Wiley-Blackwell.

Fukuyama, F. (2018). *Identity: The demand for dignity and the politics of resentment.* Farrar, Straus and Giroux.

Furman, E. (1974). *A child's parent dies: Studies in childhood bereavement.* Yale University Press.

Galatzer-Levy, I. R., & Bryant, R. A. (2013). 636,120 Ways to have posttraumatic stress disorder. *Perspectives on Psychological Science: A Journal of the Association for Psychological Science, 8*(6), 651–662.

Gardner, H. (1983). *Frames of mind: The theory of multiple intelligences.* Heinemann.

Garmezy, N. & Rutter, M. (1985). Acute reactions to stress. In M. Rutter & L. Hersov (Eds.), *Child and adolescent psychiatry: Modern approaches* (2nd ed., pp. 152–176). Blackwell.

Ghaemi, S. N. (2007). Feeling and time: The phenomenology of mood disorders, depressive realism, and existential psychotherapy. *Schizophrenia Bulletin, 33*(1), 122–130.

Ghaemi, S. N. (2010). *The rise and fall of the biopsychosocial model: Reconciling art and science in psychiatry.* Johns Hopkins University Press.

Ghaemi, S. N. (2018). *Antidepressants work for major depression! Not so fast.* https://www.medscape.com/viewarticle/897878

Gilbert, D. T., & Wilson, T. D. (2000). Miswanting: Some problems in the forecasting of future affective states. In J. P. Forgas (Ed.), *Feeling and thinking: The role of affect in social cognition* (pp. 178–197). Cambridge University Press.

Gillett, G. (1999). *The mind and its discontents: An essay in discursive psychiatry.* Oxford University Press.

Glass, A. J. (1954). Psychotherapy in the combat zone. *American Journal of Psychiatry, 110*(10), 725–731.

Glass, D. (2016, December 3). "Immoral and unethical": WorkCover needs wholesale change to restore fairness for long term injured workers. *Victorian Ombudsman.*

Goldberg, D., & Huxley, P. (1980). *Mental illness in the community: The pathway to psychiatric care.* Routledge.

Goldberg, L. R. (1993). The structure of phenotypic personality traits. *American Psychologist, 48*(1), 26–34.

Goleman, D. (1995). *Emotional intelligence.* Bantam Books.

Graeber, D., & Wengrow, D. (2021). *The dawn of everything: A new history of humanity.* Penguin UK.

Grayling, A. C. (2011). *The good book: A secular Bible.* Bloomsbury Publishing.

Grayling, A. C. (2019). *The history of philosophy.* Penguin Publishing Group.

Grice, H. P. (1975). Logic and conversation. In P. Cole & J. Morgan (Eds.), *Speech acts* (pp. 41–58). Brill.

Grice, H. P., & Strawson, P. F. (1956). In defense of a dogma. *The Philosophical Review, 65*(2), 141–158.

Grinker, R. R., & Spiegel, J. P. (1945). *Men under stress.* Blakiston.

Grinker, R. R., Werble, B., & Drye, R. C. (1968). *The borderline syndrome: A behavioral study of egofunctions.* Basic Books.

Groopman, J. E. (2007). *How doctors think.* Houghton Mifflin.

Gross, J. J. (2002). Emotion regulation: Affective, cognitive, and social consequences. *Psychophysiology, 39*(3), 281–291.

Gunderson, J. G. and Singer, M. T. (1975): Defining Borderline Personality. *American Journal of Psychiatry,* 132(1), 1-10.

Gunderson, J. G., & Zanarini, M. C. (2011). Deceptively simple—Or radical shift? *Personality and Mental Health, 5*(4), 260–262.

Guze, S. B. (1989). Biological psychiatry: Is there any other kind? *Psychological Medicine, 19*(2), 315–323.

Hall, C. S., & Lindzey, G. (1978). *Theories of personality* (3rd ed.). John Wiley & Sons.

Harari, Y. N. (2014). *Sapiens.* Random House.

Harari, Y. N. (2015). *Homo deus.* Random House.

Hari, J. (2019). *Lost connections: Why you're depressed and how to find hope.* Bloomsbury USA.

Hari, J. (2022). *Stolen focus: Why you can't pay attention.* Bloomsbury Publishing.

Harrison, A. G., Edwards, M. J., & Parker, K. C. (2007). Identifying students faking ADHD: Preliminary findings and strategies for detection. *Archives of Clinical Neuropsychology, 22*(5), 577–588.

Healy, D. (1997). *The antidepressant era.* Harvard University Press.

Healy, D. (2006). Manufacturing consensus. *Culture, Medicine and Psychiatry, 30*(2), 135– 156.

Hegel, G. W. F. (1807). *The phenomenology of spirit.* Bey Joseph Anton Goebhardt.

Heidegger, M. (1927). *Being and time* (Issue v. 8). Max Niemeyer, Verlag.

Heinrichs, M., Wagner, D., Schoch, W., Soravia, L. M., Hellhammer, D. H., & Ehlert, U. (2005). Predicting posttraumatic stress symptoms from pretraumatic risk factors: A 2year prospective follow-up study in firefighters. *The American Journal of Psychiatry, 162*(12), 2276–2286.

Herrero, A., & Flores, F. G. (2008). *The cyanobacteria: molecular biology, genomics, and evolution.* Caister Academic Press.

Hettema, J. M., Neale, M. C., Myers, J. M., Prescott, C. A., & Kendler, K. S. (2006). A population-based twin study of the relationship between neuroticism and internalizing disorders. *The American Journal of Psychiatry, 163*(5), 857–864.

Hippocrates. (1923). *Works of Hippocrates* (W. H. S. Jones & E. T. Withington, Trans.). Harvard University Press.

Hoge, C. W., & Lies, J. (2015). Posttraumatic stress disorder: Developments in assessment and treatment. *Federal Practitioner, 32*(Suppl 3), 24–28.

Hoge, C. W., Riviere, L. A., Wilk, J. E., Herrell, R. K., & Weathers, F. W. (2014). The prevalence of post-traumatic stress disorder (PTSD) in US combat soldiers: A head-tohead comparison of DSM-5 versus DSM-IV-TR symptom criteria with the PTSD checklist. *The Lancet Psychiatry, 1*(4), 269–277.

Holmes, J. (2000). Narrative in psychiatry and psychotherapy: The evidence? *Medical Humanities, 26*(2), 92–96.

Horwitz, A. V., & Wakefield, J. C. (2007). *The loss of sadness: How psychiatry transformed normal sorrow into depressive disorder.* Oxford University Press.

Howells, C. (2011). *Mortal subjects.* Wiley.

Hutton, J. S., Dudley, J., Horowitz-Kraus, T., DeWitt, T., & Holland, S. K. (2020). Associations between screen-based media use and brain white matter integrity in preschool-aged children. *Journal of the American Medical Association Pediatrics, 174*(1).

Hyman, S. E. (2011). Diagnosing the DSM: Diagnostic classification needs fundamental reform. *Cerebrum: The Dana Forum on Brain Science, 2011*, 6.

Izard, C. E. (2009). Emotion theory and research: Highlights, unanswered questions, and emerging issues. *Annual Review of Psychology, 60*, 1–25.

Jaspers, K. (1913/1997). *General psychopathology*. Johns Hopkins University Press.

Jaspers, K. (1931/1933) *Man in The Modern Age*. Routledge

Jaspers, K. (1959). *Truth and symbol*. Rowman & Littlefield.

Jaspers, K (1963) General Psychopathology, translated by J. Hoenig and Marian W. Hamilton. Chicago University Press

Jennissen, S., Huber, J., Ehrenthal, J. C., Schauenburg, H., & Dinger, U. (2018). Association between insight and outcome of psychotherapy: Systematic review and meta-analysis. *The American Journal of Psychiatry, 175*(10), 961–969.

Johnson, N. (2003). Forty years of wandering in the wasteland. *Federal Communications Law Journal, 55*(3), 521-535.

Jonas, H. (1966). *The phenomenon of life: Toward a philosophical biology*. Northwestern University Press.

Jones, E. (1946). A valedictory address. *International Journal of Psychoanalysis, 27*, 7-12.

Jones, E., Vermaas, R. H., McCartney, H., Beech, C., Palmer, I., Hyams, K., & Wessely, S. (2003). Flashbacks and post-traumatic stress disorder: The genesis of a 20th-century diagnosis. *The British Journal of Psychiatry, 182*(2), 158–163.

Jung, C. G. (1921). *Psychological types*. Rascher.

Kahneman, D. (2011). *Thinking, fast and slow*. Penguin Books Limited.

Kahneman, D., & Tversky, A. (2000). *Choices, values, and frames*. Cambridge University Press.

Kahneman, D., Sibony, O., & Sunstein, C. R. (2021). *Noise*. Harper Collins Publishers.

Kaiser, H., & Fierman, L. B. (1965). *Effective psychotherapy: The contribution of Hellmuth Kaiser*. Free Press.

Kalpakci, A., Ha, C., & Sharp, C. (2018). Differential relations of executive functioning to borderline personality disorder presentations in adolescents: Executive functioning and borderline personality disorder. *Personality and Mental Health, 12*(2), 93–106.

Kandel, E. R. (1998). A new intellectual framework for psychiatry. *The American Journal of Psychiatry, 155*(4), 457–469.

Kandel, E. R. (1998). A new intellectual framework for psychiatry. *American Journal of Psychiatry, 155*(4), 457–469.

Kandler, C., & Zapko-Willmes, A. (2017). Theoretical perspectives on the interplay of nature and nurture in personality development. In J. Specht (Ed.), *Personality development across the lifespan* (pp. 101–115). Elsevier Academic Press.

Kant, I. (1781). *The critique of pure reason*. Brian Westland.

Kant, I. (1783). *An answer to the question: What is enlightenment*. Brian Westland.

Kastenbaum, R. J. (1981). Habituation as a model of human aging. *The International Journal of Aging and Human Development, 12*(3), 159–170.

Kendall, P. C. (1998). Directing misperceptions: Researching the issues facing manual-based treatments. *Clinical Psychology: Science and Practice, 5*(3), 396–399.

Kendell, R. (1975). The concept of disease and its implications for psychiatry. *The British Journal of Psychiatry, 127*, 305–315.

Kendell, R. (1980). Diagnostic and statistical manual of mental disorders. *American Journal of Psychiatry, 137*(12), 1630–1631.

Kendell, R. E. (2002). The distinction between personality disorder and mental illness. *The British Journal of Psychiatry, 180*(2), 110–115.

Kendler, K. S. (2010). The problem: Charge to the conference. In K. Kendler, P. Sirovatka & D. Regier (Eds.), *Diagnostic issues in depression and generalized anxiety disorder: Refining the research agenda for DSM-V* (pp. 1-15). American Psychiatric Association Publishing.

Kendler, K. S. (2019). From many to one to many: The search for causes of psychiatric illness. *Journal of the American Medical Association Psychiatry, 76*(10), 1085–1091.

Kendler, K. S., & First, M. B. (2010). Alternative futures for the DSM revision process:

Iteration v. paradigm shift. *The British Journal of Psychiatry, 197*(4), 263–265.

Kendler, K. S., Abrahamsson, L., Ohlsson, H., Sundquist, J., & Sundquist, K. (2022). An extended Swedish adoption study of anxiety disorder and its cross-generational familial relationship with major depression. *American Journal of Psychiatry, 179*(9), 640–649.

Kendler, K. S., Muñoz, R. A., & Murphy, G. (2010). The development of the Feighner criteria: A historical perspective. *American Journal of Psychiatry, 167*(2), 134–142.

Kernberg, O. (1967). Borderline personality organization. *Journal of the American Psychoanalytic Association, 15*, 641–685.

Kesey, K. (1962). *One flew over the cuckoo's nest*. Viking Press.

Kessler, R. C., McLaughlin, K. A., Green, J. G., Gruber, M. J., Sampson, N. A., Zaslavsky, A. M., Aguilar-Gaxiola, S., Alhamzawi, A. O., Alonso, J., Angermeyer, M., Benjet, C., Bromet, E., Chatterji, S., de Girolamo, G., Demyttenaere, K., Fayyad, J., Florescu, S., Gal, G., Gureje, O., … Williams, D. R. (2010). Childhood adversities and adult psychopathology in the WHO World Mental Health Surveys. *The British Journal of Psychiatry: The Journal of Mental Science, 197*(5), 378–385.

Kessler, R. C., Sampson, N. A., Berglund, P., Gruber, M. J., Al-Hamzawi, A., Andrade, L., Bunting, B., Demyttenaere, K., Florescu, S., de Girolamo, G., Gureje, O., He, Y., Hu, C., Huang, Y., Karam, E., Kovess-Masfety, V., Lee, S., Levinson, D., Medina Mora, M. E., … Wilcox, M. A. (2015). Anxious and non-anxious major depressive disorder in the World Health Organization World Mental Health Surveys. *Epidemiology and Psychiatric Sciences, 24*(3), 210–226.

Kessler, R. C., Sonnega, A., Bromet, E., Hughes, M., & Nelson, C. B. (1995). Posttraumatic stress disorder in the National Comorbidity Survey. *Archives of General Psychiatry, 52*(12), 1048–1060.

Kety, S. S. (1960). A biologist examines the mind and behavior. *Science, 132*, 1861–1870.

Keynes, J. M. (1930). *Essays in Persuasion*. Brace Harcourt.

Khanna, R., & Borde, M. (1989). Mania in a five-year-old child with tuberous sclerosis. *British Journal of Psychiatry, 155*(1), 117–119.

Khanna, R., Nizamie, S. H., & Das, A. (1991). Electrical trauma, nonictal EEG changes, and mania: A case report. *The Journal of Clinical Psychiatry, 52*(6), 280.

Kierkegaard, S. (1843/2004). *Either/Or: A Fragment of life.* Penguin Books

Kierkegaard, S. (1846). *On the dedication to 'that single individual.'* Bellinger.

Kierkegaard, S. (1936). *Philosophical fragments.* Princeton University Press.

Kihlstrom, J. F., & Klein, S. B. (1997). Self-knowledge and self-awareness. *Annals of the New York Academy of Sciences, 818*(4), 4–17.

Kim, Y.-R., Tyrer, P., Lee, H.-S., Kim, S.-G., Connan, F., Kinnaird, E., Olajide, K., & Crawford, M. (2016). Schedule for personality assessment from notes and documents (SPANDOC): Preliminary validation, links to the ICD-11 classification of personality disorder and use in eating disorders. *Personality and Mental Health, 10*(2), 106–117.

Klien, E. (2020) *Why we are polarized?* Prolific Books Limited.

Klein, M. (1948). A contribution to the theory of anxiety and guilt. *The International Journal of Psychoanalysis, 29*, 114-123

Klein, M. (1975). *Love, guilt, and reparation, and other works, 1921-1945.* Hogarth Press.

Klerman, G. L. (1972). Psychotropic hedonism vs. pharmacological Calvinism. *Hastings Center Report, 2*(4), 1–3.

Knight, R. P. (1953). Borderline states. *Bulletin of the Menninger Clinic, 17*, 1–12.

Knutson, B., Wolkowitz, O. M., Cole, S. W., Chan, T., Moore, E. A., Johnson, R. C., Terpstra, J., Turner, R. A., & Reus, V. I. (1998). Selective alteration of personality and social behavior by serotonergic intervention. *The American Journal of Psychiatry, 155*(3), 373–379.

Kramer, P. (1993). *Listening to Prozac.* Viking.

Kruger, J., & Dunning, D. (1999). Unskilled and unaware of it: How difficulties in recognizing one's own incompetence lead to inflated self-assessments. *Journal of Personality and Social Psychology, 77*, 1121–1134.

Lacan, J. (1977). *The four fundamental concepts of psycho-analysis*. Norton.

Lahey, B. B., Applegate, B., Hakes, J. K., Zald, D. H., Hariri, A. R., & Rathouz, P. J. (2012). Is there a general factor of prevalent psychopathology during adulthood? *Journal of Abnormal Psychology, 121*(4), 971–977.

Lahontan, B. D. (1931). *Dialogues curieux entre l'auteur et un sauvage de bon sens qui a voyage et memoires de l'Amerique septentrionale* (2nd ed.). Gilbert Chinard.

Lazarus, N. (2020). *The Lazarus strategy: How to age well and wisely*. Hodder & Stoughton.

Lewis, A. (1934). The psychopathology of insight. *British Journal of Medical Psychology, 14*(4), 332–348.

Lewis, G., & Appleby, L. (1988). Personality disorder: The patients psychiatrists dislike. *The British Journal of Psychiatry: The Journal of Mental Science, 153*, 44–49.

Liedloff, J. (1986). *The continuum concept: In search of happiness lost*. Hachette Books.

Lifton, R. J. (1975). The postwar war. *Journal of Social Issues, 31*(4), 181–195.

Lifton, R. J. (1979). *The broken connection: On death and the continuity of life*. Simon and Schuster.

Lincoln, T. M., Lüllmann, E., & Rief, W. (2007). Correlates and long-term consequences of poor insight in patients with schizophrenia: A systematic review. *Schizophrenia Bulletin, 33*(6), 1324–1342.

Linehan, M. M. (1993). *Cognitive-behavioral treatment of borderline personality disorder*. Guilford Publications.

Loewenstein, G., Sah, S., & Cain, D. M. (2012). The unintended consequences of conflict-ofinterest disclosure. *Journal of the American Medical Association, 307*(7), 669–670.

Mann, J. J. (2005). The medical management of depression. *New England Journal of Medicine, 353*(17), 1819–1834.

Marinoff, L., & Kapklein, C. (1999). *Plato, not Prozac!: Applying philosophy to everyday problems*. Harper Collins.

Markowitz, J. C., Wright, J. H., Peeters, F., Thase, M. E., Kocsis, J. H., & Sudak, D. M. (2022). The neglected role of psychotherapy for treatment-resistant depression. *American Journal of Psychiatry, 179*(2), 90–93.

Marx, K. (1844). Contribution to the critique of Hegel's philosophy of right. *DeutschFranzösische Jahrbücher, 7*(10), 261–271.

Marx, K., Engels, F., & Waton, H. (1925). *German ideology: The materialist conception of history.* Demos Press.

Maugham, W. S. (1944). *The razor's edge: A novel.* Doubleday, Doran & Company.

Maugham, W. S. (1946). *Of human bondage, with a digression on the art of fiction* (Issue v. 88). U.S. Government Printing Office.

May, T. (2011, September 11). *The meaningfulness of lives.* https://archive.nytimes.com/opinionator.blogs.nytimes.com/2011/09/11/themeaningfulness-of-lives/

McAdams, D. P. (2015). Three lines of personality development: A conceptual itinerary. *European Psychologist, 20*(4), 252–264.

McBrearty, S., & Brooks, A. S. (2000). The revolution that wasn't: A new interpretation of the origin of modern human behavior. *Journal of Human Evolution, 39*(5), 453–563.

McFarlane, A. C. (1990). Vulnerability to posttraumatic stress disorder. In M. E. Wolf & A. D. Mosnaim (Eds.), *posttraumatic stress disorder: Etiology, phenomenology, and treatment* (pp. 3–20). American Psychiatric Association.

McGuire, M. T., Raleigh, M. J., & Johnson, C. (1983). Social dominance in adult male vervet monkeys: Behavior-biochemical relationships. *Social Science Information, 22*(2), 311–328.

McHugh, P. (1994). Psychotherapy Awry. The American Scholar, pp. 17-30

McNally, R. J. (2007). Can we solve the mysteries of the National Vietnam Veterans Readjustment Study? *Journal of Anxiety Disorders, 21*(2), 192–200.

Mencken, H. L. (1920). *Prejudices: Second series.* A. A. Knopf.

Menzies, R., & Menzies, R. (2021). *Mortals: How the fear of death shaped human society*. Allen & Unwin.

Merleau-Ponty, M. (1945). *Phénoménologie de la perception*. Gallimard.

Moffitt, T. E., Houts, R., Asherson, P., Belsky, D. W., Corcoran, D. L., Hammerle, M., Harrington, H., Hogan, S., Meier, M. H., & Polanczyk, G. V. (2015). Is adult ADHD a childhood-onset neurodevelopmental disorder? Evidence from a four-decade longitudinal cohort study. *American Journal of Psychiatry, 172*(10), 967–977.

Moncrieff, J. (2010). Psychiatric diagnosis as a political device. *Social Theory and Health, 8*(4), 370–382.

Moncrieff, J., Cooper, R. E., Stockmann, T., Amendola, S., Hengartner, M. P., & Horowitz, M. A. (2022). The serotonin theory of depression: A systematic umbrella review of the evidence. *Molecular Psychiatry*, 1–14.

Montagu, K. (1957). Catechol compounds in rat tissues and in brains of different animals. *Nature, 180*, 244–245.

Mosquera, D., & Steele, K. (2017). Complex trauma, dissociation and borderline personality disorder: Working with integration failures. *European Journal of Trauma & Dissociation, 1*(1), 63–71.

Moylan, S. (2000)

Mueller, J. (1999). *Capitalism, democracy, and Ralph's Pretty Good Grocery*. Princeton University Press.

Mulder, R., & Tyrer, P. (2019). Diagnosis and classification of personality disorders: Novel approaches. *Current Opinion in Psychiatry, 32*(1), 27–31.

Mulder, R., Horwood, J., Tyrer, P., Carter, J., & Joyce, P. (2016). Validating the proposed ICD11 domains. *Personality and Mental Health, 10*(2), 84–95.

Murphy, A., Bourke, J., Flynn, D., Kells, M., & Joyce, M. (2020). A cost-effectiveness analysis of dialectical behaviour therapy for treating individuals with borderline personality disorder in the community. *Irish Journal of Medical Science, 189*(2), 415–423.

Nagy, M. H. (1948). The child's theories concerning death. *The Pedagogical Seminary and Journal of Genetic Psychology, 73*(1), 3–27.

Nagy, M. H. (1959). *The child's view of death.* McGraw-Hill.

Nakdimen, K. A. (1981). DSM-III's multiaxial system: Political finesse. *American Journal of Psychiatry, 138*(2), 259–259.

National Institute of Mental Health. (2009). *Sequenced treatment alternatives to relieve depression.*

National Institute of Mental Health. (2022). *Any anxiety disorder.* https://www.nimh.nih.gov/health/statistics/any-anxiety-disorder

Nehamas, A. (1998). *The art of living: Socratic reflections from Plato to Foucault* (Vol. 61). University of California Press.

Nelson, K. (1993). The psychological and social origins of autobiographical memory. *Psychological Science, 4*(1), 7–14.

Nemiah, J., & Sifneos, P. (1970). Affect and fantasy in patients with psychosomatic Disorders. In O. Hill (Ed.), *Modern trends in psychosomatic medicine* (pp. 26–34). Butterworths.

Nietzsche, F. W. (1927). *Thoughts out of season part I.* George Allen and Unwin Limited.

Nietzsche, F. W. (1974). *The gay science: With a prelude in rhymes and an appendix of songs* (2nd ed.). Vintage Books.

Nietzsche, F. W., & Tille, A. (1896). *Thus spake Zarathustra: A book for all and none.*

MacMillan and Company. Office for National Statistics (2022). *Religion (2021).*

Overall, C. (2012) *Why have Children?: The Ethical Debate.* The MIT Press

Oxford Languages. (2020). Communism. In *Oxford Dictionary* (2nd ed., p. 199). Oxford University Press Australia.

Oz, F. (Director). (1991). *What about Bob?* [Film]. Touchstone Pictures.

Pam, A. (1990). A critique of the scientific status of biological psychiatry: I. Errors in methodology: II. Errors in conception. *Acta Psychiatrica Scandinavica, 82*(Suppl 382), 35–47.

Parker, J. D. A., Taylor, G. J., & Bagby, R. M. (1998). Alexithymia: Relationship with ego defense and coping styles. *Comprehensive Psychiatry, 39*(2), 91–98.

Parker, J. D. A., Taylor, G. J., & Bagby, R. M. (2001). The relationship between emotional intelligence and alexithymia. *Personality and Individual Differences, 30*(1), 107–115.

Parsons, T. (1951). Illness and the role of the physician: A sociological perspective. *American Journal of Orthopsychiatry, 21*(3), 452–460.

Paulus, M. P., & Thompson, W. K. (2018). The challenges and opportunities of small effects: The new normal in academic psychiatry. *Journal of the American Medical Association Psychiatry, 76*(4), 353–354.

Paykel, E. S. (1980). Recall and reporting of life events. *Archives of General Psychiatry, 37*(4), 485–485.

Perry, J. C., & Klerman, G. L. (1978). The borderline patient: A comparative analysis of four sets of diagnostic criteria. *Archives of General Psychiatry, 35*(2), 141–150.

Peterson, J. B. (2018). *12 rules for life: An antidote to chaos.* Penguin Books Limited.

Pettersson, E., Larsson, H., D'Onofrio, B. M., Bölte, S., & Lichtenstein, P. (2020). The general factor of psychopathology: A comparison with the general factor of intelligence with respect to magnitude and predictive validity. *World Psychiatry, 19*(2), 206–213.

Piaget, J. (1954). *The construction of reality in the child* (M. Cook, Trans.). Basic Books.

Piaget, J. (1972). Intellectual evolution from adolescence to adulthood. *Human Development, 15*(1), 1–12.Pigott HE, Dubin W, Kirsch I, et al. Call to action: RIAT

Pigott, H.E., Dubin, W, Kirsch I, et al. Call to action: RIAT Reanalysis of the sequenced treatment alternatives to relieve depression (STAR*D) study. *BMJ* March 6, 2019. Available: https://www.bmj.com/content/ 346/bmj.f2865/rr-10

Pigott, H.E., Kim, T, Colin, Xu, Kirsch, I, Amsterdam, J. (2023) What are the treatment remission, response and extent of improvement rates after up to four trials of antidepressant therapies in real-world depressed patients? A reanalysis of the STAR*D study's patient-level data with fidelity to the original research protocol. *BMJ Open* 2023;13:e063095. doi:10.1136/bmjopen-2022-063095

Pinel, P. (1806). *A treatise on insanity.* Messers Cadell & Davies, Strand.

Pinker, S. (1998). *How the mind works.* Allen Lane.

Pinker, S. (2011). *The better angels of our nature: The decline of violence in history and its causes.* Allen Lane.

Pinker, S. (2014). *The village effect: How face-to-face contact can make us healthier, happier, and smarter.* Random House Publishing Group.

Pinker, S. (2018). *Enlightenment now: the case for reason, science, humanism, and progress.* Penguin Books Limited.

Plana-Ripoll, O., Pedersen, C. B., Holtz, Y., Benros, M. E., Dalsgaard, S., de Jonge, P., Fan, C. C., Degenhardt, L., Ganna, A., Greve, A. N., Gunn, J., Iburg, K. M., Kessing, L. V., Lee, B. K., Lim, C. C. W., Mors, O., Nordentoft, M., Prior, A., Roest, A. M., … McGrath, J. J. (2019). Exploring comorbidity within mental disorders among a Danish national population. *Journal of the American Medical Association Psychiatry, 76*(3), 259–270.

Plato. (2007). *The Republic* (2nd ed.). Penguin UK.

PLoS Medicine Editors. (2012). Does conflict of interest disclosure worsen bias? *Public Library of Science Medicine, 9*(4).

Precht, R. D. (2011). *Who am I? And if so, how many?: A philosophical journey.* Scribe Publications.

Price, J., Sloman, L., RJ, G., Gilbert, P., & Rohde, P. (1994). The social competition hypothesis of depression. *The British Journal of Psychiatry, 164*(3), 309–315.

Quine, W., & Van, O. (1960). *Word and object: An inquiry into the linguistic mechanisms of objective reference.* John Wiley. Rank, O. (1924/1929). The trauma of birth in its importance for psychoanalytic therapy. *Psychoanalytic Review, 11*(3), 241–245.

Rank, O. (1936). *Truth and reality: A life history of the human will.* Knopf.

Rao, S., Heidari, P., & Broadbear, J. H. (2020). Developments in diagnosis and treatment of people with borderline personality disorder. *Current Opinion in Psychiatry*, *33*(5), 441–446.

Ratcliffe, M. (2008). *Feelings of being: Phenomenology, psychiatry and the sense of reality.* Oxford University Press.

Reed, G. M. (2018). Progress in developing a classification of personality disorders for ICD-11. *World Psychiatry*, *17*(2), 227–229.

Reed, G. M., First, M. B., Kogan, C. S., Hyman, S. E., Gureje, O., Gaebel, W., Maj, M., Stein, D. J., Maercker, A., Tyrer, P., Claudino, A., Garralda, E., Salvador-Carulla, L., Ray, R., Saunders, J. B., Dua, T., Poznyak, V., Medina-Mora, M. E., Pike, K. M., … Saxena, S. (2019). Innovations and changes in the ICD-11 classification of mental, behavioural and neurodevelopmental disorders. *World Psychiatry*, *18*(1), 3–19.

Rice, F. (2022). The intergenerational transmission of anxiety disorders and major depression. *American Journal of Psychiatry*, *179*(9), 596–598.

Richerson, P. J., Boyd, R., & Bettinger, R. L. (2001). Was agriculture impossible during the Pleistocene but mandatory during the Holocene? A climate change hypothesis. *American Antiquity*, *66*(3), 387–411.

Ricoeur, P. (1992). *Oneself as another.* University of Chicago press.

Rosenhan, D. L. (1973). On being sane in insane places. *Science*, *179*(4070), 250–258.

Rosenthal, R.L. (2013) What we counted. *American Journal of Cardiology*, 111(7), 10731075 Rosten, L. (1974). Bertrand Russell and God: A memoir. *The Saturday Review*, *23*, 25–26.

Roth, M. (1983). The aims of psychiatric treatment. In T. Helgason & European Medical Research Councils (Eds.), *Methodology in evaluation of psychiatric treatment: Proceedings of a workshop held in Vienna 10-13 June 1981* (pp. 33-55). Cambridge University Press.

Rousseau, J. J. (1762). *The social contract and discourses.* M. M. Rey.

Rush AJ, Trivedi MH, Wisniewski SR, et al. (2006) Bupropion-SR, sertraline, or venlafaxine-XR after failure of SSRIs for depression. *N Engl J Med.* 354:1231–1242

Russell, B. (1935). *In praise of idleness and other essays*. W.W. Norton.

Russell, J. A. (1980). A circumplex model of affect. *Journal of Personality and Social Psychology, 39*(1), 1161–1178.

Rutter, M. (1985). Resilience in the face of adversity: Protective factors and resistance to psychiatric disorder. *The British Journal of Psychiatry, 147*, 598–611.

Rutter, M., & Shaffer, D. (1980). DSM-III. A step forward or back in terms of the classification of child psychiatric disorders? *Journal of the American Academy of Child Psychiatry, 19*(3), 371–394.

Sadowsky, J. (2020). *The empire of depression: A new history*. Polity Press.

Salovey, P., & Mayer, J. D. (1989). Emotional intelligence. *Imagination, Cognition and Personality*, *9*(3), 185–211.

Salzman, C. D., & Fusi, S. (2010). Emotion, cognition, and mental state representation in amygdala and prefrontal cortex. *Annual Review of Neuroscience*, *33*(1), 173–202.

Sanatinia, R., Wang, D., Tyrer, P., Tyrer, H., Crawford, M., Cooper, S., Loebenberg, G., & Barrett, B. (2016). Impact of personality status on the outcomes and cost of cognitive-behavioural therapy for health anxiety. *The British Journal of Psychiatry*, *209*(3), 244–250.

Sapolsky, R. M. (2017). *Behave: The biology of humans at our best and worst*. Penguin Publishing Group.

Sartre, J. P. (1945). *L'existentialisme est un humanisme*. Nagel.

Sartre, J. P. (1952). *The age of reason*. A.A. Knopf.

Sartre, J. P. (1952/1963) *Saint Genet*. University of Minnesota Press

Sartre, J. P. (1956). *Being and nothingness: An essay in phenomenological ontology*. Taylor & Francis.

Satel, S. (2011). PTSD's diagnostic trap. *Policy Review*.

Schank, R. C., & Abelson, R. P. (1995). Knowledge and memory: The real story. In R. S. Wyer, Jr. (Ed.), *Knowledge and memory: The real story* (pp. 1–85). Lawrence Erlbaum Associates.

Schildkraut, J. J. (1965). The catecholamine hypothesis of affective disorders: A review of supporting evidence. *American Journal of Psychiatry, 122*(5), 509–522.

Schlenger, W. E., Caddell, J. M., Ebert, L., Jordan, B. K., Rourke, K. M., Wilson, D., Thalji, L., Dennis, J. M., Fairbank, J. A., & Kulka, R. A. (2002). Psychological reactions to terrorist attacks: Findings from the national study of Americans' reactions to September 11. *Journal of the American Medical Association Psychiatry, 288*(5), 581–588.

Schmideberg, M. (1959). The borderline patient. In S. Arieti (Ed.), *American handbook of psychiatry* (pp. 398–416). Basic Books.

Schrauzer, G. N., & Shrestha, K. P. (1990). Lithium in drinking water and the incidences of crimes, suicides, and arrests related to drug addictions. *Biological Trace Element Research, 25*(2), 105–113.

Seneca, L. (2007). *Seneca: Dialogues and Essays* (A new translation by John Davie) Oxford World Classics (Original work published ca. 49 A. D)

Sharp, C. (2016). Current trends in BPD research as indicative of a broader sea-change in psychiatric nosology. *Personality Disorders: Theory, Research, and Treatment, 7*(4), 334–343.

Sharp, C., Wright, A. G. C., Fowler, J. C., Frueh, B. C., Allen, J. G., Oldham, J., & Clark, L. A. (2015). The structure of personality pathology: Both general ('g') and specific ('s') factors? *Journal of Abnormal Psychology, 124*(2), 387–398.

Shatan, Chaim F. (1972, May 6). Post-Vietnam syndrome. *The New York Times,* p. 35.

Shaw, B. (1927). *Androcles and the lion.* Constable.

Shaw, P. (2018). Growing up: Evolving concepts of adult attention deficit hyperactivity disorder. *The American Journal of Psychiatry, 175*(2), 95–96.

Sibley, C. G., & Ahlquist, J. E. (1984). The phylogeny of the hominoid primates, as indicated by DNA-DNA hybridization. *Journal of Molecular Evolution, 20*(1), 2–15.

Sibley, M. H., Rohde, L. A., Swanson, J. M., Hechtman, L. T., Molina, B. S. G., Mitchell, J. T., Arnold, L. E., Caye, A., Kennedy, T. M., Roy, A., Stehli, A. (2018). Late-onset ADHD reconsidered with comprehensive repeated assessments between ages 10 and 25. *The American Journal of Psychiatry, 175*(2), 140–149.

Simon, R. I. (2002). Distinguishing trauma-associated narcissistic symptoms from posttraumatic stress disorder: A diagnostic challenge. *Harvard Review of Psychiatry, 10*(1), 28–36.

Simon, V., Czobor, P., Bálint, S., Mészáros, A., & Bitter, I. (2009). Prevalence and correlates of adult attention-deficit hyperactivity disorder: Meta-analysis. *The British Journal of Psychiatry: The Journal of Mental Science, 194*(3), 204–211.

Skodol, A. E. (2018). Impact of personality pathology on psychosocial functioning. *Current Opinion in Psychology, 21*, 33–38.

Slavney, P. R. (1991). Affective disorder: The new imperium. *Comprehensive Psychiatry, 32*(4), 295–302.

Song, P., Zha, M., Yang, Q., Zhang, Y., Li, X., & Rudan, I. (2021). The prevalence of adult attention-deficit hyperactivity disorder: A global systematic review and meta-analysis.

Journal of Global Health, 11, 2047–2978.

Southwick, S. M., Morgan, C. A., Nicolaou, A. L., & Charney, D. S. (1997). Consistency of memory for combat-related traumatic events in veterans of Operation Desert Storm. *American Journal of Psychiatry, 154*(2), 173–177.

Spearman, C. (1904). 'General intelligence,' objectively determined and measured. *The American Journal of Psychology, 15*(2), 201–293.

Sperry, R. (1981). *Some effects of disconnecting the cerebral hemispheres.* https://www.nobelprize.org/prizes/medicine/1981/sperry/25059-roger-w-sperrynobellecture-1981/

Spitzer, R. L., Endicott, J., & Robins, E. (1978). Research diagnostic criteria: Rationale and reliability. *Archives of General Psychiatry, 35*(6), 773–782.

Stein, D. J., McLaughlin, K. A., Koenen, K. C., Atwoli, L., Friedman, M. J., Hill, E. D., ... & Kessler, R. C. (2014). DSM-5 and ICD-11 definitions of posttraumatic stress disorder:

Investigating "narrow" and "broad" approaches. *Depression and Anxiety, 31*(6), 494–505.

Stein, M. B., & Rothbaum, B. O. (2018). 175 years of progress in PTSD therapeutics: Learning from the past. *The American Journal of Psychiatry, 175*(6), 508–516.

Stengel, E. (1959). Classification of mental disorders. *Bulletin of the World Health Organization, 21,* 601–663.

Stephan, A. (2012). Emotions, existential feelings, and their regulation. *Emotion Review, 4*(2), 157–162.

Sterelny, K. (2011). From hominins to humans: How sapiens became behaviourally modern. *Philosophical Transactions of the Royal Society B: Biological Sciences, 366*(1566), 809– 822.

Stossel, S. (2014). *My age of anxiety.* Random House.

Suls, J. (2001). Affect, stress, and personality. In *Handbook of affect and social cognition* (pp. 392–409). Lawrence Erlbaum Associates Publishers.

Summerfield, D. (2001). The invention of post-traumatic stress disorder and the social usefulness of a psychiatric category. *British Medical Journal, 322*(7278), 95–98.

Surís, A., Holliday, R., & North, C. S. (2016). The evolution of the classification of psychiatric disorders. *Behavioral Sciences, 6*(1), 5–15.

Survey Centre on American Life. (2021). *Family, relationships, and social life.* https://www.americansurveycenter.org/category/family-relationships-and-social-life/

Susman, W. I. (1884). 'Personality' and the making of the twentieth-century culture. Media. *Social Media & The Self.*

Susser, M., & Susser, E. (1996). Choosing a future for epidemiology: I. Eras and paradigms. *American Journal of Public Health, 86*(5), 668–673.

Swingle, M. K. (2019). *I-Minds: How and why constant connectivity is rewiring our brains and what to do about it.* New Society Publishers.

Tangney, J. P., Stuewig, J., & Mashek, D. J. (2007). Moral emotions and moral behaviour. *Annual Review of Psychology, 58,* 345–372.

Taylor, C. (1985). *Human agency and language*. Cambridge University Press.

Taylor, G. J. (2000). Recent developments in alexithymia theory and research. *Canadian Journal of Psychiatry, 45*(2), 134–142.

Taylor, G. J., Bagby, R. M., & Parker, J. D. A. (1997). *Disorders of affect regulation: Alexithymia in medical and psychiatric illness*. Cambridge University Press.

Tennyson, A. T. B. (1898). *Crossing the bar*. ER Herrick.

Tew, J., Ramon, S., Slade, M., Bird, V., Melton, J., & Le Boutillier, C. (2012). Social factors and recovery from mental health difficulties: A review of the evidence. *The British Journal of Social Work, 42*(3), 443–460.

The Lancet. (2009). A commission on climate change. *The Lancet, 373*(9676), 1659.

The Royal Australian and New Zealand College of Psychiatrists. (2016, June). *RANZCP engagement with the pharmaceutical industry*.

Thomas, J. L., Wilk, J. E., Riviere, L. A., McGurk, D., Castro, C. A., & Hoge, C. W. (2010). Prevalence of mental health problems and functional impairment among active component and National Guard soldiers 3- and 12-months following combat in Iraq. *Archives of General Psychiatry, 67*(6), 614–623.

Thompson, P. M., Giedd, J. N., Woods, R. P., MacDonald, D., Evans, A. C., & Toga, A. W. (2000). Growth patterns in the developing brain detected by using continuum mechanical tensor maps. *Nature, 404*(6774).

Tolstoy, L. N. (1886). *The death of Ivan Ilyich*. Bantam Books.

Tolstoy, L. N. (1889). *Anna Karenina*. Walter Scott.

Tomasello, M. (2010). *Origins of human communication*. MIT Press.

Tomkins, S. S. (1978). Script theory: Differential magnification of affects. *Nebraska Symposium on Motivation, 26*, 201–236.

Twenge, J. M. (2017). *IGen: Why today's super-connected kids are growing up less rebellious, more tolerant, less happy, and completely unprepared for adulthood: And what that means for the rest of us*. Atria Books.

Tyrer, P. (2017). Personality disorder: Good reasons to reclassify. *Australian & New Zealand Journal of Psychiatry, 51*(11), 1077–1078.

Tyrer, P., & Mulder, R. (2018). Dissecting the elements of borderline personality disorder. *Personality and Mental Health, 12*(2), 91–92.

Tyrer, P., & Mulder, R. (2022). *Personality disorder: From evidence to understanding.* Cambridge University Press.

Tyrer, P., Reed, G. M., & Crawford, M. J. (2015). Classification, assessment, prevalence, and effect of personality disorder. *The Lancet, 385*(9969), 717–726.

Tyrer, P., Salkovskis, P., Tyrer, H., Wang, D., Crawford, M. J., Dupont, S., Cooper, S., Green, J., Murphy, D., Smith, G., Bhogal, S., Nourmand, S., Lazarevic, V., Loebenberg, G., Evered, R., Kings, S., McNulty, A., Lisseman-Stones, Y., McAllister, S., ... Barrett, B. (2017). *Cognitive-behaviour therapy for health anxiety in medical patients (CHAMP): A randomised controlled trial with outcomes to 5 years.* NIHR Journals Library.

Tyrer, P., Tyrer, H., Yang, M., & Guo, B. (2016). Long-term impact of temporary and persistent personality disorder on anxiety and depressive disorders. *Personality and Mental Health, 10*(2), 76–83.

United Nations High Commissioner for Refugees. (1948). *Universal Declaration of Human Rights.* UN General Assembly.

United States Congress Committee on Small Business. (1967). *Competitive problems in the drug industry: Hearings before the subcommittee on monopoly of the select committee on small business, united states senate, ninetieth congress, first session on present status of competition in the pharmaceutical industry.* U.S. Government Printing Office.

Vaillant, G. E. (1984). The disadvantages of DSM-III outweigh its advantages. *The American Journal of Psychiatry, 141*(4), 542–545.

Valenstein, E. S. (1998). *Blaming the brain: The truth about drugs and mental health.* Free Press.

Van Den Berg, J. H. (1972). *A different existence: Principles of phenomenological psychopathology.* Duquesne University Press.

van Praag, H. M. (1993). Diagnosis, the rate-limiting factor of biological depression research. *Neuropsychobiology, 28*(4), 197–206.

Varela, F. J., Thompson, E., & Rosch, E. (1991). *The embodied mind: Cognitive science and human Experience*. MIT Press.

Varker, T., Cowlishaw, S., Baur, J., McFarlane, A. C., Lawrence-Wood, E., Metcalf, O., Van Hooff, M., Sadler, N., O'Donnell, M. L., Hodson, S., Benassi, H., & Forbes, D. (2022). Problem anger in veterans and military personnel: Prevalence, predictors, and associated harms of suicide and violence. *Journal of Psychiatric Research, 151*, 57–64.

Wahl, C. W. (1959). *The fear of death*. McGraw-Hill.

Wakefield, J. C. (1992). Disorder as harmful dysfunction: A conceptual critique of *DSM-III-R* 's definition of mental disorder. *Psychological Review, 99*(2), 232–247

Ward, W. (2022). *Lovers of philosophy: How the intimate lives of seven philosophers shaped modern thought*. Ockham Publishing.

Warden, D.., Rush, A. J., Trivedi, M. H., Fava, M., Wisniewski, S. R. (2007): The STAR*D project results: A comprehensive review of findings. *Current Psychiatry Reports* volume **9**, pages 449–459.

Watters, E. (2010). *Crazy like us: The globalization of the American psyche*. Simon and Schuster.

Webber, J. (2009). *The existentialism of Jean-Paul Sartre*. Routledge.

Webber, J. (2018). *Rethinking existentialism*. OUP Oxford.

Wells, H. G. (1907). *New worlds for old*. M. A. Donohue.

West, M. J., & King, A. P. (1987). Settling nature and nurture into an ontogenetic niche. *The Journal of the International Society for Developmental Psychobiology, 20*(5), 549–562.

Weston, S. J., Hill, P. L., Jackson, J. J. (2014) Personality Trait Predict the Onset of Disease. *Social, Psychological and Personality Science. Published online.*

Whitaker, R. (2010). *Anatomy of an epidemic: Magic bullets, psychiatric drugs, and the astonishing rise of mental illness in America*. Crown.

Whitwell, D. (2005). *Recovery beyond psychiatry*. Free Association Books.

Widiger, T. A., & Frances, A. J. (2002). Toward a dimensional model for the personality disorders. In P. T. Costa, Jr. & T. A. Widiger (Eds.), *Personality disorders and the fivefactor model of personality* (pp. 23–44). American Psychological Association.

Willcutt, E. G. (2012). The prevalence of DSM-IV attention-deficit/hyperactivity disorder: A meta-analytic review. *Neurotherapeutics: The Journal of the American Society for Experimental NeuroTherapeutics, 9*(3), 490–499.

Williams, J. B. (1985). The multiaxial system of DSM-III: Where did it come from and where should it go? Its origins and critiques. *Archives of General Psychiatry, 42*(2), 175–180.

Williams, T. F., Scalco, M. D., & Simms, L. J. (2018). The construct validity of general and specific dimensions of personality pathology. *Psychological Medicine, 48*(5), 834–848.

Wilson, E. O. (2012). *The social conquest of earth*. Liveright.

Will Self (2021) *A Posthumous Shock*. Harper's Magazine.

Winnicott, D., W. (1953). Transitional objects and transitional phenomena: A study of the first not-me possession. *International Journal of Psycho-Analysis, 34*, 89–97.

Wittgenstein, L. (1922). *Tractatus Logico-philosophicus*. Routledge & Kegan Paul.

Wong, K. (2012). Why humans give birth to helpless babies. *Scientific American, 28*.

World Health Organisation. (2021). *Depression*. https://www.who.int/news-room/factsheets/detail/depression.

World Health Organization. (1978). *International statistical classification of diseases and related health problems* (9th ed.).

World Health Organization. (1990). *International statistical classification of diseases and related health problems* (10th ed.).

World Health Organization. (2019). *International statistical classification of diseases and related health problems* (11th ed.).

Yalom, I. D. (1980). *Existential psychotherapy*. Basic Books.

Yalom, I. D. (1989). *Love's executioner: And other tales of psychotherapy*. Basic Books.

Yalom, I. D. (2015). *Creatures of a day: And other tales of psychotherapy*. Scribe Publications.

Yeomans, P. D., Herbert, J. D., & Forman, E. M. (2008). Symptom comparison across multiple solicitation methods among Burundians with traumatic event histories. *Journal of Traumatic Stress, 21*(2), 231–234.

Young, A. (1995). *The harmony of illusions: Inventing post-traumatic stress disorder*. Princeton University Press.

Yuanyuan et al 2022 Noise and pain

Zachar, P. (2000). Psychiatric disorders are not natural kinds. *Philosophy, Psychiatry & Psychology, 7*(3), 167–182.

Zanarini, M. C. (2009). Psychotherapy of borderline personality disorder. *Acta Psychiatrica Scandinavica, 120*(5), 373–377.

Zanarini, M. C., Frankenburg, F. R., Reich, D. B., & Fitzmaurice, G. (2010). Time to attainment of recovery from borderline personality disorder and stability of recovery: A 10-year prospective follow-up study. *The American Journal of Psychiatry, 167*(6), 663–667.

Zanarini, M. C., Frankenburg, F. R., Reich, D. B., & Fitzmaurice, G. (2012). Attainment and stability of sustained symptomatic remission and recovery among patients with borderline personality disorder and axis II comparison subjects: A 16-year prospective follow-up study. *The American Journal of Psychiatry, 169*(5), 476–483.

Zaner, R. M. (1998). *Ethics and the clinical encounter*. Prentice Hall.

Zhou, W., Ye, C., Wang, H., Mao, Y., Zhang, W., Liu, A., Yang, C.-L., Li, T., Hayashi, L., & Zhao, W. (2022). Sound induces analgesia through corticothalamic circuits. *Science, 377*(6602), 198–204.

Zisook, S., Shuchter, S. R., Pedrelli, P., Sable, J., & Deaciuc, S. C. (2001). Bupropion sustained release for bereavement: Results of an open trial. *Journal of Clinical Psychiatry, 62*(4), 227–230.

ACKNOWLEDGEMENT

I grew up in a family with modest financial means. My father (Kameshwar) and his three brothers (Kali, Kamal and Kumareshwar) lived in a joint family system for most of my childhood. There were eight boys and eight girls in my generation. Birthdays and festivities occurred at frequent intervals. As the family size grew the house kept getting extended, kitchens separated, but the four families remained remarkably close.

There was abundance of love and care. Education and knowledge were valued and encouraged. We were a family that loved to talk. Discussions were open and frank. Friends of the family would drop in all the time and gossip over cups of tea and snacks. Kids were allowed to be around and well welcome to participate in the discussion.

My parents remained the primary motivating force in my life. I had long arguments over matters related to God and religion with my dad. He was a man of deep faith. To his credit, he would never get angry at my 'impertinence.' My mother (Krishna) was quite stoic. She was quietly assertive. My parents had immense belief and pride in me.

I would like to acknowledge Professor B. G. Gupta who would often praise my writings in English. One day I expressed my doubts and pointed out that I have been quoting extensively from the books on History of English Literature from my fathers' bookshelves. His words still ring in my ears: "Rakesh, if you think that one day you will write something that no one has ever written, you will be forever disappointed. The main thing is not where you got an idea from; what matters is how you bring many ideas together to make your point." Those words provided me lot of confidence then and ever since.

I see the book as more of a compilation and crystallization of my reading and experience as a psychiatrist, rather than any profound wisdom. As Nietzsche rightly said: "All knowledge was interpretation and that there was no 'original' non-interpreted text."

Soon after joining medicine, I decided that my future was in psychiatry. I was interested in the whole person and not just their illness. I was also interested in literature and philosophy. My introduction to serious philosophy started much later, but even in my childhood one of my uncles' (Kumareshwar), a primary care physician, lovingly called me a *philosopher*. His influence on my life has been quite significant.

Over the years Prof. R. P. N. Singh, my first mentor and guide in psychiatry has been a major source of inspiration. A very well read and extremely articulate man, he fired my imagination and provided me all the encouragement at every stage of my career until his sad demise in 1998. My first research work (part of the requirement for M.D. in psychiatry) was an "Observations on patients with terminal illness and attitude of the staff and relatives caring for the patient" under the guidance of Prof. Singh.

Prof P. S. V. N. Sharma has been a considerable influence in my growth as a psychiatrist. I consider him as one of the best teachers in psychiatry that I have ever seen. My regular brainstorming with colleagues for a decade at the Central Institute of Psychiatry in India were very stimulating. Colleagues who had a significant impact included L. N. Sharma, P. S. V. N. Sharma, Samshul Haque Nizamie, Vinod Sinha, and S. K. Mattoo.

Two months at the NIMH, Bethesda with Thomas Wehr and Norman Rosenthal were very stimulating. I also managed to briefly meet Robert Post, Janice Egeland, and several other distinguished researchers. A weekend in Iowa was marked by a few hours with George Winokur and Nancy Andreasen. A month with Robert Spitzer while on a WHO fellowship to US in 1992 brought about a significant shift in my thinking.

A chance acquaintance with Prof. Phil Mitchell (who was visiting NIMH from Sydney) led to my move to Australia in 1995 to make first Bendigo and later Melbourne my new home. After moving to Australia, the two people who became my new mentors were John Bomford and Chris Lorbati.

Over the last many years my two peer review groups have played a significant role in shaping my thoughts. Members of the groups include David Hickingbotham, Rod Smith, Kerry Mack, Ray Murphy, Samir Ibrahim, Surya Tipernini, Yoganand Bellakere, Simon Croke, Sam Asadi, Pralay Majumdar, Viren Kothari, Saji Damodaran, Sathya Rao, Shashi Verma, Nitin Dharwarkar, Hillol Das, Sri Vadassaeri, and Pradeep Chabra. Graham Burrows, Malcolm Hopwood, Anne Buist, and Ravi Bhat have been a source of support and inspiration.

My various long conversations with my late father-in-law (Rajeshwar Tandon) an ophthalmologist with knowledge of encyclopaedic proportions provided me with many important insights. Namita (my wife with a PhD in psychology) has been a constant motivating person in my life. She often comes with counterpoints that helps me to think even more broadly. One of my most valued brainstorming friend over the last several years, is my son (Rahul) who is a young psychiatrist. He has already demonstrated immense potential. His research and publications have been of immense help. He has also helped with the process of the publication of this book. Reetika (my daughter and a Juris Doctor) who has had experience as assistant to the editor of a journal in public law has helped me in editing the book. I must also acknowledge the contributions of Christie (my daughter in law who works passionately towards creating an environmentally friendly urban development) and Karan (my soon to be son-in-law and a Juris Doctor). Namita and I feel more secure when 'under the supervision of the kids.' They are our technology gurus too.

I like to acknowledge my very dear grandson Jaival (three-year-old) with his beautiful eyes and a lovely smile. He is the latest link to the chain of our conjoint family lines. I would love him to live a life better than the generations before.

John Timlin played an especially key role of an editor in refining and polishing the manuscript to bring it to publication standard. It was one of those random events which led to our chance meeting, and he very graciously agreed to help. His meticulous editing skills have been effective. He was also instrumental in seeking the help from Edward Harari, a psychiatrist of great repute to comment on the manuscript. This enabled me to iron out some lacunas in the writing. Despite their health problems people like John and Ed remain committed to the cause of helping inexperienced writers to reach their goals.

www.ingramcontent.com/pod-product-compliance
Ingram Content Group UK Ltd.
Pitfield, Milton Keynes, MK11 3LW, UK
UKHW062310290726
14090UKWH00018B/978

9 798897 440016